278
Current Topics in Microbiology and Immunology

Springer-Verlag Berlin Heidelberg GmbH

D.R. SALOMON · C. Wilson (Eds.)

Xeno-transplantation

With 22 Figures and 17 Tables

Springer

Daniel R. Salomon, M.D.
The Scripps Research Institute
Department of Molecular and Experimental Medicine
MEM 55, 10550 North Torrey Pines Road, La Jolla, CA 92037, USA
e-mail: dsalomon@scripps.edu

Carolyn Wilson, M.D.
U.S. Food and Drug Administration
Division of Cellular and Gene Therapies
Center for Biologics Evaluation and Research, FDA
Building 29B, Room 2NN11
8800 Rockville Pike, HFM-530, Bethesda, MD 20892, USA
e-mail: wilsonc@cber.fda.gov

Cover Illustration by C. Wilson:
Shown on the front cover is a fluorescent confocal micrograph (630x) of HEK 293 cells productively infected with PERV-A (strain 14/220, provided by Clive Patience, Immerge Therapeutics). Cells were immunostained as follows: 1) Green = Goat anti-simian sarcoma-associated virus gp70 (which cross-reacts with PERV gp70 envelope) followed by a FITC donkey-anti-goat anti-serum (Jackson ImmunoResearch Laboratories, Inc., West Grove, PA); 2) Red = Mouse monoclonal anti-human golgin-97 (Molecular Probes, Eugene, OR) followed by a Texas Red donkey-anti-mouse anti-serum (Jackson ImmunoResearch Laboratories, Inc., West Grove, PA); and 3) Blue = Topro-3, a fluorescent stain for the cell nucleus (Molecular Probes, Eugene, OR).

ISSN 0070-217X

ISBN 978-3-642-62431-5 ISBN 978-3-642-55541-1 (eBook)

DOI 10.1007/978-3-642-55541-1

Library of Congress Catalog Card Number 72-152360

http://www.springer.de

Originally published by Springer-Verlag Berlin Heidelberg New York in 2003
Softcover reprint of the hardcover 1st edition 2003

Typesetting: Stürtz AG, Würzburg
Cover Design: Design & Production GmbH, Heidelberg
Production Editor: Angélique Gcouta, Berlin
Printed on acid-free paper SPIN: 10835211 27/3020 5 4 3 2 1 0

Forward

The advent of transplantation surgery has heralded significant advances in medical therapy. The limiting factor is no longer the technical surgical procedure but the accompanying suppression of the recipient's immune response that is often required and the availability or lack of availability of donor tissues/cells for transplantation. One approach to this dilemma is the use of donor tissues from non-human species. The "Certain Promise and Uncertain Peril" of xenotransplantation as addressed by Robin Weiss in several of his earlier thoughtful papers sets the foundation for this debate. The issues of this debate are clearly addressed by eight knowledgeable workers in the area who participate in this interesting and important scientific and ethical discussion as co-ordinated by the guest editors of this volume, Daniel Salomon from the Department of Molecular and Experimental Medicine at The Scripps Research Institute, and Carolyn Wilson of the United States Food and Drug Administration. Both Drs. Salomon and Wilson have credentials in and have explored this ongoing debate at the scientific and administrative level and are aware of the germane issues encompassing this field. As such this volume will provide a necessary background for those interested in understanding the pros and cons of this medical dilemma.

Michael B.A. Oldstone
La Jolla, California

Preface

The purpose of the present book is to provide the reader with a series of discussions updating a number of critical issues raised by clinical trials of animal cells, tissues and organs transplanted into humans — xenotransplantation. Obviously the primary focus is on issues of potential infectious disease exposure raised by xenotransplantation. However, where necessary, we have included appropriate discussions of the immunological barriers in xenotransplantation to help the reader understand the various immunosuppressive strategies that will be required for successful clinical trials. A key point is that any consideration of infectious disease risks in this area must be seen in the context of fully and aggressively immunosuppressed patients.

A few general ideas are appropriate to consider here so as to help provide the reader with a perspective.

Infectious disease risks are part of living in our world. The movement of pathogens from animal reservoirs to human beings is a regular phenomenon. Therefore, it is important to start by considering what kind of infectious disease risks are the specific issues for xenotransplantation. In other words, to phrase the questions in a proper perspective we need to ask: "What are the incremental risks of moving animal pathogens to humans which are created by xenotransplantation?"

Many animal-to-human infections comprise the natural life cycle of certain pathogens (i.e., malaria or West Nile fever) that move regularly through animal and human hosts. Infection of human hosts with animal-borne pathogens due to close living contact such as happens with hunting, animal husbandry, food preparation and food contamination are often referred to as zoonoses or zoonotic infections (i.e., Ebola, Hanta virus and any number of parasitic infections endemic to animals). These forms of infectious disease have really little or nothing to do with our risk concerns for xenotransplantation. Basically, an animal herd designated as suitable for harvesting tissues or organs will be derived and maintained under conditions in which known zoonotic agents will be eliminated from the herd. Indeed, considerable work has been done worldwide in collaboration with many experts in infectious disease and veterinary medicine to establish a set of guidelines for maintaining and screening animal herds suitable for xenotransplantation (for an example of what has been done in the United States, see *"Guideline on Infectious Disease Issues in Xenotransplantation"* http://www.fda.gov/cber/gdlns/xenophs1000.htm).

In contrast, the infection of a human patient specifically by xenotransplantation is referred to as a xenogeneic infection or xenozoonosis. Xenogeneic animal-to-human infections will largely involve potential pathogens contained in animal tissues that would not normally spread to humans but could be carried over in the process of transplanting tissues or organs (i.e., porcine CMV or exogenous retroviruses in nonhuman primates). The donor animals will not be sick at the time of transplantation and in many instances the pathogen will not produce disease in the donor animal but only in the recipient human patient. The central example for xenotransplantation is the potential of transmitting endogenous retroviruses such as porcine endogenous retrovirus (PERV) from pigs to humans. Endogenous retroviruses have been incorporated into the donor animal's germ line and therefore cannot be eliminated. In most cases, endogenous retroviruses do not produce any pathology in the host animal. Nonetheless, porcine endogenous retroviruses retain the ability to infect the cells and tissues of other species including humans. This then is a good example of the risk of xenotransplantation that is the issue at hand.

At the beginning of any clinical trial is a decision based on risk versus benefit. Simply put, if xenotransplantation has no chance of benefit then even the smallest risk is unacceptable. Unfortunately, there has been a series of scientific setbacks in xenotransplantation over the last 5 years. Specifically, the preclinical large animal experiments transplanting genetically engineered pig hearts and kidneys into monkeys and baboons have not demonstrated survival of the xenografts beyond weeks to a few months. Also, a very well-designed trial of implanting pig fetal neural cells into patients with neurological disease was not successful. As a consequence, the current situation for xenotransplantation suggests little benefit and, thus, infinite risk. Therefore, some critics have concluded that there is no future to this procedure and further considerations of risk are unnecessary. We reject this view as short sighted.

Xenotransplantation, like many endeavors at the cutting edges of medical science, has tremendous potential. The critical donor organ shortage for human transplantation is such that thousands of patients die each year waiting for a transplant, and millions of patients with diabetes that could benefit from a successful islet transplant will wait for their chance at the few thousand usable pancreata available each year. Therefore, it would be ridiculous to ignore the tremendous impetus to solve the problems and make xenotransplantation successful. History cautions us to take the longer view where the temporary ups and downs of progress eventually lead to success. Thus, no one is likely to abandon the search for a cancer cure that has eluded us many decades longer than xenotransplantation despite investment of substantially more resources. In other words, xenotransplantation research will continue. In fact, a series of 12 children with juvenile onset diabetes mellitus underwent pig islet transplantation in Mexico last year and a report of successful pig liver cell transplantation has come out of China. In the United States, a number of small clinical xenotransplantation trials are underway using various pig cells, some in devices. Therefore, clinical trials in xenotransplantation are reality, not fantasy. That some of these trials are being done in other countries where regulatory oversight and scientific resources are limited is even greater reason for concern.

Risk also has several unique elements that are necessary to consider for xenotransplantation. The classic risk for a clinical trial is based on concerns for the individual patient. For example, a risk could be a side effect of a new drug or an unexpected, adverse reaction. In xenotransplantation, the individual risk could be that the organ is rejected or never works properly. From a xenogeneic infectious disease viewpoint, the individual risk could be that a xenotransplant transmits an animal pathogen and results in a human illness. In the case of an endogenous retrovirus this could be a form of cancer such as lymphoma or leukemia. Individual risk can be dealt with by proper informed consent. While this is an imperfect procedure, it is one that has been reviewed and continuously refined in clinical trials for many years. The interesting element of risk in xenotransplantation is public risk — the potential that a xenogeneic pathogen will start in the patient and then spread to close contacts, medical professionals and the public. There is no instrument like an informed consent document to deal with public risk. Thus, while a patient dying of liver failure could make an informed decision to personally accept the risks of a pig liver transplant, neither this patient nor the family could ever accept any risk for transmission of a pathogen from the pig liver to the public. At present, it is the nature of the public health risk in xenotransplantation that is a major issue.

From our view, the only way to deal responsibly with the public health risk of xenotransplantation is to engage in a wide-ranging, science-based, public discussion of this risk. Thus, the present volume reviews what is known at this time about a number of potential xenogeneic risks and attempts wherever possible to point in the favored directions for future research. The hardest thing to define is an unknown risk. Thus it is one thing to be faced with the current AIDS pandemic and search originally to identify the new pathogen (i.e., HIV) and then develop strategies to control, treat and cure the disease. It is entirely another thing to be faced with a theoretical risk of a theoretical infection. Nonetheless, that is the current state of affairs in xenotransplantation. It does not change our responsibility to the public to do everything possible to insure the safe conduct of any clinical xenotransplant trial including those that are already underway. In this respect, we believe that more scientific knowledge is necessary to inform any debate of risk in xenotransplantation. With knowledge the risks can be placed in a proper context and science-based evaluations of risk versus benefit can be made for xenotransplantation clinical trials.

May 2003 Daniel R. Salomon and Carolyn A. Wilson

List of Contents

Genetic Modification of Xenografts
J.L. Platt 1

Public Health Risks – Patient vs. Society in an Emerging Field
L.E. Chapman 23

Cross-Species Infections
R.A. Weiss 47

Non-Human Primate Herpesviruses: Importance for Xenotransplantation
M.G. Michaels 73

Understanding Xenotransplantation Risks from Non-Human Primate Retroviruses
J.S. Allan 101

Exogenous Porcine Viruses
P.S. Paul, P. Halbur, B. Janke, H. Joo, P. Nawagitgul, J. Singh, and S. Sorden 125

Swine Hepatitis E Virus: Cross-Species Infection and Risk in Xenotransplantation
X.J. Meng 185

Molecular Cloning and Functional Characterization of Infectious PERV and Development of Diagnostic Tests
M. Niebert and R.R. Tönjes 217

Xenotransplantation – Federal Regulatory Considerations
E.T. Bloom 239

Subject Index 253

List of Contributors

(Their addresses can be found at the beginning of their respective chapters)

ALLAN, J.S. 101

BLOOM, E.T. 239

CHAPMAN, L.E. 23

HALBUR, P. 125

JANKE, B. 125

JOO, H. 125

MENG, X.J. 185

MICHAELS, M.G. 73

NAWAGITGUL, P. 125

NIEBERT, M. 217

PAUL, P.S. 125

PLATT, J.L. 1

SINGH, J. 125

SORDEN, S. 125

TÖNJES, R.R. 217

WEISS, R.A. 47

Genetic Modification of Xenografts

J. L. Platt

Transplantation Biology and the Departments of Surgery,
Immunology and Pediatrics, Medical Sciences Building 2-66, Mayo Clinic,
200 1st Street S.W., Rochester, MN 55905, USA
E-mail: Platt.jeffrey@mayo.edu

1 Introduction: A Rationale for Xenotransplantation 2

2 The Hurdles to Xenotransplantation 3

3 The Immunological Hurdles to Xenotransplantation of Organs 5
3.1 Hyperacute Rejection 6

4 Acute Vascular Rejection. 7

5 Genetic Engineering of Donor Antigen 8

6 Accommodation 10

7 How Can Genetic Engineering Be Applied to Accommodation? 10

8 Chronic Rejection 11

9 Physiologic Hurdles to Xenotransplantation 12

10 Infection. 13

11 Comments on Genetic Engineering for Xenotransplantation 13

12 Concluding Remarks 15

References. 16

Abstract For nearly a century, xenotransplantation has been seen as a potential approach to replacing organs and tissues damaged by disease. Until recently, however, the application of xenotransplantation has seemed only a remote possibility. What has changed this perspective is the advent of genetic engineering of large animals; that is, the ability to add genes to and remove genes from lines of animals that could provide an enduring source of tissues and organs for clinical application. Genetic engineering could address the immunologic, physiologic and infectious barriers to xenotransplantation, and could allow xenotransplantation to provide a source of cells with defined and even controlled expression of exogenous genes. This communication will consider one perspective on the application of genetic engineering in xenotransplantation.

1 Introduction: A Rationale for Xenotransplantation

Xenotransplantation could have an impact on at least three aspects of medicine. The first, and some would say the preeminent aspect, is as a means of overcoming a severe shortage of human donor organs for the treatment of organ failure. Dimensions of this organ shortage and the significant need that could be addressed by xenotransplantation have been discussed in detail elsewhere (Evans 2001; Evans et al. 1992). The second aspect relates to the possibility that a xenogeneic organ would not be susceptible to infection by a 'human' virus and thus the xenograft might resist injury caused by such viruses. Based on this consideration, xenotransplantation has been proposed as an approach to the treatment of hepatitis (Starzl et al. 1993) and AIDS (Mueller et al. 1999). The third and, as of yet, unexplored aspect relates to a means of delivering genes for therapeutic purposes, thus overcoming some of the limitations of 'conventional' gene therapy (Platt 1998). Genes introduced into animals can be expressed at high levels, potentially under conditions subject to regulation; whereas, genes delivered by human cells or directly into a human subject may not be expressed at such high levels or may not be subject to regulation.

If the rationale for xenotransplantation is compelling, the hurdles are at least equally so. These hurdles include: (a) the immune response of the recipient against the graft; (b) the physiologic limitations of organs or tissues functioning in a xenogeneic environment; and (c) the possibility of transferring an infectious agent from the graft to the recipient. This author and others have discussed these limitations in detail (Auchincloss 1988; Auchincloss and Sachs 1998; Cascalho and Platt 2001; Platt 1998).

This communication will consider how genetic engineering can address the hurdles to xenotransplantation and, conversely, how xenotransplantation can be used for genetic engineering. The subject of genetic engineering in xenotransplantation is now too broad to consider in a brief essay such as this one, and, therefore, the goal will be to convey the author's overall approach to these issues, rather than a detailed exposition.

Table 1 Classification of xenografts

Type of xenograft (example)	Type of vascular supply	Microenvironment	Types of rejection
Isolated cells (hepatocytes, bone marrow)	Neovascularization	Recipient	Cellular and Primary non-function
Free tissue (pancreatic islets, skin)	Neovascularization + anastomosis of donor and recipient vessels	Donor and recipient	Cellular and Primary non-function
Organ (kidney, heart)	Primary anastomosis of donor and recipient vessels	Donor	Cellular and Vascular

2 The Hurdles to Xenotransplantation

The preeminent hurdle to xenotransplantation appears to be the immune response of the recipient against the graft. The biological hurdles depend predominantly on the type of transplant undertaken. Table 1 lists the various types of transplants. Transplants consisting of isolated cells such as hepatocytes receive a vascular supply through the in-growth of blood vessels of the recipient. Although the survival of isolated cells and the in-growth of recipient blood vessels may depend on the compatibility of growth factors, cytokines and hormones between the donor and the recipient (Gritsch et al. 1994; Hammer 1998), the hurdles to cellular xenotransplantation appear to be surprisingly modest. The 'modest' hurdle to cellular transplantation reflects, in part, that the blood vessels of the recipient provide a barrier between the immune system of the recipient and the xenotransplant (Nagayasu and Platt 1998).

The first hurdle to cellular xenotransplants may be 'primary nonfunction' (Kaufman et al. 1990). The cause of primary nonfunction is uncertain but may include such factors as the compatibility of the microenvironment of the recipient with donor cells, the ability of the graft to promote angiogenesis, and early inflammatory and cellular immune reactions with the graft. Until the molecular basis for primary nonfunction of xenografts can be established, genetic engineering cannot be offered as a solution to the problem. However, to the extent that the hurdle of primary nonfunction can be overcome by increasing the size of the graft

(Kaufman et al. 1990), xenotransplantation may offer a more feasible approach than allotransplantation.

The principal immune hurdle to the transplantation of isolated cells is cellular rejection. The primacy of this hurdle is suggested by the work of Gunsalus et al. (1997) and Deacon et al. (1997). Deacon et al. demonstrated that porcine hepatocytes could be transplanted into rabbits successfully if the rabbits were treated with cyclosporin A, and that porcine substantia nigra cells could be transplanted into human subjects with Parkinson's disease treated with immunosuppressive drugs. Recent studies by Nagata et al. (2003) suggest that the threshold for successful xenotransplantation of hepatocytes may be even lower; that is, xenogeneic hepatocytes may survive and function even in the absence of immunosuppression.

The biological hurdles to xenotransplantation of free tissues such as pancreatic islets and skin also appear to include primary nonfunction and cellular rejection. In this case, as in the case of cellular transplants, specific approaches to genetic engineering may have to await the elucidation of a molecular basis of these conditions. However, some have suggested that survival of tissue transplants, especially of pancreatic islets, may be limiting. In this case, one might consider introducing 'survival' genes, such as Bcl-2, to prevent apoptosis of cells in the transplant.

The transplantation of xenogeneic organs is not evidently limited by primary nonfunction or incompatibilities of the microenvironment, but rather by the action of the immune system of the recipient on blood vessels in the donor organ. This action gives rise to a series of vascular diseases or vascular types of rejection listed in Fig. 1. Much of the focus in the field of xenotransplantation has been on understanding the basis for vascular rejection and developing strategies, including genetic engineering, for overcoming that problem. Because much is known about the molecular basis of vascular rejection, the sections that follow will focus on this issue in some detail. The point of this discussion, however, is to emphasize the opportunities and limitations of genetic engineering in xenotransplantation, rather than to provide a prescription for an optimal approach to that end.

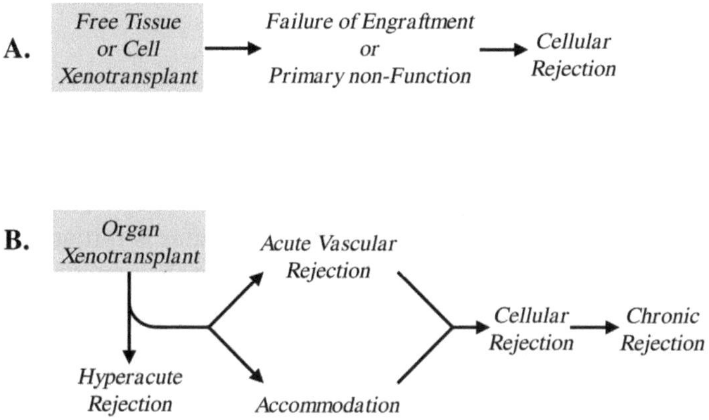

Fig. 1A, B The immunological response to xenotransplantation. The immune response to xenotransplantation can be classified according to whether the graft consists of isolated cells or free tissues, such as islets of Langerhans or of a primarily vascularized organ such as the kidney or heart. **A** Free tissue grafts are subject to failure caused by primary nonfunction, failure of neovascularization or failure of the microenvironment to support the survival and function of the foreign tissue. If the free tissue or isolated cells engraft, they are then subject to cellular or humoral rejection. **B** Vascularized organ grafts are subject to hyperacute and acute vascular rejection caused by the action of antidonor antibodies on donor endothelium. If hyperacute or acute vascular rejection is averted, the graft may undergo accommodation, a condition in which the graft appears to resist injury despite the return of antidonor antibodies to the circulation and the presence of an intact complement system. A vascularized organ graft may also be subject to cellular rejection and chronic rejection more or less like the corresponding types of rejection observed in allografts. (Adapted from *Graft* 1:19–24, 1998, with permission from *Landes Bioscience* and *Graft*)

3
The Immunological Hurdles to Xenotransplantation of Organs

Figure 1 lists various vascular diseases of organ transplants. These diseases are especially common and severe in xenotransplants, but all are seen with some frequency in allotransplants (transplants between different individuals of the same species).

3.1 Hyperacute Rejection

An organ transplanted between disparate species is subject to immediate or hyperacute rejection, which can destroy the organ within minutes to a few hours of reperfusion by the recipient's blood (Perper and Najarian 1966). Hyperacute rejection of porcine organs by primates is initiated by complement-fixing xenoreactive antibodies that bind to the endothelium of the newly transplanted organ and activate the complement system (Platt et al. 1991). In humans, xenoreactive antibodies against lower mammals are directed against Galα1–3Gal (Sandrin et al. 1993; Starzl et al. 1993), a saccharide synthesized by New World monkeys and lower mammals but not by humans, apes and Old World monkeys (Galili et al. 1987). The critical event for the development of hyperacute rejection appears to be the rapid assembly of terminal complement complexes (Brauer et al. 1993; Dalmasso et al. 1992; Platt et al. 1990b). Over a decade ago, the author and colleagues suggested that xenografts might be especially susceptible to hyperacute rejection because of incompatibility between 'complement-regulatory proteins' such as human decay accelerating factor (DAF), CD59 and membrane co-factor protein expressed in the graft with the complement system of the recipient (Dalmasso et al. 1991; Platt et al. 1990a). If the control of human complement in a porcine organ is ineffective, allowing massive activation of complement in graft blood vessels, then the problem might be solved if complement-regulatory proteins compatible with the recipient were expressed in the graft (Platt et al. 1990a). We tested this concept using pigs genetically engineered to express human DAF and CD59 (McCurry et al. 1995). Even though these human proteins were expressed only transiently and at a very low level in pigs, the expression of the proteins dramatically prevented hyperacute rejection (Byrne et al. 1997; McCurry et al. 1995). Subsequent work by the author and by others (Bhatti et al. 1999; Cozzi et al. 1997; Schmoeckel et al. 1997; Zaidi et al. 1998) confirmed this concept. Of these, the use of genetically engineered pigs is now a standard approach to preventing hyperacute rejection of organ xenografts.

Listed in Table 2 are various approaches to preventing hyperacute rejection. Because the target of xenoreactive antibodies that trigger hyperacute rejection, Galα1–3Gal, is known, another potential approach to preventing this process would be to genetically engineer pigs in such a way that expression of that antigen is decreased or abolished. That sub-

Table 2 Approaches to prevention of hyperacute rejection

Approach	Example	References
Depletion of xenoreactive antibodies	Column absorption	Cooper et al. 1988; Lin et al. 1997
Inhibition of complement	Cobra venom factor, sCR1	Leventhal et al. 1993; Pruitt et al. 1994
Genetic engineering for the expression of complement regulatory proteins	DAF, CD59, MCP	Cozzi et al. 1997; Diamond et al. 2001; McCurry et al. 1995
Genetic engineering to decrease antigen expression[a]	H transferase	Sharma et al. 1996

[a] This approach is proposed but not yet proven.

ject will be discussed in detail below, rather than here, since the control of complement as discussed above and depletion of xenoreactive antibodies as demonstrated by Cooper et al. (1988) and others (Lin et al. 1997; Sachs and Sablinski 1995) have already been shown to be effective for that end.

4
Acute Vascular Rejection

When hyperacute rejection is prevented, an organ xenograft becomes subject to acute vascular rejection. The author originally described acute vascular rejection and named it as such because the resemblance of that process to what once was called 'acute vascular rejection of allotransplants' (Leventhal et al. 1993b; Magee et al. 1995). Others have referred to this process as 'delayed xenograft rejection' (Bach et al. 1996; Kobayashi et al. 1996). Acute vascular rejection may be seen over a period of days to weeks after transplantation (and occasionally later in the case of allografts) and is characterized by focal ischemia and thrombosis (Magee et al. 1995; Nagayasu et al. 2000).

A number of potential causes of acute vascular rejection have been advanced; some of these are listed in Table 3. Although acute vascular rejection may be multifaceted and complex in its pathogenesis, most evidence suggests that acute vascular rejection is caused by the on-going interaction of xenoreactive antibodies with donor blood vessels (Lin et al. 1998). This interaction may cause the activation of donor endotheli-

Table 3 Potential causes of acute vascular rejection

Potential cause	References
Xenoreactive antibodies	Lin et al. 1998
Complement	Cozzi et al. 1997
Platelets	Bustos et al. 2001
Macrophages	Blakely et al. 1994
Natural killer cells	Artrip et al. 1999
Molecular incompatibilities	Bach et al. 1996

Table 4 Approaches to prevention of acute vascular rejection

Approach	References
Tolerance	Sachs and Sablinski 1995
Decrease antigen expression	Sandrin and McKenzie 1999
Accommodation	Platt 1998

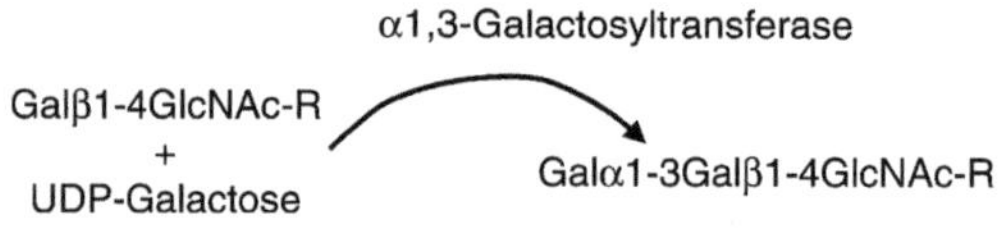

Fig. 2 Synthesis of Galα1,3Gal, the major xenogeneic antigen. In porcine cells, α1,3-galactosyltransferase catalyzes the addition of a terminal galactose to a subterminal *N*-acetyl lactosamine (*Galβ1,4GlcNAc*) to produce the carbohydrate moiety Galα1,3Galβ1,4GlcNAc

um and, thus, a prothrombotic diathesis. Potential solutions to the problem of acute vascular rejection are listed in Table 4. These solutions include the induction of immunological tolerance, the decrease in expression of donor antigens, and the induction of accommodation. Because the latter two might be brought about by genetic engineering of donors, they will be considered here in some detail.

5 Genetic Engineering of Donor Antigen

Recent studies in the author's laboratory have suggested that the main antigen recognized early in the course of the immune reaction giving rise to acute vascular rejection of xenografts is Galα1–3Gal, the same antigen recognized by antibodies causing hyperacute rejection (Lin et al.

2000). Thus, attempts to prevent acute vascular rejection might focus on this antigen. Figure 2 shows the biochemical reaction, giving rise to the synthesis of Galα1–3Gal. Because embryonic stem cells are not available for pigs as they are for mice, early approaches to lowering expression of Galα1–3Gal have focused on perturbing this biochemical pathway (Platt 1998). These approaches have included the expression of glycosyltransferases, such as H-transferase, which would compete with α1-3galactosyltransferase for catalyzing determination of saccharide chains (Artrip et al. 1999; Chen et al. 1998; Sandrin et al. 1995; Sharma et al. 1996) and expression of α-galactosidase, which would cleave the terminal sugar from the mature chain (Osman et al. 1997). Although these approaches have been effective in decreasing expression of Galα1–3Gal in vitro and to some extent in transgenic mice, none have succeeded in completely eliminating Galα1–3Gal in pigs. Since recent studies by Parker et al. (2001) suggested that expression of Galα1–3Gal would have to be decreased by at least 98% to prevent acute vascular rejection, virtually complete elimination of the antigen must be the goal of genetic engineering, and accordingly, the aforementioned approaches have not been successful.

Recent success in the cloning of pigs has provided an alternative strategy for modifying expression of Galα1–3Gal (Betthauser et al. 2000; Onishi et al. 2000; Polejaeva et al. 2000). Cloning allows, potentially, the 'knocking out' of genes by homologous recombination in cultured cells. Nuclei from the genetically-modified cultured cells can be transferred to an enucleated egg, which can be used to generate an embryo (Lai et al. 2002; Dai et al. 2002; Phelps et al. 2002). By these means, cloning has been used to knock out α1,3galactosyltransferase. Although some have advocated targeting α1,3galactosyltransferase to eliminate hyperacute rejection, this problem is more easily addressed by other means. A better use of this technology would be to address acute vascular rejection. However, if knocking out α1,3galactosyltransferase were to prove useful for the problem of acute vascular rejection, it would probably not provide a solution to the problem. The reason for this is that xenotransplants produce a variety of antigens against which antibodies may form that can cause acute vascular rejection and, therefore, eliminating one antigen is unlikely to solve this problem. Thus, when organs are transplanted between nonhuman primate species, acute vascular rejection occurs even though the donor of the transplant does not express Galα1–3Gal. How many other antigens in pigs might be targets of antibodies causing acute vascular rejection is, as of yet, unknown. In any case, it seems reasonable to conclude that cloning of pigs and homologous recombination might be useful but will probably not be a solution for the problem of acute vascular rejection of xenografts.

6
Accommodation

The author and colleagues were the first to observe accommodation as a distinct syndrome in kidney allografts carried out across ABO blood group barriers (Bannett et al. 1989; Chopek et al. 1987; Platt et al. 1990a). It was found that the temporary depletion of recipient antibodies against blood group A and/or B antigens could allow the enduring transplantation of an incompatible kidney, even if those antibodies returned to the circulation. This phenomenon was later called accommodation and the suggestion was made that it could be useful in xenotransplantation. Studies in pig-to-primate xenografts have suggested that accommodation can occur in xenografts and may be a useful approach to preventing acute vascular rejection (Lin et al. 2000).

Experiments in rodents suggest that accommodation is associated with expression of genes such as *Bcl-2* that inhibit apoptosis, genes such as hemoxygenase-1 (HO-1) that confer protection against toxic injury (Bach et al. 1997; Delikouras et al. 2001) and genes such as CD59 that inhibit complement-mediated lysis (Dalmasso et al. 2000). Xenografts with targeted disruption of HO-1 are subject to severe vascular injury and may not be capable of accommodation. Hence, HO-1 may be necessary for establishment or accommodation (Soares et al. 1998). However, expression of these genes may not be sufficient for accommodation as grafts with increased expression of HO-1 and/or CD59 may still undergo acute vascular rejection (Diamond et al. 1996; Dean et al. 2001).

7
How Can Genetic Engineering Be Applied to Accommodation?

Accommodation has been ascribed to a change in antigen (Yuzawa et al. 1995), a change in antibody (Yu et al. 1996), or a change in the xenograft leading to resistance to humoral mediated injury as discussed above. Based on work in rodents associating accommodation with expression of protective genes, such as HO-1, some would suggest that expression

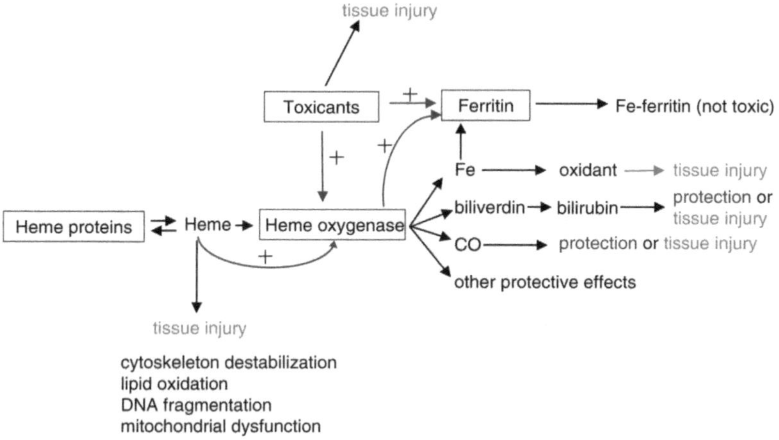

Fig. 3 Heme oxygenase in tissue injury and protection. Under conditions of oxidative stress, heme, an Fe-containing prosthetic group, may be released from heme proteins whereupon it induces cellular injury. Heme oxygenase, induced by endotoxin, oxidants and cytokines, protects against tissue injury by: metabolizing heme; fostering the synthesis of the Fe-sequestering protein ferritin; producing carbon monoxide (*CO*), which is vasodilatory; promoting the production of bilirubin, an antioxidant; and triggering cellular protection through pathways as yet undefined. However, each of the products generated by the action of heme oxygenase on heme-Fe, CO and bilirubin may cause injury in certain circumstances. For example, Fe catalyzes oxidant reactions, CO may poison heme proteins and bilirubin may injure lipid bilayers. (Reprinted from *Nature Medicine* 4:1364–1365, 1998, with permission)

of this or other genes might be helpful in inducing accommodation. Figure 3 shows potential mechanisms by which HO-1 may protect tissues. However, anecdotal studies suggest that induced expression of HO-1 may not afford sufficient protection to prevent graft injury, but this approach has not been adequately tested. Because HO-1 and other protective genes might also induce cellular injury, we have suggested that application of this approach to xenotransplantation may require a critical balance or a fine-tuning (Platt and Nath 1998).

8 Chronic Rejection

Chronic rejection is the major cause of loss of clinical allografts. It is thought that chronic rejection would also improve a major hurdle to xenotransplantation (Hancock et al. 1998; Platt 1998). The cause and molecular basis for chronic rejection is uncertain, although some studies have pointed to a potential role of antidonor antibodies (Hancock et al. 1998). If antidonor antibodies leading to chronic rejection were to prove a serious impediment to xenotransplantation of organs, then the approaches given above in the discussion of acute vascular rejection might also apply to chronic rejection. On the other hand, if chronic rejection were to be caused by factors in the donor, such as age (Halloran et al. 1999), ischemia, or inflammation (Nagano et al. 1997; Waaga et al. 2000), then a xenograft might prove less susceptible to chronic rejection than an allograft. In any case, the point to be emphasized here is that applying genetic engineering to this problem can best be accomplished as a means of testing pathogenetic factors or overcoming specific molecular defects deduced by other means.

9 Physiologic Hurdles to Xenotransplantation

Although serious concerns have been raised about the prospect of physiologic hurdles to xenotransplantation, studies in recent years have suggested that xenografted kidneys (Zaidi et al. 1998), hearts (Waterworth et al. 1998) and lungs (Daggett et al. 1998) might function nearly as well, if not as well, as the corresponding organ allografts. On the other hand, there is more reason to believe that livers transplanted between disparate species might not function adequately to meet the metabolic demands of the recipient or might even induce pathophysiologic changes in the recipient (Calne et al. 1968, 1970; Kanai and Platt 2000; Valdivia et al. 1994). Although some recent studies have tempered this concern (Gunsalus et al. 1997; Ramirez et al. 2000), it seems likely that hepatic xenografts would suffer from or induce at least some physiologic defects. However, if one or if a few enzymes were found to be deficient, the genes for these enzymes might be expressed in transgenic animals. Of greater concern, however, is the possibility that proteins produced by the xenograft might interfere with metabolic cascades in the recipient. For example, von Willebrand factor, which might be secreted by the liver of the pig (Holzknecht et al. 2001), has been shown to induce spontaneous aggregation of human platelets (Mazzucato et al. 1996). As another example, porcine thrombin might interact inefficiently with human thrombinmodulin (Jurd et al. 1996; Lawson and Platt 1996). As still another example, porcine complement might be activated on human cells (Platt 2001).

In any of these circumstances, simply expressing the human gene in a pig would not be sufficient. Rather, eliminating the porcine gene at the same time that the human gene was induced by homologous recombination, i.e. gene knock-in, might address the problem. Gene knock-in has been accomplished in cloned sheep (McCreath et al. 2000), but not yet in cloned pigs.

10
Infection

The possibility of transferring infection from the xenograft source to the recipient, and then more broadly into society, is viewed as a major hurdle to xenotransplantation (Chapman et al. 1995). Because the animals used as the source of xenografts can be bred and manipulated in various ways to eliminate most, if not all, known zoonotic agents, the xenograft might well pose a lower risk of infection than an allograft. However, endogenous retroviruses, such as the porcine endogenous retrovirus (Patience et al. 1997), or new and yet unidentified agents might not be excluded by this means. If such agents were deemed to be impediments to xenotransplantation, then genetic engineering might be applied with some advantage. In the specific case of retroviruses, it might be possible to express some genes, which, in principle, could limit activation or replication of the virus. On the other hand, because the use of animals allows the introduction of genes into the germline, it might be possible to exploit approaches that have failed in the treatment of human viruses. Further, if an endogenous retrovirus was to prove to be an impediment to xenotransplantation, critical genetic sequences of that virus might be 'knocked out' by homologous recombination in the course of cloning of pigs.

11
Comments on Genetic Engineering for Xenotransplantation

Xenotransplantation offers, in principle, a full range of opportunities for application of gene transfer and genetic engineering. Examples of each have been given above and are listed in Table 5. Gene transfer by conventional means is relatively inexpensive and avoids the breeding of animals. It also avoids introduction of genes that are lethal in a fetus, conventional gene transfer potentially allows the specific targeting of the or-

Table 5 Genetic engineering in xenotransplantation: conventional gene therapy versus transgenic therapy versus cloning

	Conventional gene therapy	Conventional transgenic techniques	Cloning
Delivery	Vector or vehicle required	Injection of genetic material directly into pronuclei of fertilized egg	Transfection of cultured somatic cells
Expression	Dependent on ability of each cell to take up genetic material	Genetic material introduced into the germline, leading to expression in a line of animals	Genetic material introduced into the germline, leading to expression in a line of animals
	Requires treatment for every transplant or recipient May require repeated treatment	One manipulation	One manipulation
Immunogenicity	Delivery vehicle or transgene may be immunogenic in donor or recipient	The transgene may elicit immune response only in the recipient	The transgene may elicit immune response only in the recipient
Target of genetic manipulation	The recipient and the graft may be transduced	Genetic manipulation of the donor only	Genetic manipulation of the donor only
Genetic manipulation	Gene addition Dominant negative	Gene addition Dominant negative	Gene addition Dominant negative Gene knock out

gan or tissue to be transplanted through xenotransplantation. Because gene transfer is carried out in the animal source, approaches might be used that would pose an unacceptable risk in a human subject. However, conventional gene transfer might not allow controlled, high level and enduring expression of the exogenous gene and might fail to achieve expression of the gene in all cells, such as endothelial cells, in which expression is needed.

'Conventional' engineering of animals involves the introduction of a gene construct by microinjection or other means in a fertilized egg (Logan and Martin 1994). Integration of the construct occurs randomly in the genome and in a small percentage of injected eggs. Testing the offspring and breeding desired lines of animals is expensive but feasible for commercial purposes. Thus, conventional transgenic techniques have been applied with success, as discussed above. Another advantage of this technique is that the gene expression occurs in the germline, although expression may be lost over ensuing generations. One disadvantage of conventional transgenic techniques, however, is that the site of integration of the extrinsic gene(s) is random, and, as a result, expression may be subject to control by endogenous regulatory regions of DNA. Another disadvantage is that, in the absence of embryonic cells, the technique cannot be used to 'knock out' genes. A third limitation is that only a limited length of intact DNA can be introduced. This last limitation, in turn, imposes a limitation on the number of loci that can be modified without overreaching the limitations of breeding.

Cloning of pigs and other animals is achieved by transferring the nucleus into an enucleated egg or embryo. Various approaches to the cloning of pigs have been reported (Onishi et al. 2000; Polejaeva et al. 2000). Because the nucleus to be transferred can be taken from cultured cells, there exists the possibility of specific modification. By introducing genetic material into a great many cultured cells and selecting the cells in which desired modifications have occurred, it becomes possible to carry out homologous recombination and/or to introduce DNA at many loci. Hence, cloning overcomes the main limitation of conventional genetic engineering. Cloning, however, is less efficient and more expensive than conventional transgenic techniques and may give rise to offspring that are not so vigorous. Gene knockout has yet to be reported in cloned pigs.

12
Concluding Remarks

The experience of the author and others in genetic engineering for xenotransplantation would suggest some lessons of potential value. The first lesson is to undertake only those genetic manipulations that rigorous experiments would suggest are essential for success. Unnecessary manipulations not only increase the expense and the difficulty of applying genetic engineering, such manipulations may obscure results achieved for reasons given below. Genetic manipulations are generally tested in rodents first. However, not all lessons learned from rodents have proved applicable in pigs and nonhuman primates.

A second lesson is that nearly every genetic manipulation is likely to have an unpredictable outcome. Some manipulations will not work as predicted, others will induce compensatory changes that may be worse than the unmanipulated condition.

The third lesson is that the rationale for each change and the judgment regarding the benefits should be founded on in vivo experiments and preferably on transplants. For example, in vitro studies would suggest that natural killer cells and incompatibility of coagulation proteins would have a profound effect on organ xenografts (Inverardi et al. 1992; Itescu et al. 1997; Malyguine et al. 1997). However, neither the influx of natural killer cells nor unwanted coagulation is the inevitable outcome of organ xenotransplantation; indeed, natural killer cells may be absent in rejecting xenografts (Magee et al. 1995; Nagayasu et al. 2000). Regardless of the value of these lessons, it would seem inevitable that genetic manipulation for xenotransplantation, whether effective or ineffective, will teach much about the cellular and molecular basis of tissue injury and disease and thus will lead to still more incisive strategies for the treatment of disease.

Acknowledgements. Supported by grants from the National Institutes of Health.

References

Artrip JH, Kwiatkowski P, Michler RE, et al. 1999 Target cell susceptibility to lysis by human natural killer cells is augmented by alpha(1,3)-galactosyltransferase and reduced by alpha(1, 2)-fucosyltransferase. J Biol Chem 274:10717–10722

Auchincloss H, Jr. 1988 Xenogeneic transplantation. Transplantation 46:1-20

Auchincloss Jr. H, and Sachs DH 1998 Xenogeneic transplantation. Annu Rev Immunol 16:433–470

Bach FH, Ferran C, Hechenleitner P, et al. 1997 Accommodation of vascularized xenografts: expression of 'protective genes' by donor endothelial cells in a host Th2 cytokine environment. Nat Med 3:196–204

Bach FH, Winkler H, Ferran C, et al. 1996 Delayed xenograft rejection. Immunol Today 17:379–384

Bannett AD, McAlack RF, Morris M, et al. 1989 ABO incompatible renal transplantation: a qualitative analysis of native endothelial tissue ABO antigens after transplant. Transplant Proc 21:783–785

Betthauser J, Forsberg E, Augenstein M, et al. 2000 Production of cloned pigs from in vitro systems. Nat Biotechnol 18:1055–1059

Bhatti FNK, Schmoeckel M, Zaidi A, et al. 1999 Three-month survival of HDAFF transgenic pig hearts transplanted into primates. Transplant Proc 31:958

Blakely ML, Van Der Werf WJ, Berndt MC, et al. 1994 Activation of intragraft endothelial and mononuclear cells during discordant xenograft rejection. Transplantation 58:1059–1066

Brauer RB, Baldwin III WM, Daha MR, et al. 1993 Use of C6-deficient rats to evaluate the mechanism of hyperacute rejection of discordant cardiac xenografts. J Immunol 151:7240–7248

Bustos M, Saadi S, and Platt JL (2001) Platelet-mediated activation of endothelial cells: implications for the pathogenesis of transplant rejection. Transplantation 72:509–515

Byrne GW, McCurry KR, Martin MJ, et al. 1997 Transgenic pigs expressing human CD59 and decay-accelerating factor produce an intrinsic barrier to complement-mediated damage. Transplantation 63:149–155

Calne RY, Davis DR, Pena JR, et al. 1970 Hepatic allografts and xenografts in primates. Lancet 1:103–106

Calne RY, White HJO, Herbertson BM, et al. 1968 Pig-to-baboon liver xenografts. Lancet 1:1176–1178

Cascalho M, and Platt JL 2001 The immunological barrier to xenotransplantation. Immunity 14:437–446

Chapman LE, Folks TM, Salomon DR, et al. 1995 Xenotransplantation and xenogeneic infections. New Eng J Med 333:1498–1501

Chen CG, Salvaris EJ, Romanella M, et al. 1998 Transgenic expression of human alpha1,2-fucosyltransferase (H-transferase) prolongs mouse heart survival in an ex vivo model of xenograft rejection. Transplantation 65:832–837

Chopek MW, Simmons RL, and Platt JL 1987 ABO-incompatible renal transplantation: initial immunopathologic evaluation. Transplant Proc 19:4553–4557

Cooper DKC, Human PA, Lexer G, et al. 1988 Effects of cyclosporine and antibody adsorption on pig cardiac xenograft survival in the baboon. J Heart Transpl 7:238–246

Cozzi E, Yannoutsos N, Langford GA, et al. 1997 Effect of transgenic expression of human decay-accelerating factor on the inhibition of hyperacute rejection of pig organs. 2nd ed. In Xenotransplantation: the transplantation of organs and tissues between species. Cooper DKC, Kemp E, Platt JL, et al., editors. Springer, Berlin. 665–682

Daggett CW, Yeatman M, Lodge AJ, et al. 1998 Total respiratory support from swine lungs in primate recipients. J Thorac Cardiovasc Surg 115:19–27

Dai Y, Vaught TD, Boone J, Chen S, Phelps CJ, Ball S, Monahan JA, Jobst PM, McCreath KJ, Lamborn AE, Cowell JL, Wells KD, Colman A, Polejaeva IA, Ayares DL 2002 Nature Biotechnology 20:251–255

Dalmasso AP, Benson BA, Johnson JS, et al. 2000 Resistance against the membrane attack complex of complement induced in porcine endothelial cells with a Gal alpha(1–3)Gal binding lectin: up-regulation of CD59 expression. J Immunol 164:3764–3773

Dalmasso AP, Vercellotti GM, Fischel RJ, et al. 1992 Mechanism of complement activation in the hyperacute rejection of porcine organs transplanted into primate recipients. Am J Pathol 140:1157–1166

Dalmasso AP, Vercellotti GM, Platt JL, et al. 1991 Inhibition of complement-mediated endothelial cell cytotoxicity by decay accelerating factor: potential for prevention of xenograft hyperacute rejection. Transplantation 52:530–533

Deacon T, Schumacher J, Dinsmore J, et al. 1997 Histological evidence of fetal pig neural cell survival after transplantation into a patient with Parkinson's disease. Nat Med 3:350–353

Dean PG, Kim DY, Ninova, et al. 2001 Induction of Heme oxygenase-1 with cobalt protoporphyrin fails to prolong hamster-to-rat kidney xenograft survival. (Abstract 1266). Am J Transplant 1[Suppl 1]:456

Delikouras A, Hayes M, Malde P, et al. (2001) Nitric oxide-mediated expression of Bcl- 2 and Bcl-xl and protection from TNFα -mediated apoptosis in porcine endothelial cells after exposure to low concentrations of xenoreactive natural antibody. Transplantation

Diamond LE, McCurry KR, Oldham ER, et al. 1996 Characterization of transgenic pigs expressing functionally active human CD59 on cardiac endothelium. Transplantation 61:1241–1249

Diamond LE, Quinn CM, Martin MJ, et al. 2001 A human CD46 transgenic pig model system for the study of discordant xenotransplantation. Transplantation 71:132–142

Evans RW 2001 Coming to terms with reality: why xenotransplantation is a necessity. In Xenotransplantation. Platt JL, editor. ASM Press, Washington, D. C. 29–51

Evans RW, Orians CE, and Ascher NL 1992 The potential supply of organ donors: an assessment of the efficiency of organ procurement efforts in the United States. JAMA 267:239–246

Galili U, Clark MR, Shohet SB, et al. 1987 Evolutionary relationship between the natural anti-Gal antibody and the Gal α1–3Gal epitope in primates. Proc Natl Acad Sci USA 84:1369–1373

Gritsch HA, Glaser RM, Emery DW, et al. 1994 The importance of nonimmune factors in reconstitution by discordant xenogeneic hematopoietic cells. Transplantation 57:906–917

Gunsalus JR, Brady DA, Coulter SM, et al. 1997 Reduction of serum cholesterol in watanabe rabbits by xenogeneic hepatocellular transplantation. Nat Med 3:48–53

Halloran PF, Melk A, and Barth C 1999 Rethinking chronic allograft nephropathy: the concept of accelerated senescence. J Am Soc Nephrol 10:167–181

Hammer C 1998 Physiological obstacles after xenotransplantation. Ann N Y Acad Sci 862:19–27

Hancock WW, Buelow R, Sayegh MH, et al. 1998 Antibody-induced transplant arteriosclerosis is prevented by graft expression of anti-oxidant and anti-apoptotic genes. Nat Med 4:1392–1396

Holzknecht ZE, Coombes S, Blocher BA, et al. 2001 Immune complex formation after xenotransplantation: evidence of type III as well as type II immune reactions provide clues to pathophysiology. Am J Pathol 158:627–637

Inverardi L, Samaja M, Motterlini R, et al. 1992 Early recognition of a discordant xenogeneic organ by human circulating lymphocytes. J Immunol 149:1416–1423

Itescu S, Artrip JH, Kwiatkowski PA, et al. 1997 Lysis of pig endothelium by IL-2 activated human natural killer cells is inhibited by swine and human major histocompatibility complex (MHC) class I gene products. Ann Transplant 2:14–20

Jurd KM, Gibbs RV, and Hunt BJ 1996 Activation of human prothrombin by porcine aortic endothelial cells–a potential barrier to pig to human xenotransplantation. Blood Coagul Fibrinolysis 7:336–343

Kanai N, and Platt JL 2000 Xenotransplantation of the liver. Clinics in Liver Disease 4:731–746

Kaufman DB, Platt JL, Rabe F, et al. 1990 Differential roles of Mac-1+ cells, and CD4+ and CD8+ T lymphocytes in primary nonfunction and classic rejection of islet allografts. J Exp Med 172:291–302

Kobayashi T, Taniguchi S, Ye Y, et al. 1996 Delayed xenograft rejection in C3-depleted discordant (pig-to-baboon) cardiac xenografts treated with cobra venom factor. Transplant Proc 28:560

Lai L, Prather RS 2002 Progress in producing knockout models for xenotransplantation by nuclean transfer. Annals of Medicine 34:501–506

Lawson JH, and Platt JL 1996 Molecular barriers to xenotransplantation. Transplantation 62:303–310

Leventhal JR, Dalmasso AP, Cromwell JW, et al. 1993a Prolongation of cardiac xenograft survival by depletion of complement. Transplantation 55:857–866

Leventhal JR, Matas AJ, Sun LH, et al. 1993b The immunopathology of cardiac xenograft rejection in the guinea pig-to-rat model. Transplantation 56:1-8

Lin SS, Hanaway MJ, Gonzalez-Stawinski GV, et al. 2000 The role of anti-Galα1–3Gal antibodies in acute vascular rejection and accommodation of xenografts. Transplantation (Rapid Communication) 70:1667–1674

Lin SS, Kooyman DL, Daniels LJ, et al. 1997 The role of natural anti-Galα1–3Gal antibodies in hyperacute rejection of pig-to-baboon cardiac xenotransplants. Transpl Immunol 5:212–218

Lin SS, Weidner BC, Byrne GW, et al. 1998 The role of antibodies in acute vascular rejection of pig-to-baboon cardiac transplants. J Clin Invest 101:1745–1756

Logan JS, and Martin MJ 1994 Transgenic swine as a recombinant production system for human hemoglobin. Methods Enzymol 231:435–445

Magee JC, Collins BH, Harland RC, et al. 1995 Immunoglobulin prevents complement mediated hyperacute rejection in swine-to-primate xenotransplantation. J Clin Invest 96:2404–2412

Malyguine AM, Saadi S, Holzknecht RA, et al. 1997 Induction of procoagulant function in porcine endothelial cells by human NK cells. J Immunol 159:4659–4664

Mazzucato M, De Marco L, Pradella P, et al. 1996 Porcine von Willebrand factor binding to human platelet GPIb induces transmembrane calcium influx. Thromb Haemost 75:655–660

McCreath KJ, Howcroft J, Campbell KHS, et al. 2000 Production of gene-targeted sheep by nuclear transfer from cultured somatic cells. Nature 405:1066–1069

McCurry KR, Kooyman DL, Alvarado CG, et al. 1995 Human complement regulatory proteins protect swine-to-primate cardiac xenografts from humoral injury. Nat Med 1:423–427

Mueller YM, Davenport C, and Ildstad ST 1999 Xenotransplantation: application of disease resistance. Clin Exp Pharmacol Physiol 26:1009–1012

Nagano H, Mitchell RN, Taylor MK, et al. 1997 Interferon-gamma deficiency prevents coronary arteriosclerosis but not myocardial rejection in transplanted mouse hearts. J Clin Invest 100:550–557

Nagata H, Ito M, Cai J, Edge AS, Platt JL, Fox IJ 2003 Treatment of cirrhosis and liver failure in rats by hepatocyte xenotransplantation. Gastroenterology 124:422–431

Nagayasu T, and Platt JL 1998 Progress in xenotransplantation. Graft 1:19–24

Nagayasu T, Saadi S, Holzknecht RA, et al. 2000 Expression of tissue factor mRNA in cardiac xenografts: clues to the pathogenesis of acute vascular rejection. Transplantation 69:475–482

Onishi A, Iwamoto M, Akita T, et al. 2000 Pig cloning by microinjection of fetal fibroblast nuclei. Science 289:1188–1190

Osman N, McKenzie IF, Ostenried K, et al. 1997 Combined transgenic expression of alpha-galactosidase and alpha1,2-fucosyltransferase leads to optimal reduction in the major xenoepitope Galalpha(1,3)Gal. Proc Natl Acad Sci 94:14677–14682

Parker W, Lin SS, and Platt JL 2001 Antigen expression in xenotransplantation: how low must it go? Transplantation 71:313–319

Patience C, Takeuchi Y, and Weiss RA 1997 Infection of human cells by an endogenous retrovirus of pigs. Nat Med 3:282–286

Perper RJ, and Najarian JS 1966 Experimental renal heterotransplantation. I. In widely divergent species. Transplantation 4:377–388

Phelps CJ, Koike C, Vaught TD, Boone J, Wells KD, Chen SH, Ball S, Specht SM, Polejaeva IA, Monahan JA, Jobst PM, Sharma SB, Lamborn AE, Varst AS, Moore M, Demetris AJ, Rudert WA, Bottino R, Bertera S, Trucco M, Starzl TE, Dai Y, Hyares DL 2003 Production of α1,3-galactosyltransferase-deficient pigs. Science 299:411–414

Platt JL 1998 New directions for organ transplantation. Nature 392 (Suppl): 11–17

Platt JL 2001 Xenotransplantation of the liver: is more complement control needed? Liver Transpl 7(10):933–934

Platt JL, Fischel RJ, Matas AJ, et al. 1991 Immunopathology of hyperacute xenograft rejection in a swine-to-primate model. Transplantation 52:214–220

Platt JL, and Nath KA 1998 Heme oxygenase: protective gene or Trojan horse. Nat Med 4:1364–1365

Platt JL, Vercellotti GM, Dalmasso AP, et al. 1990a Transplantation of discordant xenografts: a review of progress. Immunol Today 11:450–456

Platt JL, Vercellotti GM, Lindman BJ, et al. 1990b Release of heparan sulfate from endothelial cells: implications for the pathogenesis of hyperacute rejection. J Exp Med 171:1363–1368

Polejaeva IA, Chen S, Vaught TD, et al. 2000 Cloned piglets produced by nuclear transfer from adult somatic cells. Nature 407:86–90

Pruitt SK, Kirk AD, Bollinger RR, et al. 1994 The effect of soluble complement receptor type 1 on hyperacute rejection of porcine xenografts. Transplantation 57:363–370

Ramirez P, Chavez R, Majado M, et al. 2000 Life-supporting human complement regulator decay accelerating factor transgenic pig liver xenograft maintains the metabolic function and coagulation in the nonhuman primate for up to 8 days. Transplantation 70:989–998

Sachs DH, and Sablinski T 1995 Tolerance across discordant xenogeneic barriers. Xenotransplantation 2:234–239

Sandrin MS, Fodor WL, Mouhtouris E, et al. 1995 Enzymatic remodelling of the carbohydrate surface of a xenogeneic cell substantially reduces human antibody binding and complement-mediated cytolysis. Nat Med 1:1261–1267

Sandrin MS, and McKenzie IF 1999 Recent advances in xenotransplantation. Curr Opin Immunol 11:527–531

Sandrin MS, Vaughan HA, Dabkowski PL, et al. 1993 Anti-pig IgM antibodies in human serum react predominantly with Galα(1,3)Gal epitopes. Proc Natl Acad Sci 90:11391–11395

Schmoeckel M, Bhatti FNK, Zaidi A, et al. 1997 Xenotransplantation of pig organs transgenic for human DAF: an update. Transplant Proc 29:3157–3158

Sharma A, Okabe JF, Birch P, et al. 1996 Reduction in the level of Gal (α1,3) Gal in transgenic mice and pigs by the expression of an α(1,2) fucosyltransferase. Proc Natl Acad Sci 93:7190–7195

Soares MP, Lin Y, Anrather J, et al. 1998 Expression of heme oxygenase-1 can determine cardiac xenograft survival. Nat Med 4:1073–1077

Starzl TE, Fung J, Tzakis A, et al. 1993 Baboon-to-human liver transplantation. Lancet 341:65–71

Valdivia LA, Fung JJ, Demetris AJ, et al. 1994 Donor species complement after liver xenotransplantation. Transplantation 57:918–922

Waaga AM, Gasser M, Laskowski I, et al. 2000 Mechanisms of chronic rejection. Curr Opin Immunol 12:517–521

Waterworth PD, Dunning J, Tolan M, et al. 1998 Life-supporting pig-to-baboon heart xenotransplantation. J Heart Lung Transplant 17:1201–1207

Yu PB, Holzknecht ZE, Bruno D, et al. 1996 Modulation of natural IgM binding and complement activation by natural IgG antibodies. J Immunol 157:5163–5168

Yuzawa Y, Brett J, Fukatsu A, et al. 1995 Interaction of antibody with forssman antigen in guinea pigs. Am J Pathol 146:1260–1272

Zaidi A, Schmoeckel M, Bhatti F, et al. 1998 Life-supporting pig-to-primate renal xenotransplantation using genetically modified donors. Transplantation 65:1584–1590

Xenotransplantation: Public Health Risks—Patient vs. Society in an Emerging Field

L. E. Chapman

CDC, 1600 Clifton Road, Mailstop A-12, Atlanta, GA 30333, USA
E-mail: lec3@cdc.gov

1	Background—Xenotransplantation in Historical Perspective	24
1.1	What Constitutes Xenotransplantation in this Millennium?	25
2	Framing the Safety Issues Impacting Public Policy Development	26
3	Xenotransplantation as a Public Policy Controversy	30
3.1	Viewpoints on Ethical Imperatives	30
4	Reexamining Existing Assumptions	32
4.1	Does Xenotransplantation Pose a Unique Risk?	32
4.2	Is Xenotransplantation More Dangerous than Other Routes of Exposure?	33
4.3	Can the Risk Associated with Xenotransplantation Be Quantified?	35
4.4	Do Endogenous Retroviruses Represent a Significant Risk?	36
5	Summary and Future Directions	38
References		39

Abstract Xenotransplantation is a public health concern because it has the potential to infect human recipients with zoonotic and other infectious agents that are not endemic in human populations, thereby potentially introducing new infections to the human community. From this perspective, xenotransplantation clinical trials combine a potential benefit for individual recipients with a potential risk to the human community. However, the potential for benefit also extends beyond the individual recipient to society as a whole, a fact infrequently recognized in discussions of this topic. Further, diseases neither endemic in human communities nor recognized as classic zoonoses are introduced into humans periodically through routine interactions between human and nonhuman animals. Thus, xenotransplantation is one of multiple potential routes by which infectious agents of nonhuman origin may enter human ecosystems. The intentional and controlled nature of xenotransplantation exposures enables implementation of measures to minimize associated biohazards. Development of guidelines and implementation of regulatory oversight of xenotransplantation clinical trials in most nations where such research occurs has promoted a standard level of practice in the field and markedly reduced the risk of xenotransplant-introduced infection compared to the situation in 1995.

1 Background—Xenotransplantation in Historical Perspective

Xenotransplantation—attempts to use living biological material from nonhuman animals in humans for therapeutic purposes—has been the recent focus of both interest and controversy. Attempts to replace failing human organs with substitutes harvested from nonhuman animals predate an understanding of modern immunology. In the days before either availability of dialysis or an understanding of the scientific basis of immune rejection kidneys from rabbits and sheep were transplanted into children dying of Bright's disease in vain attempts to sustain life. Extracts from glands of nonhuman animals were touted as cures for failing potency or other aspects of bodily decline associated with aging. Inevitably these failed, and as a basic understanding of immune response developed such efforts by serious researchers declined.

Over the past half century, advances in understanding of immunology and physiology, combined with technical innovations, resulted in a revolution in the ameliorative powers of allotransplantation (transplantation of organs and tissues among humans). However, a critical shortage of human donors continues to limit the benefits (United Network for Organ Sharing 1997). The demonstrated ability to overcome immunologic hurdles that initially prohibited allotransplantation and the demonstrated ameliorative power of transplant medicine combined with the shortage of available human donor biologic material have combined to again raise interest in xenotransplantation (Auchincloss 1988).

In the early 1960s, prior to either the availability of universal dialysis or the widespread use of human cadaver kidneys for transplantation when renal failure was often a fatal disease, researchers at Tulane Medical Center transplanted chimpanzee kidneys into humans with renal failure with limited success. One recipient survived for 9 months with functioning chimpanzee kidneys intact, thus initiating the modern era of xenotransplantation in the USA (Reemtsma 1969). A series of attempts to transplant whole nonhuman animal organs (primarily from nonhuman primates or pigs) into humans followed without notable success, and efforts to develop whole organ xenotransplantation currently remain stalled at the preclinical stage (Xenotransplantation Subcommittee of the Biological Response Modifiers Advisory Committee to the US Food and Drug Administration 1999). However, a variety of creative attempts to develop cellular or tissue xenotransplantation products have shown enough promise to progress to clinical trials in the USA.

Optimism about and funding for xenotransplantation experimentation have fluctuated over the years, influenced by advances in science or disappointments in clinical trial attempts. The clearly superior potential of biologic products over mechanical devices as therapeutic replacements for failing innate biologic function of humans has sustained a recurring return to xenotransplantation as an area of promise for therapeutic advancement. Advances in stem cell research and cloning technology, both current centers of controversy, may one day enable production of tailor made biologic replacement parts for humans that avoid the innate liabilities that the immunologic and physiologic distances between species impose (Kind and Colman 1999; Fischer 2000). Short of delivery on potential in these areas of innovation, xenotransplantation continues to emit a siren call for biomedical researchers who hope to contribute to paradigm shifts in the therapeutic potential of modern medicine for disease that results when human organs fail.

1.1 What Constitutes Xenotransplantation in this Millennium?

By the beginning of this millennium, the range of envisioned potential therapeutic uses for living biologic material from nonhuman animals extended well beyond the concept of replacement parts for human organs in short supply. In recent years the majority of proposed clinical xenotransplantation trials use cellular preparations, often immunoprotected in some manner, and attempt to ameliorate disease other than by replacement of whole organs. Use of some types of cellular xenotransplantation products currently in clinical trials under the oversight of the Food and Drug Administration (FDA) in the USA are discussed below.

The US Public Health Service (PHS) defines xenotransplantation as any procedure that involves the transplantation, implantation, or infusion into a human recipient of either: (a) live cells, tissues, or organs from a nonhuman animal source; or (b) human body fluids, cells tissues, or organs that have had ex vivo contact with live nonhuman animal cells, tissues, or organs (US Public Health Service 2001). A single term that encompasses the living material used in all categories of xenotransplantation, 'xenotransplantation product', is now used to refer to the live cells, tissues, or organs (whether human or nonhuman) used in xenotransplantation.

Clinical trials in the USA have implanted porcine neurologic cells into the central nervous system of patients with degenerative neurologic disorders, such as Parkinson's disease and Huntington's disease (Fink et al. 2000). Patients with fulminant hepatic failure have been supported with blood perfused through devices containing porcine hepatocytes (Chari et al 1994). Human epidermal cells cultured ex vivo on a murine cell line have been used to replace missing skin in severely burned patients (Dapolito and Auchincloss 2000). Attempts to functionally cure diabetes using injections or implantation of porcine pancreatic cell preparations have been explored in clinical trials in Europe and in preclinical animal studies in the USA (Groth et al. 1994; Zhang et al. 2000). Preclinical studies have explored xenografting of porcine neuronal cells into rodents, raising hopes that porcine neuronal cells might some day be used for axonal regeneration of neurons involved in spinal cord injuries (Imaizumi et al. 2000). Increasing numbers of humans participants in clinical trials are alive months to years after receiving cellular transplantation products that have survived in situ for prolonged periods of time (Fink et al. 2000; Chari et al. 1994; Dapolito and Auchincloss 2000; Groth et al. 1994; Zhang et al. 2000; Heneine et al. 1998; Patience et al. 1998; Paradis et al. 1999).

2 Framing the Safety Issues Impacting Public Policy Development

Inevitably, advances in medicine and science are accompanied by associated unintended consequences. The transmission of both metastatic cancer and infectious pathogens through allotransplantation has been well documented (Eastlund 1995; Simonds 1993). Serious complications, including graft rejection or death, that can result from infections derived from transplanted allografts in immunosuppressed transplant recipients are routinely recognized (Gerstenkorn et al. 2001; LeBlanc et al. 1998).

Transplantation of xenogeneic cells, tissues, or organs inevitably also has the potential to transfer infectious agents from the source to the recipient. However, in this setting the receiving animal is human, and the source animal is not. This adds a complexity not present in allotransplantation where the donor-to-recipient loop does not cross species lines.

Xenotransplantation may serve to transmit classic zoonoses (infectious diseases transmissible across species lines) to xenotransplantation product recipients. The intimacy of interaction between health care workers and both patients and patient bodily fluids exceeds that of most communal human activities. The introduction of a zoonotic infection into a single hospitalized patient provides a nidus for potential dissemination of a nosocomial outbreak of zoonotic disease. Such nosocomial outbreaks have been documented with a variety of zoonoses, including a variety of viral hemorrhagic fevers (WHO 1978; Burney et al. 1980; Suleiman et al. 1980; Swanepoel et al. 1987).

Of more concern is that the unique facilitating circumstances of xenotransplantation may allow infectious agents not recognized to cross species barriers under normal circumstances to breech host defenses and establish infections in recipients of xenogeneic biologic materials. The terms xenosis and xenozoonosis have been proposed to describe infections such as these introduced into humans through procedures involving xenogeneic tissue (Fishman 1994; Michaels and Simmons 1994).

Experience with zoonotic disease suggests that mechanisms of evolutionary adaptation are inherent in both pathogens and their natural hosts. The pathogenic potential of an infection is a function of the relationship developed between the host and the infecting agent; the biologic features of both are contributory (Woolhouse et al. 2000; Weiss 2001). Thus, the pathogenic potential of an infection may be changed when an infecting microbe is transmitted from its natural host into a new species.

This change may manifest abruptly when the host environment changes in the absence of alteration in the microbe. An example is the Hantavirus pulmonary syndrome that results when an unmodified sin nombre virus is transmitted from an asymptomatic persistently infected rodent into a human (Chapman et al. 2002). Nearly half of all human cases of Hantavirus pulmonary syndrome are fatal. Another example is the acquired immunodeficiency syndrome (AIDS) that accompanies human immunodeficiency virus (HIV) infection of humans, contrasted with the disease-free state of chimpanzees infected with simian immunodeficiency virus (SIV), the progenitor virus of HIV.

The cumulative body of science addressing the origin of the HIV pandemic suggests that multiple SIVs that were nonpathogenic in their natural host, were transmitted to individual humans through injuries or other exposures. Evidence supports introduction of SIV counterparts of HIV type 1 and HIV type 2 into human populations at least seven times (Hahn et al. 2000). At least one cross-species transmission resulted in a persistent infection and secondary transmission among humans eventually responsible for the majority of pandemic human infections with HIV-1 group M viruses (Hahn et al. 2000). By the turn of the millennium, HIV was an established endemic human infection and no longer a zoonosis.

Alternatively, abrupt changes in the biologic properties of viruses may occur through recombination (i.e., gene reassortment) between human and animal strains during passage of a virus adapted to one species through cells of another species. Such changes may modulate infectivity, pathogenicity, and transmissibility in an unpredictable manner. New influenza viral variants with pandemic potential for humans are recognized intermittently, and probably originate from cross-species infections that provide opportunity for reassortment of genes between human and porcine, avian, or other species influenza during passage through another host (Brown 2000). The avian influenza that resulted in 18 human infections (six of them fatal) in Hong Kong in 1997 is a recent example of such phenomenon (Subbarao and Katz 2000). The Swine influenza pandemic of 1918–19, estimated to have been responsible for 40 million human deaths worldwide, is a more distant example (Oxford 2000).

Changes in the infectivity and pathogenicity of an infecting agent may evolve quietly over time through a process of serial mutations resulting in viral adaptation, influenced by the addition or removal of selective pressures associated with the change in host species (Chapman and Fishman 1997). Specific selective pressures might include preexisting immunity or exposure to antiviral agents. Recombination between distinct viral lineages co-infecting a single animal are not rare events in nature, and can lead to altered tropism, virulence, and drug resistance patterns.

Pharmacologic immunosuppression will frequently accompany xenotransplantation. Persistent replication in immunocompromised hosts of viruses that characteristically produce short nonpersistent infections in immune competent hosts has been described (Klimov et al 1995; Rocha et al 199135, 36). Whenever persistent viral replication occurs, viral mutants will accumulate over time. As a result, the viral population shed late in the course of any persistent viral infection may have different biologic characteristics from the progenitor viral variant that originated the infection. Temporal modulation of viral virulence in association with the evolution of viral variants occurs and accounts for the attenuation of pathogenicity of a passaged virus compared to wild-type. This potential for attenuation has been exploited in the development of live viral vaccines. However, the potential for accumulation of variants with augmented pathogenicity also exists.

In some instances, such as non-zoonotic bacteria, the microbes associated with the source animal may intrinsically differ little from those present in the human or the human health care environment. Nevertheless, the introduction of such bacteria may not be entirely inconsequential. For instance, patterns of antibiotic usage in animal husbandry differ from those in human medicine (Gorbach 2001). Introduction of bacteria from animal husbandry environments into human health care settings may also introduce unanticipated patterns of antibiotic resistance, mandating vigilance.

Studies of recipients of historic xenotransplants have removed these concerns from the realm of the merely theoretical. Simian foamy virus (SFV) and baboon endogenous retrovirus were identified in microchimeric baboon cells in distal anatomic sites of two recipients of baboon livers weeks after transplantation (Allan et al 1998). Studies have also identified baboon cytomegalovirus (CMV) in the white blood cells of one recipient of a baboon liver transplant, although whether this indicates baboon CMV infection of human cells or simply expression of baboon CMV from persistently infected microchimeric baboon lymphocytes remains undetermined (Michaels et al 2001).

In summary, xenotransplantation is a public health concern because it has the potential to infect human recipients with zoonotic and other infectious agents that are not endemic in human populations, thereby potentially introducing new infections to the human community (xenogeneic infection). From this perspective, xenotransplantation clinical trials combine a potential benefit for individual recipients with a potential risk to the human community.

3 Xenotransplantation as a Public Policy Controversy

Respect for biohazards potentially associated with xenotransplantation has generated a great deal of concern among both lay people and scientists (Chapman et al 1995; Bach et al 1998). In the past, individual prominent scientists, lay persons, and the Council of Europe called for a moratorium on clinical trials. In December 1998 the international Campaign for Responsible Transplantation petitioned the Secretary of the US Department of Health and Human Services for rulemaking to prohibit xenotransplantation in the USA. That petition was denied in December 1999.

The lessons learned from the experience with zoonotic disease in general, and the AIDS pandemic in particular, do argue that there are sufficient infectious risks inherent in xenotransplantation to justify a reasonable degree of concern. Scientists and policy makers in this field labor on the horns of a dilemma resulting from the inextricable wedding of uncertain collective risk to the potential benefit for both individuals and society as discussed below. Protecting the human community from infectious risks associated with xenotransplantation differs from protecting them from the risk of meningococcal disease and is more analogous to gene therapy experience: a potential benefit is accompanied by a need for public safeguards. Planning for these infectious risks should be incorporated into the development of any clinical strategy involving the use of xenogeneic tissue in humans.

3.1 Viewpoints on Ethical Imperatives

The difficulties of applying basic principles of biomedical ethics such as beneficence, non-maleficence, autonomy and justice to both the individual and to the community are manifest. Ethical thinkers have wrestled with the potential for conflict between the right of a dying patient to the only available treatment and the right of the community to avoid being exposed to an unknown and possibly nonexistent threat of infection (Aluwihare 1999). Much interest has focused on the responsibility of individual patients to the community, including discussion of whether compliance with post-transplantation surveillance could be coerced and whether consideration should be given to contracts that bind patients in advance to follow up, regardless of any later wavering on the part of the individuals (Daar 1999). Others have focused on the responsibility of the community to the individual patient. The National Academy of Sciences, Institute of Medicine Workshop on Xenotransplantation, for instance, argued that we diminish our own humanity if we, as a community, are unwilling to accept some level of risk for the sake of those among us whose suffering is evident and potentially ameliorable (Institute of Medicine 1996). At least one ethicist has attempted to look at risks and benefits associated with xenotransplantation through reasoning influenced by a cognizance of the evolutionary theories of Darwin. Donnelley's premise is that ethical reasoning in the arena of evolutionary biology should attempt to operate with a recognition of complex cascades of multiplying cause and effect, and reject both the possibility of perfection and the inherent limitations of attempts at ethical reasoning that assume straight-line cause and effect (Donnelley 1999).

In the end, the responsibilities and benefits of both the individuals and the larger community to which they belong are intertwined. Xenotransplantation does in fact hold a potential for risk but also for benefit both individual recipients and to society as a whole.

That benefit may extend beyond the individual recipient, a fact too often unrecognized or unacknowledged in discussions of this topic, can be illustrated by even a limited examination of one proposed application for xenotransplantation: attempts to functionally cure juvenile onset type 1 diabetes mellitus using porcine pancreatic islets. The cost of the disease burden of juvenile onset diabetes has a tremendous impact on society. In 1998 diabetes mellitus was the seventh leading cause of death in the USA. Diabetes accounted for 24.7 deaths and 176.8 years of productive life lost before age 75 per 100,000 population (Eberhardt et al 2001). Despite ongoing efforts at research and therapeutic innovation, this impact has not diminished significantly since 1950. In 1999 in the USA diabetes was responsible for 96,000 hospitalizations with an average duration of 6 days each (Eberhardt et al 2001). Human diabetes has long been managed by intermittent injections of porcine insulin. If early onset diabetes could be functionally cured by implanting porcine pancreatic islets, the cost savings to society in both dollars and years of productive life would be significant.

4 Reexamining Existing Assumptions

Is there a potential for a xenogeneic infection to constitute a threat to the general public health? The simple answer is 'yes'. But the more cogent question may not be 'Does xenotransplantation present a risk to society?' but rather 'Does xenotransplantation pose a unique risk to society?' The answer to this question manifestly is 'no'.

4.1 Does Xenotransplantation Pose a Unique Risk?

Disease neither endemic in human communities or recognized as classic zoonoses are introduced into humans periodically through routine interactions between human and nonhuman animals during husbandry, hunting, and other activities. Recent examples include Nipah virus encephalitis in humans involved in pig husbandry in Malaysia in 1999 (Parashar et al 2000); avian influenza in humans in Hong Kong, 1997 (Subbarao and Katz 2000); atypical Creutzfeldt–Jakob disease in beef eaters in Britain in 1994 (Belay 1999); Ebola in an ethnologist who conducted a necropsy on a wild chimpanzee in Cote d'Ivoire, West Africa in 1994 (Formenty et al 1999); and swine influenza in visitors to and exhibitors of pigs in a county fair in Wisconsin in 1988 (Wells et al 1991). Biomedical research activities are rich sources of opportunity for acute human infections with non-endemic agents. Examples include infections of persons occupationally exposed to nonhuman primates with SIV, SFV, cercopithecine herpes virus 1, and Marburg virus (Khabbaz et al 1994; Heneine et al 1998; CDC 1998; Martini 1969). Xenotransplantation is one of a growing number of therapeutic bioproducts that provide opportunity for human exposure to infections agents originating from nonhuman animals. SV40, a polyomavirus, was first isolated from rhesus monkey kidney cells used for polio vaccine stocks in the 1950s, when a generational cohort of children seroconverted to SV40 after polio vaccination (Strickler et al 1998). The Centers for Disease Control and Prevention (CDC), FDA, and the United States Department of Agriculture laboratories recently investigated the significance of avian retroviral activity in measles vaccine stock and of porcine parvovirus and porcine endogenous retrovirus (PERV) in porcine factor VIII (Heneine et al 2001; Hussain et al 2001; Johnson and Heneine 2001; Tsang et al 1999).

Further, historical data argue that many diseases currently endemic in human populations were originally introduced through cross-species infections from nonhuman animals. The evidentiary links arguing that HIV-2 came into humans as cross-species transmission of SIV from sooty mangabey monkeys in West Africa (Hirsch et al 1989), and that HIV-1 originated in humans as cross-species transmission of SIV from chimpanzees (Hahn et al 2000) have already been mentioned. Comparative genomic analysis of the human tapeworm and other species of *Taenia* suggest that the human tapeworms evolved from parasites that originally colonized East African herbivores and utilized lions and hyenas as their final host. These ancestral tapeworms were probably introduced into humans who consumed scavenged or hunted meat in East Africa. A *Taenia* species specialized to utilize humans as the final host probably evolved hundreds of thousands of years prior to completion of the current life cycle, utilizing pigs and cows as intermediate hosts (Hoberg et al 2001). Similarly, comparative genomic analysis of *Yersinia* species suggests that *Y. pestis*, the agent of the bubonic plague that decimated the Roman Empire in 542 a.d. and Europe in 1347, is a recently emerged clone of *Y. pseudotuberculosis*, a bacterium that is shed in rodent feces and causes only mild disease in humans (Achtman et al 1999). All these introductions of new diseases into the human community through cross-species infections occurred without host-defense breeching interventions such as xenotransplantation and prior to the advent of frequent intimate exposures of humans to nonhuman animals through biomedical research activities or therapeutic products derived from biologic materials originating from nonhuman species.

Xenotransplantation, therefore, is just one of multiple potential entry points by which infectious agents of nonhuman origin enter human ecosystems.

4.2
Is Xenotransplantation More Dangerous than Other Routes of Exposure?

Prior to 1995, unscreened domestic farm pigs, baboons from large unscreened open breeding colonies, or even feral nonhuman primates were considered appropriate sources for xenotransplantation products. These practices carried a risk of introducing xenogeneic infections via xenotransplantation that was high compared to other potential exposures, such as exposure through animal husbandry activities where host barrier protections were rarely breeched. Regulatory oversight of xenotransplantation clinical trials in the USA and most nations where such research is proceeding currently excludes the use of products from nonhuman primates and enforces adherence to public health guidelines on husbandry of source animals, pretransplantation screening and posttransplantation surveillance. This oversight ensures a standard level of practice in the field and markedly reduces the risk of xenotransplant-introduced infection compared to the situation in 1995. The implications for safety of this evolution in practice should not be ignored in discussions of the relative safety of xenotransplantation clinical trials.

Yes, breeches of normal host defenses, exogenous immunosuppression of the human recipient, and modifications of the source animal that may have the unintended side effect of facilitating the ability of viruses contained within the xenotransplantation product to evade host defenses all conspire to increase the likelihood that microbes unable to infect humans under normal conditions may be able to create persistent productive infections in the xenotransplant setting. However, the husbandry and screening practices outlined in the PHS Guideline on Infectious Disease Issues in Xenotransplantation and other guidances, if enforced, decrease the probability that exogenous infectious agents will be contained in xenotransplantation products to almost negligible levels (U.S. Public Health Service 2001; Health Canada 1999; Health Council of the Netherlands 1998; Subcommission of Xenotransplantation of the Permanent Commission of the Transplants of the Interterritorial Council of the National Health System 1998; Swedish Committee on Xenotransplantation 1999; United Kingdom Department of Health 1997; Transplantation Society of Australia and New Zealand Inc. 1998; Council of Europe 1997; WHO 1998). The rigorous husbandry and screening procedures result in source animals that have a defined lifetime of exposures to infections, and that are therefore much less likely than either feral animals or human donors to transmit infection to recipients of xenotransplantation products. Arguably under those circumstances, xenotransplantation in fact provides a lower level of risk of introducing cross-species infections than do other activities such as frequent intimate exposure to nonhuman primates through biomedical research activities. Presently, the risk of introduction of infection via contamination of the product, as happens with artificial heart valves and hardware incorporated into humans through orthopedic procedures, probably exceeds the risk of transfer of inherent agents via xenotransplantation, provided existing guidances are closely followed.

4.3 Can the Risk Associated with Xenotransplantation Be Quantified?

Caution should be exercised regarding assumptions of both safety and risk until the science is adequate to establish a solid basis for risk assessment. However, knowledgeable observers have always argued that the risk of introduction of a new pandemic through xenotransplantation was low, but never the less worthy of respect due to the potential impact on society if it occurred (Stoye and Coffin 1995; Stoye 1997, 1998; Stoye et al 1998; Murphy 1996). Progress in policy development has reduced the level of risk compared to that associated with the unregulated field in 1995. Progress in science has provided some basis for estimates of risks. Combined, these advances allow greater confidence in the reasonableness of proceeding with limited clinical trials, provided the trials are accompanied by appropriate safeguards and there is reasonable basis for expectation of benefit to the participants (Stoye 1999).

The risk that human recipients will be infected with exogenous viruses and other identifiable infectious agents can be reduced to negligible levels by limiting the geographic origin and life-long contacts of potential source animals combined with adequate pretransplant screening of the source animal, the colony from which it is chosen, and the xenotransplantation product itself. Pretransplant elimination of known zoonoses through development of specified pathogen free (SPF) colonies is quite feasible with pigs, and SPF facilities and husbandry techniques adequate to exclude known exogenous viruses will probably also exclude unrecognized exogenous viruses. Therefore safety can be increased enormously by limiting source animal selection to closed SPF herds where the presence of infectious agents will be largely limited to endogenous retroviruses and unrecognized transplacentally transmitted agents.

Post-transplantation surveillance will remain necessary to identify infectious agents that were transplanted with the xenotransplantation product because either they were not known to exist (e.g., porcine hepatitis E prior to 1997), they were known to exist but our diagnostic tools were inadequate to detect them (e.g., prions), or they could not be removed from the xenograft (e.g., endogenous retroviruses).

These interventions are all currently practiced in association with clinical trials in nations where such practices are regulated (U.S. Public Health Service 2001; Health Canada 1999; Health Council of the Netherlands 1998; Subcommission of Xenotransplantation of the Permanent Commission of the Transplants of the Interterritorial Council of the National Health System 1998; Swedish Committee on Xenotransplantation 1999; United Kingdom Department of Health 1997; Transplantation Society of Australia and New Zealand Inc. 1998; Council of Europe 1997; WHO 1998). Careful adherence to existing guidances should minimize or eliminate risks of recipient infection with exogeneous infectious agents. Endogenous retroviruses remain as an under-characterized concern. However, much progress has been made in characterizing the ability of these entities to create active infections in human hosts.

4.4 Do Endogenous Retroviruses Represent a Significant Risk?

Hypothesized to represent 'fossil remnants' of exogenous retroviruses once capable of causing active infection in the host species, endogenous retroviruses exist as inactive and usually defective proviral DNA integrated into the germline of all mammals adequately studied to date, including humans and all species considered as potential source animals for xenotransplantation. Many of these endogenous retroviruses can express infectious virus, but are no longer capable of causing active infection in the host species. Some expressed viruses are xenotropic, meaning that they are able to infect cell lines from other species. Endogenous retroviruses of both pigs and baboons can infect human cell lines in vitro (Deinhardt 1980; Patience et al 1997; Wilson et al 1998). Thus, all xenotransplantation products from any species may contain benign genomic DNA that, on transfer into a human host, may express infectious retrovirus capable of creating active persistent infection. The significance of this innate infectious potential of animal tissue devoid of any identifiable exogenous microorganisms has been the subject of much concern and scientific inquiry over the past 5 years.

Recent scientific investigations have attempted to define the significance of endogenous retroviruses of pigs, currently the preferred source animal for xenotransplantation. Three variants of PERV have been shown to be expressed from multiple porcine cell lines, as well as from primary porcine tissue (Patience et al 1997; Wilson et al 1998; Armstrong et al 1971; Strandstrom et al 1974; Todaro et al 1974). The capacity for PERV released from both porcine cell lines and primary porcine cells to productively infect both cell lines and primary cells from humans has also been established (Patience et al 1997; Wilson et al 1998). Amplification of PERV DNA in severely immunodeficient murine recipients of porcine pancreatic islet cells has been demonstrated, but only within tissue compartments that contain microchimeric porcine cells (Van der Laan et al 2000). These observations may represent abortive, asymptomatic PERV infection of the murine host, and could support concerns that PERV expressed from porcine xenotransplantation products may be able to infect the human recipients. However, these data could also be interpreted to support suspicions of some investigators that the clinical and public health consequences of putative PERV infections of xenotransplantation recipients, if such infections occurred, might be limited and inconsequential. Alternative hypotheses regarding proper interpretation of these findings remain untested to date. Further research is needed to allow proper interpretation of the significance of this report.

Since October 1997, when evidence that PERV could infect human cells in vitro emerged, the FDA has required all sponsors of porcine xenotransplantation product trials to develop adequate assays to test such products for infectious virus and to monitor recipients for PERV infections. To date, limited studies of 202 humans exposed to pig cells and tissues have produced no clinical or laboratory evidence of PERV infection (Heneine et al 1998; Patience et al 1998; Paradis et al 1999; Schumacher et al 2000; Pitkin and Mullon 1999). However, persons who had undergone transient hemoperfusion through pig spleens showed evidence of persistent microchimerism with porcine cells surviving up to 8 years later (Paradis et al 1999).

It may be possible to intervene clinically in ways that further diminish the risk of human infection. An emerging literature demonstrates that the engineering of xenotransplantation products as well as duration and nature of exposure may influence the risk of recipient exposure to PERV. Artificial liver dialysis devices, currently in use in clinical protocols, contain porcine hepatocytes encased within hollow fiber membranes. Extraluminal samples from devices made with membranes with mathematically predicted pore sizes of 5 nm and 10 nm could not infect human cell lines, while the extraluminal samples from devices made with mixed cellulose fibers with 200 nm porosity were infective. Thus, experiments show that pore size, membrane composition, and duration of exposure influence the risk of recipient exposure to PERV during bioartificial liver therapy (Nyberg et al. 1999). Reasoning by analogy from the phylogenetic proximity between PERV and feline leukemia virus, it has been hypothesized that peritransplant use of antiretroviral drugs may increase the selective pressure towards abortive rather than persistent infection, and that protective pretransplantation immunization of human recipients may be possible (Qari et al. 2001; D. Onions, Q-one Biotech, Glasgow, Scotland, unpublished results). Recent reports of the identification of pig strains that may exhibit diminished PERV expression combined with successful cloning of pigs suggest other avenues of exploration (Oldmixon et al. 2000).

More studies are needed before the risk posed by the existence of endogenous retroviruses can be definitively quantified. Continued surveillance for evidence of human infections resulting from endogenous retroviruses, archiving of biological materials as insurance if future public health investigations are needed, and further exploration of animal models and engineering innovations are warranted. However, the cumulative science to date is very reassuring, and points the way to additional modifications that may further decrease the low level of clinical risk that currently appears to be associated with human exposure to nonhuman cells and tissue containing endogenous retroviruses.

5
Summary and Future Directions

Xenotransplantation protocols should not progress into clinical trials until convincing preclinical evidence supports a probability of real benefit to individuals. However, at that point current science supports the reasonableness of limited trials performed under regulatory oversight, provided that public safeguards with stable funding and infrastructure are in place at the onset of the clinical trials.

Progress in the development of evidence based public policy will require continuing research in critical areas combined with periodic syntheses/critiques of the existing knowledge base. The initial investigations described here are a promising beginning to what must be a laboriously developed multiphase process. The presence or absence of endogenous retrovirus infection in larger numbers of these recipients must be explored to develop a database with which to quantify the risk of xenogeneic infections. Continued efforts to define the validity of existing diagnostic assays, to develop new assays, and to characterize the risk associated with specific infectious agents will enhance the safety of the community as xenotransplantation moves from research to clinical trials. The development of national and/or international registries and harmonization of efforts to allow comparability of collected information and collective analysis would be very valuable. The development of stable funding and infrastructures for central archiving would further enhance safety. Existing public policies can then be refined in light of new knowledge.

New diseases and newly discovered viruses and other pathogens will continue to emerge. Knowledgeable observers have argued that the risk to the public from xenotransplantation may be exaggerated when compared to that from other types of ongoing exposures such as occupational risk of exposure to simian retroviruses among animal workers and researchers (Murphy 1996; Stoye 1999). While we cannot control what happens in nature, xenotransplantation is an intentional exposure that occurs under controlled circumstances. The intentional and controlled nature of these exposures enables us to implement measures to minimize the biohazard associated with xenotransplantation.

References

Achtman M, Zurth K, Morelli G, Torrea G, Guiyoule A, Carniel E (1999) Yersinia pestis, the cause of plague, is a recently emerged clone of Yersinia pseudotuberculosis. Proceedings of the National Academy of Sciences of the United States of America 96:14043–8

Allan JS, Broussard SR, Michaels MG, Starzl TE, Leighton KL, Whitehead EM, Comuzzie AG, Lanford RE, Leland MM, Switzer WM, Heneine W (1998) Amplification of simian retroviral sequences from human recipients of baboon liver transplants. AIDS Research & Human Retroviruses 14:821–4

Aluwihare A.P.R (1999) New problems beget new solutions. Bull of the WHO 77: 64–5

Armstrong JA, Porterfield JS, De Madrid AT (1971) C-type virus particles in pig kidney cell lines. J. Gen Virol. 10:195–8

Auchincloss Jr. H (1988) Xenogeneic Transplantation: A review. Transplantation 46:1–20

Bach FH, Fishman JA, Daniels N, et al (1998) Uncertainty in xenotransplantation: individual benefit versus collective risk. Nat Med 4:141–44

Belay ED (1999) Transmissible spongiform encephalopathies in humans. Annual Review of Microbiology 53:283–314

Brown EG (2000) Influenza virus genetics. Biomedicine & Pharmacotherapy. 54:196–209

Burney MI, Ghafoor A, Saleen M, Webb PA, Casals J (1980) Nosocomial outbreak of viral hemorrhagiv fever caused by Crimean Hemorrhagiv Fever-congo virus in Pakistan, January 1976. Am J Trop Med Hyg 29:941–7

CDC (1998) Fatal Cercopithecine herpesvirus 1 (B virus) infection following a mucocutaneous exposure and interim recommendations for worker protection. MMWR—Morbidity & Mortality Weekly Report 47:1073–6

Chair's draft report of the June 3–4, 1999 meeting of the Xenotransplantation Subcommittee of the Biological Response Modifyers Advisory Committee to the U.S. Food and Drug Administration. Accessible on Internet at http://www.fda.gov/ohrms/dockets/ac/cber99.htm#Biological

Chapman LE and Fishman JA (1997) Xenotransplantation and Infectious Diseases. In: Xenotransplantation: The Transplantation of Organs and Tissues Between Species, Edition 2. Edited by Cooper D.K.C., Kemp E., Platt J.L., White D.J. Springer-Verlag Berlin Heidelberg New York. pp 736–48

Chapman LE, B Ellis PhD, FT Koster MD, M Sotir MPH, T.G. Ksiazak, D.V.M., PhD, G Mertz MD, PE Rollin MD, KF Baum MD, AT Pavia MD, JC Christenson MD, PJ Rubin MD, HM Jolson MD, RE Behrman MD, AS Khan MD, LJ Wilson Bell MD, GL Simpson MD, M Carroll MD, J Hawk, RC Holman MS, CJ Peters MD, and the Ribavirin Study Group (2002) Discriminators between hantavirus-infected and hantavirus-negative persons enrolled in an open label trial of intravenous ribavirin for presumptive hantavirus pulmonary syndrome. Clinical Infectious Diseases In press, June 2001, anticipated release January 2001

Chapman LE, Folks TM, Salomon DR, Patterson AP, Eggerman TL, Noguichi PD (1995) Xenotransplantation and Xenogeneic Infections. New England Journal of Medicine 333:1498–1501

Chari RS, Collins BH, Magee JC, DiMaio JM, Kirk AD, Harland RC, McCann RL Platt JL, and Meyers WC (1994) Brief report: treatment of hepatic failure with ex vivo pig-liver perfusion followed by liver transplantation. New England Journal of Medicine 331:234–7

Council of Europe (1997) Recommendation on xenotransplantation, September 1997 (Internet:<htt//www.cm.coe.int/ta/rec/1997/97r15.html>)

Daar AS (1999) Xenotransplantation: informed consent / contract and patient surveillance. Biomedical Ethics 4:87–91

Dapolito G, Auchincloss H, Jr (2000) Report of the Food and Drug Administration Subcommittee on Xenotransplantation: meeting of 13 January 2000, Center for Biologics Evaluation and Research. Xenotransplantation 7:75–9

Deinhardt F (1980) Biology of primate retroviruses. In: Klein G, ed. Viral oncology. New York: Raven Press, 357–98

Donnelley S (1999) The Moral Landscape of Xenotransplantation. Presented at Cold Spring Harbor, New York on May 12, 1999 and University College, Oxford University, United Kingdom on September 17, 1999

Eastlund T (1995) Infectious disease transmission through cel, tissue, and organ transplantation: reducing the risk through donor selection. Cell Transplant 4:455–77

Eberhardt MS, Ingram DD, Makuc DM, et al (2001) Urban and Rural Health Chartbook. Health, United States, 2001. Hyatesville, Maryland: National Center for Health Statistics

Fink JS, Schumacher JM, Ellias SL, Palmer P, Saint-Hilaire M, Shannon K, Penn R, Starr P, VanHorne C, Knott HS, Dempsey PK, Fischman AJ, Raineri R, Manhart C, Dinsmore J, Isacson O (2000) Porcine xenografts in Parkinson's disease and Huntington's disease patients: preliminary results. Cell. Transplant. 9:273–8

Fischer JS (2000) Five little piggies going to market. Will clones be a source of organs for humans? US News & World Report 128:51

Fishman JA (1994) Miniature swine as organ donors for man: strategic for prevention of xenotransplant-associated infections. Xenotransplantation 1:27–57

Formenty P, Hatz C, LeGuenno B, Stoll A, Rogenmoser P, Widner A (1999) Human infection due to Ebola Virus, subtype Cote d'Ivoire: clinical and biologic presentation. Journal of Infectious Diseases 179:S48–53

Gerstenkorn C, Jackson G, Di Franco F, Thomusch O, Talbot D (2001) Outcome of PTLD in renal and liver allograft recipients. Transplantation Proceedings 33:2469–72

Gorbach SL (2001) Antimicrobial use in animal feed–time to stop. New England Journal of Medicine 345:1202–3

Groth CG, Korsgren O, Tibell A, Tollemar J, Moller E, Bolinder J, Ostman J, Reinholt FP, Hellerstrom C, and Andersson A (1994) Transplantation of porcine fetal pancreas to diabetic patients. Lancet 344:1402–4

Hahn BH, Shaw GM, De Cock KM, Sharp PM (2000) AIDS as a zoonosis: Scientific and Public health Implications. Science 287:607–14

Health Canada (1999) Proposed Canadian standard for xenotransplantation. The Expert Working Group on Xenotransplantation. July 1999 (Available on the Internet: www.hc-sc.gc.ca/hpb-dgps/therapeut/zfiles/english/btox/standards/xeno_std_e.html)

Health Council of the Netherlands (1998) Committee on Xenotransplantation. xenotransplantation. Rijswijk, The Netherlands: Health Council of The Netherlands, 1998; publication no. 1998/01E

Heneine W, Switzer WM, Sandstrom P, Brown J, Vedipuri S, Shable CA, Khan AS, Lerche NW, Schweizer M, Neumann-Haefelin D, Chapman LE, Folks TM (1998) Identification of a human population infected with simian foamy viruses. Nature Medicine 4:403–7

Heneine W, Switzer WM, Soucie JM, Evatt BL, Shanmugam V, Rosales GV, Matthews A, Sandstrom P, Folks TM (2001) Evidence of porcine endogenous retroviruses in porcine factor VIII and evaluation of transmission to recipients with hemophilia. Journal of Infectious Diseases 183:648–52

Heneine W, Tibell A, Switzer WM, Sandstrom P, Rosales GV, Matthews A, Korsgren O, Chapman LE, Folks TM, Groth CG (1998) No evidence of infection with the porcine endogenous retrovirus in human recipients of porcine islet cell xenografts. Lancet 352:695–9

Hirsch VM, Olmsted RA, Murphey-Corb M, Purcell RH, Johnson PR (1989) An African primate lentivirus (SIVsm) closely related to HIV-2. Nature 339:389–92

Hoberg EP, Alkire NL, de Queiroz A, Jones A (2001) Out of Africa: origins of the Taenia tapeworms in humans. Proceedings of the Royal Society of London—Series B: Biological Sciences 268:781–7

Hussain AI, Shanmugam V, Switzer WM, Tsang SX, Fadly A, Thea D, Helfand R, Bellini WJ, Folks TM, Heneine W (2001) Lack of evidence of endogenous avian leukosis virus and endogenous avian retrovirus transmission to measles, mumps, and rubella vaccine recipients. Emerging Infectious Diseases 7:66–72

Imaizumi T, Lankford KL, Burton WV, Fodor WL, Kocsis JD (2000) Xenotransplantation of pig olfactory ensheathing cells promotes axonal regeneration in rat spinal cord. Nature Biotechnology 18:949–53

Institute of Medicine (1996) Xenotransplantation: Science, Ethics, and Public Policy. National Academy Press, Washington, D.C

Johnson JA, Heneine W (2001) Characterization of endogenous avian leukosis viruses in chicken embryonic fibroblast substrates used in production of measles and mumps vaccines. Journal of Virology 75:3605–12

Khabbaz RF, Heneine W, George JR, Parekh B, Rowe T, Woods T, Switzer WM, McClure HM, Murphey-Corb M, Folks TM (1994) Brief report: infection of a laboratory worker with simian immunodeficiency virus. New England Journal of Medicine 330:172–7

Kind A, Colman A (1999) Therapeutic cloning: needs and prospects. Seminars in Cell & Developmental Biology 10:279–86

Klimov AI, Rocha E, Hayden FG, et al (1995) Prolonged shedding of amantadine-resistant influenza A viruses by immunodeficient patients: detection by polymerase chain reaction-restriction analysis. J Infect Dis 172:1352–5

LeBlanc MH, Boudriau S, Doyle D, Gagnon A, Beaudoin D, Coulombe D, Gleeton O, Kingma JG Jr., Boutet M (1998) Epstein-Barr virus mediated graft rejection in heart transplant patients: implication of the cardiac cytoskeleton. Transplantation Proceedings 30:918–24

Martini GA (1969) Marburg agent disease: in man. Trans R Soc Trop Med Hug 63:295–302

Michaels MG, Jenkins FJ, St George K, Nalesnik MA, Starzl TE, Rinaldo CR Jr (2001) Detection of infectious baboon cytomegalovirus after baboon-to-human liver xenotransplantation. Journal of Virology 75:2825–8

Michaels MG, Simmons RL (1994) Xenotransplant-associated zoonoses: strategies for prevention. Transplantation 57:1–7

Murphy FA (1996) The public health risk of animal organ and tissue transplantation into humans. Science 273:746–7

Nyberg SL, Hibbs JR, Hardin JA, Germer JJ, Persing DH (1999) Transfer of porcine endogenous retrovirus across hollow fiber membranes: significance to a bioartificial liver. Transplantation 67:1251–5

Oldmixon B, Wood J, Ericsson T, White-Scharf M, Patience C (2000) Absence of human-tropic endogenous retroviruses in inbred miniature swine. Presented at: 12th International Workshop of Retroviral Pathogenesis; October 30, 2000; Annapolis, Maryland

Oxford JS (2000) Influenza A pandemic of the 20th century with special reference to 1918: virology, pathology and epidemiology. Reviews in Medical Virology 10:119–33

Paradis K, Langford G, Long Z, Heneine W, Sandstrom P, Switzer WM, Chapman LE, Lockey C, Onions D, the Xen 111 Study Group, Otto E (1999) Search for cross species transmission of porcine endogenous retrovirus in patients treated with living pig tissue. Science 285:1236–41

Parashar UD, Sunn LM, Ong F, Mounts AW, Arif MT, Ksiazek TG, Kamaluddin MA, Mustafa AN, Kaur H, Ding LM, Othman G, Radzi HM, Kitsutani PT, Stockton PC, Arokiasamy J, Gary HE Jr, Anderson LJ (2000) Case-control study of risk factors for human infection with a new zoonotic paramyxovirus, Nipah virus, during a 1998–1999 outbreak of severe encephalitis in Malaysia. Journal of Infectious Diseases 181:1755–9

Patience C, Patton GS, Takeuchi Y, Weiss RA, McClure MO, Rydberg L, Breimer ME (1998) No evidence of pig DNA or retroviral infection in patients with short-term extracorporeal connection to pig kidneys. Lancet 352:699–701

Patience C, Takeuchi Y, Weiss RA (1997) Infection of human cells by an endogenous retrovirus of pigs. Nature Medicine 3:282–6

Pitkin Z, Mullon C (1999) Evidence of absence of porcine endogenous retrovirus (PERV) infection in patients treated with a bioartificial liver support system. Artif Organs 23:829–33

Qari SH, Magre S, Garcia-Lerma JG, Hussain AI, Takeuchi Y, Patience C, Weiss RA, Heneine W (2001) Susceptibility of the porcine endogenous retrovirus to reverse transcriptase and protease inhibitors. Journal of Virology 75:1048–53

Reemtsma K (1969) Renal heterotransplantation from nonhuman primates to man. Ann NY Acad Sci 162:412

Rocha E, Cox NJ, Black RA, et al (1991) Antigenic and genetic variation in influenza A (H1N1) virus isolates recovered from a persistently infected immunodeficient child. J Virol 65:2340–50

Schumacher JM, Elias SA, Palmer EP, et al (2000) Transplantation of embryonic porcine mesencephalic tissue in patients with PD. Neurology 54:1042–50

Simonds RH (1993) HIV transmission by organ and tissue transplantation. AIDS 7:Suppl 2:S35-S38

Stoye JP, Coffin JM (1995) The dangers of xenotransplantation. Nature Medicine 11:1100

Stoye JP, Le Tissier P, Takeuchi Y, Patience C, Weiss RA (1998) Endogenous retroviruses: a potential problem for xenotransplantation? Annals of the New York Academy of Sciences 862:67–74

Stoye JP (1997) Xenotransplantation. Proviruses pose potential problems. Nature 386:126–7

Stoye JP (1998) No clear answers on safety of pigs as tissue donor source. Lancet 352:666–7

Stoye JP (1999) The pathogenic potential of endogenous retroviruses: a skeptical view. Trends in Microbiology 7:430

Strandstrom H, Vejalainen P, Moenning V, Hunsmann G, Schwartz H, Schafer W (1974) C-type particles produced by a permanent cell line from a leukemic pig. 1. Origin and properties of the host cells and some evidence of the occurrence of C-type-like particles. Virology 57:175–8

Strickler HD, Rosenberg PS, Devesa SS, Hertel J, Fraumeni JF Jr., Goedert JJ (1998) Contamination of poliovirus vaccines with simian virus 40 (1953–1963) and subsequent cancer rates. JAMA 279:292–5

Subbarao K, Katz J (2000) Avian influenza viruses infecting humans. Cellular & Molecular Life Science 57:1770–84

Subcommission of Xenotransplantation of the Permanent Commission of Transplants of the Interterritorial Council of the National Health System (1998) Xenotransplantation: recommendations for the regulation of these activities in Spain. Available in Spanish or English translation from: Organizacion Nacional de Transplantes, C/ Sinesio Delgado, 8, 28029 Madrid, Tel: (44) 91 314 24 06; Fax: (44) 91 314 29 69; E-mail: bmiranda@msc.es

Suleiman MN, Muscat-Baron JM, Harries JR, et al (1980) Congo/Crimean haemorrhagic fever in Dubai:an outbreak at the Rashid Hospital. Lancet 2:939–41

Swanepoel R, Shepherd AH, Leman PA, et al (1987) Epidemiologic and clinical features of Crimean-Congo hemorrhagiv fever in southern Africa. Am J Trop Med Hyg 36:120–32

Swedish Committee on Xenotransplantation (1999) From one species to another – transplantation from animals to humans. A report by the Swedish Committee on Xenotransplantation, Stockholm. Swedish Government Official Report No. 1999:120. Ministry of health and Social Affairs. The complete report in Swedish or a short version (Summary and Statutory Proposals) in English are available upon request from: Stefan Reimer, Secretary, The Swedish committee on xenotransplantation, P.O. Box 187, S-201 21 MALMO, Sweden. E-mail: stefan.reimer@hsb.dom.se

Todaro GJ, Beneveniste RE, Lieber MM, Sherr CJ (1974) Characterization of a type C virus released from the porcine cell line PK (15). Virology 58:65–74

Transplantation Society of Australia and New Zealand, Inc (1998) Xenotransplantation: a report to the Research Committee (Public Health and Medical), the National health and medical Research council, from an Ad Hoc Working Party, August 1998. Revised December 1998 (Internet:<http://www.racp.edu.au/tsanz/xenomain.htm>)

Tsang SX, Switzer WM, Shanmugam V, Johnson HA, Goldsmith C, Wright A, Fadly A, Thea D, Jaffe H, Folks TM, Heneine W (1999) Evidence of avian leukosis virus subgroup E and endogenous avian virus in measles and mumps vaccines derived from chicken cells: investigation of transmission to vaccine recipients. Journal of Virology 73:5843–51

U.S. Public Health Service (2001) PHS Guideline on Infectious Disease Issues In Xenotransplantation. MMWR Recommendations and Reports. 50 (RR-15):1–46

United Kingdom Department of Health (1997) The Government Response to "Animal Tissues into Humans." The report of the Advisory Group on the Ethics of Xenotransplantation. The Stationary Office, London, January 1997 (Further information is available on the United Kingdom Xenotransplantation Interim Regulatory Authority (UKXIRA) website: <http://www.doh.gov.uk/ukxira.htm>)

United Network for Organ Sharing (1997). Data highlights from the 1997 Annual Report: The U.S. Scientific Registry of Transplant Recipients and the Organ Procurement and Transplantation Network – Transplant data: 1988–1996. U.S. Department of Health and Human Services, Rockville, MD

Van der Laan LJW, Lockey C, Griffeth BC, et al (2000) Infection by porcine endogenous retrovirus after islet xenotransplantation in SCID mice. Nature 407:90–4

Weiss RA (2001) The Leeuwenhoek Lecture 2001. Animal origins of human infectious disease. Philosophical Transactions of the Royal Society of London—Series B: Biological Sciences. 356:957–77

Wells DL, Hopfensperger DJ, Arden NH, Harmon MW, Davis JP, Tipple MA, Schonberger LB (1991) Swine influenza virus infections. Transmission from ill pigs to humans at a Wisconsin agricultural fair and subsequent probable person-to-person transmission. JAMA 265:478–81

WHO (1978) Ebola haemorrhagic fever in Zaire, 1976. Bull World Health Organ 56:271–93

Wilson CA, Wong S, Muller J, et. al (1998) Type C retrovirus released from porcine primary peripheral blood mononuclear cells infects human cells. J Virol 72:3082–3087

Woolhouse MEJ, Taylor LH, Haydon DT (2000) Population Biology of Multihost Pathogens. Science 292:1109–1112

World Health Organization (1998) Xenotransplantation: guidance on infectious disease prevention and management. World health Organization, Geneva, Switzerland, November 1998 (document WHO/EMC/ZOO/98.1; available from Division of Emerging and Other Communicable Diseases Surveillance and Control, World Health Organization, 1211 Geneva 27, Switzerland) (Internet:<http://www.who.int/emc-documents/zoonoses/whoemczoo981c.html>)

Zhang Z, Bedard E, Luo Y, Wang H, Deng S, Kelvin D, Zhong R (2000) Animal models in xenotransplantation. Exp. Opin. Invest. Drugs 9:2051–68

Cross-Species Infections

R. A. Weiss

Department of Immunology and Molecular Pathology,
Windeyer Institute of Medical Sciences, University College London,
46 Cleveland Street, London, W1T 4JF, UK
E-mail: r.weiss@ucl.ac.uk

1 Introduction 48

2 Family Heirlooms and New Acquisitions 48
2.1 Heirlooms 49
2.2 Zoonoses 49
2.3 Acquisitions 51

3 The Colombian Exchange 53

4 Cross-Infection Between Host Species 56

5 Virulence and Cross-Species Infection 58

6 Possible New Zoonotic Hazards 61

7 Iatrogenic Sources of Infection 62
7.1 Vaccines, Vaccination and Biologicals 63
7.2 Xenotransplantation 64

8 Concluding Remarks 66

References 67

Abstract Animals have always been a major source of human infectious disease. Some infections like rabies are recognized as primary zoonoses caused in each case by direct animal-to-human transmission, whereas others like measles become independently sustained within the human population so that the causative virus has diverged from its morbillivirus progenitor in ruminants. Recent examples of direct zoonoses are variant Creutzfeldt–Jakob disease arising from bovine spongiform encephalopathy, and the H5N1 avian influenza outbreak in Hong Kong. Recent epidemic diseases of animal origin are the 1918–1919 influenza pandemic, and the acquired immune deficiency syndrome pandemic caused by human immunodeficiency virus. Some retroviruses move into and out of the chromosomal DNA of the host germline, so that they may oscillate between being an avirulent inherited Mendelian trait in one species and an infectious pathogen in another. Cross-species viral and other infections are reviewed historically with respect to the evolution of virulence and the concern about iatrogenic enhancement of cross-species transfer by medical procedures akin to xenotransplantation.

1
Introduction

The prospect of clinical xenotransplantation—the grafting of animal cells, tissues and organs into humans—has rightly raised concerns about xenografts serving as an unwitting and unfortunate source of zoonotic infection. Such animal-to-human transfer of a pathogen poses a potential risk of causing iatrogenic illness to the xenograft recipient. Moreover, if the pathogen were to spread to the patient's contacts, or to take off epidemically, it would become a threat to the community at large, raising a rather different risk–benefit appraisal to that for the individual transplant recipient.

In order to place the infection hazards of xenotransplantation in perspective, it seems opportune to review cross-species infection by pathogens more generally. I shall argue that the pervasive evidence for natural transfer of microbes to new host species indicates that the risk of cross-species infection occurring through xenotransplantation is far from unique. On the other hand, that is no reason for complacency. The readiness of infections to traffic between hosts is attested by novel zoonoses such as variant Creutzfeldt–Jakob disease transmitted from cattle with bovine spongiform encephalopathy, and by new epidemics like acquired immune deficiency syndrome caused by the human immunodeficiency virus, emanating from a lentivirus of apes.

2
Family Heirlooms and New Acquisitions

In his ecological commentary on human health and disease, McMichael (2001) calls the microbes that have co-evolved with the human species our 'family heirlooms', whereas those that have come from animals are 'new acquisitions'.

2.1 Heirlooms

These are the parasites and commensal micro-organisms that have colonized the host ever since it diverged from other host species. For humans, the co-evolving microbes are, in the main, persistent virus infections such as most if not all the herpesviruses, and papovaviruses including the skin and genital papillomaviruses, and the SV40-related agents, BK and JC. Different genotypes may diversify with their hosts, as we have recently tracked for human herpesvirus 8 in Sephardi and Ashkenazi Jews (Davidovici et al. 2001), although exchange also takes place with host population mixing. Maximum likelihood phylogenetic reconstruction can be used to estimate demographic history of an infection within a host species, e.g., HIV (Pybus et al. 2000), and host parasite co-speciation (Huelsenbeck et al. 1997).

The ultimate in co-evolution is the endogenous retrovirus integrated in the germ-line of the host (Boeke and Stoye 1997). Thus relatives of porcine endogenous retrovirus (PERV) are present in the DNA of all old world pig species studied, but are absent from new world peccaries, suggesting a 30-million-year sojourn among the *Suidae* (Patience et al. 2001). It seems extraordinary that such ancient germ-line proviruses can emerge as potentially infectious viruses, yet such endogenous retroviruses can and do cross host species as exemplified in Fig. 1. Recent analyses of endogenous DNA related to the murine leukemia virus genus (gamma-retroviruses including PERV) show large discontinuities between host and viral phylogenies (Martin et al. 1999, 2001), indicating that cross-species transfer has occurred on numerous occasions during mammalian evolution.

2.2 Zoonoses

Approximately 300 different viruses, rickettsia, bacteria, fungi, protozoa and helminth parasites are known to infect humans as zoonoses, including 42 from pigs (McNeill 1976; Palmer et al. 1998). Some recent zoonotic outbreaks are listed in Table 1. They occur in many developed or developing countries, come from wild or domestic animals, and transfer via diverse routes. Many zoonoses do not spread further than the index patient. This is usually the case with rabies, which as been recognized

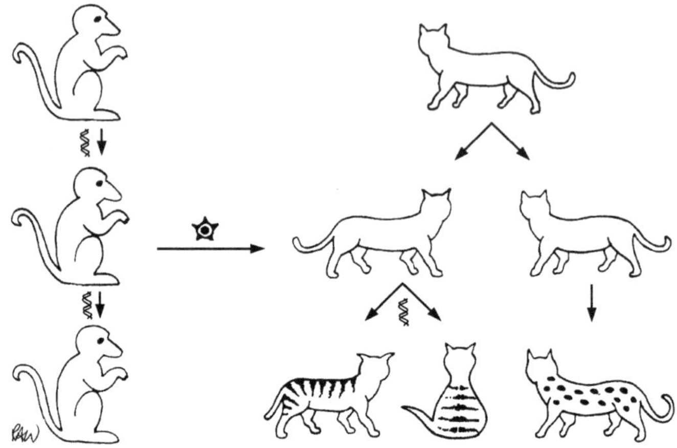

Fig. 1 Transmission of retrovirus from the baboon germ-line to that of cats. Baboon endogenous virus (BaEV) is expressed at high load as infectious virions in the placenta, which was perhaps once scavenged by a cat. The virus colonized the germ-line of cats after the Asian spotted species of *Felis* diverged from tabby African, Mediterranean and European species (Benveniste and Todaro 1974). BaEV itself is a recombinant between a β-retrovirus (its *env* gene) and a γ-retrovirus (its *gag* and *pol* genes) (Boeke and Stoye 1997) and the cat has inherited the chimeric virus. (Reproduced with permission from Weiss and Wain-Hobson 2001)

since ancient times (Oldstone 1998), and also, we hope, with vCJD, an entirely new disease in humans just as BSE is novel in cattle. Others, like Lassa fever, and Ebola and Marburg viruses can be highly contagious for close contacts and carers but have soon petered out rather than becoming permanently established in the human population. A 1996 outbreak of Ebola virus infection in Gabon resulted in the death of 21 among 37 persons who handled the flesh of a dead chimpanzee before it was cooked as bushmeat (Mahy 1998). The Hantavirus outbreak in Southwest USA was an example of multiple zoonoses from *Peromyscus*, the deer mouse, without human-to-human infection (Morse 1994), whereas a related Hantavirus in Argentina showed evidence of limited human-to-human transmission (Wells et al. 1997). We may regard these zoonotic infections as 'temporary exhibits', borrowed from the animals that represent the long-term reservoir necessary for the microbe's survival.

Table 1 Examples of zoonotic outbreaks in the past 25 years

Microbe	Reservoir	Vector or intermediate	Location	Year
Ebolavirus	Unknown	Unknown	Sudan/Zaire	1976
			Zaire (DRC)	1995
		Chimpanzee	Gabon	1996
			Uganda	2000
Lassa fever	Rodent	None	Liberia	1977
			Sierra Leone	1997
S. enteriditis	Chicken	Eggs	UK	1988
Hantavirus	Rodent	None	SW USA	1993
			Argentina	1996
Plague	Rodent	Flea	India	1993
VEE	Horse	Mosquito	Mexico	1995
CCH fever	Sheep, hare	Tick	Bulgaria	1994
Typhus	Rodent	Louse	Bosnia	1995
			Burundi	1996
E. coli O157	Cattle	Food	UK	1996
BSE/vCJD	Cattle	Food	UK	1996
West Nile	Bird	Mosquito	New York	1999
Hendravirus	Bat	Horse	Australia	1997
Influenza H5N1	Duck, quail	Chicken	Hong Kong	1997
Nipahvirus	Bat	Pig	Malaysia	1998
Influenza H9N2	Chicken	None	Hong Kong	1999
Monkeypox	Monkeys	None	Zaire (DRC)	2000

CCH, Crimean-Congo hemorrhagic fever virus; VEE, Venezuelan equine encephalitis virus; BSE, bovine spongiform encephalopathy; vCJD, variant Creutzfeldt-Jakob disease; DRC, Democratic Republic of Congo.

2.3 Acquisitions

The 'new acquisitions' are the microbes that we have encountered and held on to during our social evolution of the last 12,000 years or so. In fact, humankind's progress since the last ice age from isolated bands of hunter-gatherers to a global population of over six billion has allowed us to become astonishingly 'nouveaux riches' with respect to infectious pathogens (McMichael 2001). Diamond (1997) argues that a large proportion of these microbes have been acquired from the animals we have domesticated, or which in Budiansky's (1997) view have opted for do-

Table 2 Examples of human infectious diseases acquired from animals

Disease	Microbe	Animal source	Estimated date of crossover[a]
Malaria (*P. vivax*)	Parasite	Monkey	~8000 BCE
Measles	Virus	Sheep or goat	~6000 BCE
Smallpox	Virus	Horse or cow	>2000 BCE
Tuberculosis	*Mycobacterium*	Ruminant	>1000 BCE
Typhus	Rickettsia	Rodent	430 BCE
			1492 CE
Plague	Bacterium	Rodent	541 CE
			1347 CE
			1665 CE
Dengue fever	Virus	Monkey	~1000 CE
Sleeping sickness	Parasite	Ruminant	<1500 CE
Yellow fever	Virus	Monkey	1641 CE
Influenza	Virus	Bird, pig	1918 CE
AIDS/HIV-1	Virus	Chimpanzee	~1931 CE
AIDS/HIV-2	Virus	Monkey	20th Century

[a] The dates shown are estimates of initial crossover, or dates of specific transfers. BCE, before Christian era; CE, Christian era. For example, the dates for typhus are the plague of Athens described by Thucydides and the siege of Granada; but that for yellow fever is its introduction into the Americas.

mestication, to which I would add fellow travelers like rats, and genuinely wild animals like monkeys.

Table 2 provides examples of human infectious disease of animal origin. These include microbes such as measles virus which has diverged from its likely morbillivirus progenitor, rindepest, to become established as a distinctive virus circulating exclusively among humans. Other epidemic diseases now specific to humans that originally crossed from domestic herd or flock animals include smallpox, influenza, mumps, and tuberculosis. *Mycobacterium tuberculosis* is now distinct from *M. bovis,* though the latter remains an infectious hazard to humans. In contrast, *M. avium paratuberculosis,* is an enteric infection of cattle also present in milk and might be linked to Crohn's disease in humans as a zoonosis (Hermon-Taylor et al. 2000). The lesson of acquisition is that the animal source and route of original cross-over is varied, sometimes uncertain, often unexpected.

Thus infectious microbes, and viruses in particular, evolve in diverse ways (Domingo et al. 1999). New epidemics, outbreaks and sporadic cas-

Table 3 Examples of emerging virus infections in pigs

a. Long-established infections newly emerging to human knowledge
Porcine endogenous retroviruses, A, B and C[a]
Porcine hepatitis E[a]
Porcine circovirus type 1
Porcine β and γ herpesviruses
b. Novel porcine infections acquired from other host species
African swine fever
Nipah virus[a]
Avian influenza[a]
Porcine circovirus type 2
c. Re-emerging epidemic infections
Foot and mouth disease
Swine vesicular disease
Classical swine fever
Swine influenza[a]
Porcine rotavirus

[a] Potential to infect humans.

es of infectious disease are often grouped together under the fashionable term 'emerging infections'. These may be emerging for different reasons, as exemplified in Table 3 for virus infections of pigs, the species of most relevance to xenotransplantation.

3
The Colombian Exchange

The conditions for colonization and spread of an infectious disease when it is introduced into a naïve host population that has not previously gained any adaptive immunity or genetic host resistance is analogous in several ways to cross-species infection. The Colombian exchange refers to the immense consequences to the ecology, economy and public health that followed Columbus' voyages to America. Let us take the example of measles.

Because it is not normally a persistent infection, measles requires a sufficient size of host population to maintain its reproductive rate, $R_0>1$ (Anderson and May 1992), meaning that on average, an infected person must pass the infection on to at least one other. Since recovery from measles provides life-long immunity from re-infection in human societies, where measles is endemic outbreaks occur in infants with a periodicity reflecting the size and fecundity of the host population (Anderson and May 1992). But when measles reaches naïve populations, such as native Americans following the Conquistadors, it infects adults and children alike with lethal consequences (Oldstone 1998). McNeill (1976) estimates that the North American indigenous population fell from over 30 million to less than 3 million during the sixteenth century, largely because of smallpox and measles epidemics. Infection of naïve populations elsewhere caused similar catastrophes, leading Darwin to note in 1836, "Wherever the European has trod, death seems to pursue the aboriginal" (Darwin 2001).

The reason why European explorers and colonizers like Columbus, Cook and Vancouver exported far more diseases than they imported was that the major contiguous populations of Africa, Asia and Europe had already experienced them. In contrast, communities which had started with smaller founder populations, such as those on Pacific islands and the migrant populations that crossed the Bering Straits, were either too small initially to sustain nonpersistent infections, or had become isolated from other populations before humans acquired them from animals. Thus the ancestors of present day Australian aborigines, for example, reached their destination at least 40,000 years ago, and then remained isolated during the period when farming and large populations developed in Mesopotamia, the Indus Valley and Southern China.

Even when crowded civilizations developed, such as the pre-Colombian Mayans, Aztecs and Incas, they were relatively free of infectious disease. Tuberculosis may have been present, and also pinta, related to syphilis, though the notion that Columbus brought syphilis back from Hispaniola is hotly disputed (Quétel 1990). It is true that syphilis first broke out in 1493 in Spain soon after Columbus's return from his first voyage, and then, following the siege of Naples in 1495, it spread disastrously across Europe and Asia, reaching Japan in 1505. But yaws, caused by a closely related treponeme spirochete was already present in Africa. Typhus similarly spread across Europe following the siege of Granada in 1492 when more than 17,000 Spanish troops fell to the disease before wresting the city from the Moors (Zinsser 1934). Typhus, a rodent rickettsial zoonosis, spread onward among humans via lice, continues to be a salient disease of war and prison camps. It is no coincidence that the most recent reported outbreaks arose in Burundi and Congo among Rwandan refugees, and in the Balkans during the Serbian war in Bosnia (Raoult et al. 1997).

Plague is another epidemic disease of zoonotic origin that crops up from time to time and was formerly impossible to control (Ziegler 1970). The Plague bacillus, *Yersinia pestis,* occurs naturally in burrowing rodents in the Central Asian steppes. The outbreak that reached Europe in 1347 as the Black Death probably resulted from the black rat (*Rattus rattus*) migrating from India to newly infest the caravan routes that were already well established across Central Asia between China and the Near East. *Y. pestis* adapted to the black rat's flea (*Xenopsylla*, literally 'foreign flea') and the rest is history—and also inspired writing. Great diarists like Ibn Battuta (Gibb 1999) and Boccaccio (1995) in the fourteenth century, and Pepys (1995) and Defoe (1999) in the seventeenth century wrote movingly about contemporary plague epidemics. Ships carried the rats, fleas and plague worldwide. Once plague colonized humans, the bubonic form was transmitted by human fleas, the septicemic form by lice and fleas and the pneumonic form by aerosol droplets. Following the San Francisco earthquake in 1906, *Y. pestis* went underground again by colonizing chipmunks and ground squirrels, spreading eastwards as far as the Rocky Mountains. Plague is now endemic in burrowing rodents in Arizona and New Mexico, similar in ecology to its origin in marmots of the Gobi Desert. Because the fleas of these rodents are largely confined to the young in the nest, only isolated cases of human infection occur among campers.

Another disease of the Colombian exchange was yellow fever. This virus had to await the establishment of suitable mosquito vectors (*Aedes aegypti*) to become established in the New World, and thus it did not become epidemic in the Americas until 1641, more than a century after smallpox and measles wrought such devastation. 'Yellow jack' remained a seasonal threat until the role of the mosquito vector was proven 102 years ago (Oldstone 1998). Interestingly, as with the plague bacillus, humans were the means by which yellow fever virus spread from one wild animal reservoir to a new one. Long endemic in African monkeys, yellow fever virus colonized New World monkeys after its transport by ship in humans.

Other flaviviruses have shown similar feats of migration. Dengue fever probably had an East African origin in monkeys, but has spread worldwide as an exclusively human infection alongside the dispersion of its vector, *Aedes aegypti*, which thrives in semi-urban environments (Jacobs 2000). West Nile virus is but the latest westward bound Colombian exchange, appearing in the Western Hemisphere for the first time in New

York in 1999 (Lanciotti et al. 1999). It infects birds and *Culex pipiens* is its major vector. No-one knows how West Nile virus crossed the Atlantic: was it first imported to the USA by migratory birds (Rappole et al. 2000), or by an infected human flying with a valid ticket, or by a stowaway mosquito boarding a similar flight?

The post-Colombian agricultural experience was a genuine two-way exchange: such staple foods as maize, potatoes, tomatoes, and peppers came from the New World while wheat and beef went West. Yet it is difficult to pin down a single infectious disease that crossed the Atlantic eastbound to become epidemic or endemic in the Old World. Diamond (1997) argues that fewer infectious diseases originated in the New World because far fewer species of animals were domesticated. While Diamond's reasoning is quite persuasive, one must also query why the few zoonotic diseases of the New World have not spread. Chargas' disease came from guinea-pigs (cavies) and is spread by bugs. It is endemic in tropical South America but has never taken off in the parts of Africa and Europe where similar bugs abound. Diamond (1997) may also over-emphasize domestic animals as a source of human infectious disease, considering the number of microbes acquired from wild rodents and primates (Table 2).

4
Cross-Infection Between Host Species

The fertile ground for pandemic spread in naïve host populations also applies to cross-species infections, once the pathogen gains a firm foothold in the new species together with fitness for transmissibility. In humans this was evident from the 1918/19 'Spanish' influenza pandemic, which probably arose as a reassortant strain of influenza in pigs from mammalian and avian parent strains (Laver et al. 2000; Oxford 2000). On the other hand, the recent outbreak of avian H5N1 influenza in Hong Kong was equally virulent to the infected individual, but not being reassorted, was ill-adapted to onward transmission between humans (Horimoto and Kawaoka 2001; Webster et al. 2000).

The human immunodeficiency viruses are new acquisitions that we are most unlikely to eradicate; once acquired, they are here to stay. HIV-2 is derived from the Simian immunodeficiency virus of sooty mangabeys (SIVsm) and may have crossed to humans on numerous occasions without onward transmission (Gao et al. 1992), yet some strains became infectious. SIVmac in macaques also originated from SIVsm, presumably when these Asian and African species of monkey were housed together in the same primate facilities in the USA. Similarly, HIV-1 groups M, N and O each appear to come from a separate cross-over events from chimpanzee SIVcpz to human (Gao et al. 1999). While each group of HIV-1 has become locally endemic, only group M thus far has given rise to the global pandemic of AIDS (Hahn et al. 2000).

There are many examples of animal-to-animal cross species infections resulting in outbreaks of novel disease or epidemics. A morbillivirus related to canine distemper, the phocine distemper virus, devastated seal populations in the North Sea, Baltic Sea and Atlantic (Osterhaus 1989). Mediterranean dolphins and porpoises experienced an epidemic of a distinct cetid distemper strain (Barrett et al. 1993). In Lake Baikal, 8,000 km distant from the North Atlantic epidemic, seals succumbed to a separate interspecies transmission of the canine distemper virus itself (Osterhaus 1989), as did lions in Africa (Harder et al. 1995). The sudden, global dispersion of canine parvovirus, possibly from a feline source, resulted in one strain following rapidly on another (Parrish 1999). Given that animal parvoviruses can utilize the human transferrin receptor (Parker et al. 2001) to infect erythroblasts, the porcine parvovirus should be regarded as a potential hazard in xenotransplantation.

Myxoma virus endemic in New World cotton-tailed rabbits became epidemic in Old World rabbits, and was deliberately introduced to control the rabbit population in Australia in the 1950s (Fenner and Fantoni 1999). A novel calicivirus is being similarly exploited for biological control of rabbits today (Fenner and Fantoni 1999; White et al. 2001), as they have evolved disease resistance to myxomatosis. The exotic calicivirus causing vesicular exanthema in swine may have a reservoir in marine mammals such as sea lions (Prato et al. 1974) A new porcine circovirus (type 2) was recognized in domestic pigs in 1991 and comes from an unknown origin rather as the parvovirus did among dogs 20 years earlier. It is of obvious concern in xenotransplantation, although there is no evidence to date of human infection (Allan et al. 2000).

5 Virulence and Cross-Species Infection

It is difficult to predict whether the virulence of a pathogen will be increased or decreased upon crossing to a new host species. "The received wisdom, set forth in most medical texts and elsewhere, is that 'successful' or 'well-adapted' parasites are relatively harmless to their hosts", wrote Anderson and May (1992). These authors show, however, that while the long-equilibrated infectious agent may well become attenuated, this general assumption is not valid because the probability of onward transmission of a microbe is affected by its virulence, according to the formula for its basic reproductive rate (R_o):

$$R_o = \frac{\beta(\alpha, N)N}{\alpha + \mu + v(\alpha)}$$

where α is the disease-induced host mortality rate, β is the transmission coefficient, v is the recovery rate, μ is the mortality rate for all causes, and N is the total population size. If neither transmission rate nor recovery rate depend on virulence, then R_o is maximized by making α infinitesimal, i.e., nonpathogenic.

Epidemics in new populations tend to diminish in virulence over time (Lederberg 2000; Lipsitch and Moxon 1997) as was seen following the introduction of myxoma virus in Australian rabbits (Fenner and Fantoni 1999; Frank 1996). Girolamo Frascotoro, who first defined infectious diseases without knowing about microbes, wrote his treatises on syphilis in 1530 and on contagion in 1546. He noted the lessening mortality in the syphilis epidemic among afflicted persons between 1495 and 1530 (Quetel 1990). Yet some evolutionary biologists tend to interpret the majority of pathological symptoms in the host as adaptive features of the microbe to promote its transmission (Ewald 1994). Some symptoms of disease are indeed precisely adapted to aid transmission of the microbe and hence maximize R_o, e.g., coughing and sneezing, diarrhea, skin pocks, genital sores and for rabies, aggression. Some disease symptoms, such as fever, are part of the host's innate response to overcome infection, or in hepatitis C virus (HCV) and lymphocytic choriomeningitis virus (LCMV), may result from the adaptive immune response as an immunopathologic reaction. Other symptoms, such as paralysis in polio, or immune deficiency and dementia in AIDS, play no direct role in transmis-

Table 4 Examples of changes in virulence upon crossing host species

Microbe	Old host	New host	Virulence
Myxoma virus	Cotton-tail rabbit	European rabbit	Mild→lethal
Cowpox virus	Cattle	Human	Medium→mild
Herpesvirus A	African elephant	Indian elephant	Mild→lethal
Herpesvirus B	Rhesus monkey	Human	Mild→lethal
Lentivirus SIVcpz	Chimpanzee	Human	Mild→lethal
Lentivirus SIVsm	Sooty mangabey	Human	None→lethal
		Macaque	None→lethal
Yellow fever virus	Monkey	Human	Mild→severe
Distemper virus	Dog	Seal	Severe→lethal
Influenza H5N1	Bird	Human	Lethal→lethal
Sindbis virus	Bird	Human	Severe→none[a]
Lassa fever virus	Rodent	Human	Mild→lethal
LCMV	Rodent	Human	Medium→none
Bornavirus	Horse, sheep	Human	Severe→mild
Psittacosis	Bird	Human	Severe→severe
Anthrax	Ruminant	Human	Severe→lethal
E. coli O157	Ruminant	Human	None→severe
Trypansoma cruzi	Rodent	Human	None→severe
Trypansoma brucei	Antelope	Cattle	None→severe
		Human	None→severe
Toxoplasma gondii	Cat	Human	Mild→none[a]

[a] Except when immunosuppressed.

sion, but are the consequences of bearing a high pathogen load, which in turn helps transmission (Clarke 2001; Levy 1998; Perelson et al. 1996). Short-term selection within an infected host may increase virulence if there is competition between variants (Lipsitch and Moxon 1997), e.g., with HIV and other high-load RNA viruses.

Multiple factors including immune status, time and dose of infection, and genetic variation of both host and parasite affect the virulence of a pathogen. Some evolutionary biologists argue that well-adapted host–parasite relationships tend toward increasing virulence (Ebert and Hamilton 1996; Ewald 1994). Yet within a host species as in cross-species infection, infection of a naïve population, e.g., with measles, can lead to severe mortality in adults, whereas in an experienced population, the epidemics which are largely restricted to infants have less severe effects on the population as a whole. Delayed infections by Epstein–Barr virus and polio virus tend to be more virulent than infection in infancy, which may explain the emergence of glandular fever and paralytic polio in the mid twentieth century as mainly middle class epidemics.

Microbes are frequently mild or nonpathogenic in their natural host species and lethal in their new host (Table 4). Avirulent myxoma virus of American cotton-tail rabbits became the deadly epidemic of European rabbits (Fenner and Fantoni 1999). A mild endotheliotropic herpesvirus infection of African elephants kills Asian elephants and possibly vice versa (Richman et al. 1999). Herpesvirus B causes nothing worse than cold sores in Rhesus monkeys but leads to a lethal encephalopathy in humans (Palmer et al. 1998). SIVsm appears harmless in sooty mangabeys yet causes AIDS in humans and macaques. These examples are a further reason not to be complacent about xenotransplantation; what might be a harmless commensal in the source animal may cause severe disease on crossing the species barrier.

With bacterial infections, the emerging knowledge based on comparative genomics should encourage a radical reappraisal of transmission dynamics in relation to virulence (Weinstock 2000; Wren 2000). Whole sets of 'virulence' genes encoding toxins or adhesion proteins may cross microbial species, affecting pathogenicity. Again, one should be wary of simplistically relating virulence factors to transmission. For example, the natural host for *Escherichia coli* O157 is cattle, in which it is readily transmissible but not pathogenic, although it causes severe enteric disease in humans.

Changing hosts and serial transmission in 'unnatural' hosts often diminishes pathogenicity. Pasteur's success in immunizing against rabies and anthrax was based on this principle (Brock 1975). Similarly, the vaccine strains of polio virus types 1, 2 and 3 were attenuated through serial passage (Sabin et al. 1954), and yellow fever virus (Theiler and Smith 1937) and measles virus became attenuated through passage in eggs. We need to gain a greater understanding of virulence determinants in microbes, the ways they evade or delay immunity, and how immune responses differ from host to host (Nowak and Bangham 1996). The lack of lentivirus disease in SIV-infected African monkey species, for example, may relate to less activation of immune cells than in humans (Dalgleish et al. 1999).

Changes in virulence upon crossing host species can be modeled (Frank and Jeffrey 2001) but not always foreseen (Table 4). With two related arenaviruses of rodents, Lassa fever is often lethal upon transfer to humans, whereas lymphocytic choriomeningitis virus infection occurs more frequently but passes unnoticed. While some animal pathogens that can infect humans seldom cause disease, others are pathogenic in both the old and new hosts. The H5N1 avian influenza virus was deadly and highly transmissible among chickens in the crowded conditions of Hong Kong's markets; it was equally lethal but luckily without onward transmission among the crowded human residents. On the other hand, we are, of course, far more aware of catastrophic zoonoses than the infections that never spread (Ebert and Hamilton 1996). There is likely to be a large ascertainment bias towards detecting an increase in virulence upon species cross-over, because the ones that are nonpathogenic are seldom studied, e.g., avian Sindbis virus in humans. Among the 300 or so known zoonoses (Palmer et al. 1998), many cause severe symptoms only in immunosuppressed people, again having implications for xenotransplantation.

6
Possible New Zoonotic Hazards

With our long history of acquiring infections from animals, it might be thought that humans have exhausted the possibilities for novel infections. But new situations combined with chance, serendipitous events will always allow the unexpected to occur, and zoonoses are no exception. "If there is any conceivable way a germ can travel from one species to another, some microbe will find it" wrote the demographic historian William McNeill (McNeill 1976), and that includes xenotransplantation.

Humankind's own dominion over environmental change will affect the future spectrum of human infectious disease (McMichael 2001). The ecological changes occurring with global warming may allow vector-borne infections to spread to novel regions (Desowitz 1997), though we should remember that it is less than a century since malaria was eradicated from the UK, northern Europe and Siberia. Trans-continental travel allows infected and infectious persons to traverse large distances and climatic regions within hours. Habitat destruction may release novel infections, such as Nipah virus from fruit-bats (flying foxes) in Malaysia crossing species to domestic pigs and thence to humans, or Ebola fever outbreaks in Africa. On the other hand, nature conservation may allow animal reservoirs to burgeon, as seen with growing deer and tick populations in the USA aiding the spread of Lyme disease to humans. The prion wasting disease of mule-deer in the Rockies may also have put hunters at risk of a form of CJD. Intensive farming of livestock and industrial food-processing practices have led to increased risks of a variety of food-borne zoonoses, such as *Salmonella entiriditis* from chickens, *E. coli* O157 from cattle, and vCJD from BSE contaminated meat pies and hamburgers.

The changing human condition may also allow novel infections to arise from the environment as well as from animals. Thus Legionnaire's disease arose when we unwittingly built ideal warm, humid, aerated incubators: the cooling towers, air conditioners and jacuzzis that serve as 'artificial lungs' for *Legionella's* adaptation to colonize our lungs. Many species of nontuberculous *Mycobacteria* exist as free-living microbes in the soil, but several of them can become parastic in immunocompromised humans and animals (Shafer and Sierra 1992). Given the appropriate conditions, *Legionnella* and some of these *Mycobacteria* conceivably could evolve from 'opportunistic parasitism' to 'obligate parasitism'. I have argued elsewhere (Weiss 2001) that opportunistic microbes either from animals or the environment might more readily adapt, spread infectiously and become obligate in a novel host species if a significant proportion of the host population were immunocompromised. In this respect the advent of AIDS may be unique in the annals of host–parasite evolution.

7
Iatrogenic Sources of Infection

Iatrogenic diseases are those caused in the course of medical (or veterinary) treatment. The meaning could be broadened to include nosocomial sources of infection generally, and the fact that hospitals are the most frequent reservoir of methicillin-resistant *Staphylococcus aureus*. Indeed, the evolution of antibiotic resistance in bacteria, or chloroquin resistance in *Plasmodium falciparum* may be regarded as community health hazards resulting from innumerable beneficial treatments of individuals. This paradox that a benefit to individual patients may harm the population at large is resonant in the debate about xenotransplantation.

7.1 Vaccines, Vaccination and Biologicals

A well known concern over iatrogenic infection is the contamination of vaccines by viruses, and the contamination of the injecting equipment used to deliver vaccines. One veterinary example was the widespread dispersion of bovine leukosis virus (BLV) in cattle herds immunized again tuberculosis or brucellosis. By multiple use of syringes and needles a single infected animal could be the source of a BLV epidemic (Burny et al. 1980). There was speculation that canine parvovirus arose from feline parvovirus contamination of a distemper vaccine propagated in feline cells, though sequence analysis of the viral genomes does not uphold such a view (Truyen et al. 1998).

Similar parenteral spread of infection through contaminated needles or biologicals has caused numerous cases of human infection and mortality. Patients with hemophilia became almost universally infected with HCV through contaminated clotting factor pools. Iatrogenic infection by hepatitis B virus and by HIV in the same type of patient was hardly less dire before screening for these viruses was introduced.

Avoiding cross-species infection via contamination of biological and vaccines also needs great vigilance. Murine hybridoma cultures harvested for medicinal monoclonal antibodies may contain xenotropic retroviruses capable of infecting human cells (Weiss 1982). Human vaccines grown in eggs or chick embryo fibroblasts used to contain avian leukosis viruses (Harris et al. 1966) and still contain avian endogenous retroviral particles (Boni et al. 1996; Johnson and Heneine 2001), although there is no epidemiological evidence of transmission to humans (Hussain et al. 2001). SV40 undoubtedly contaminated early batches of inactivated and live attenuated poliovirus batches through its presence in macaque kidney cell substrates used for vaccine manufacture (Sweet and Hilleman 1960). While there is no evidence for an increase in cancer incidence in vaccines (Carroll-Pankhurst et al. 2001; Shah and Nathanson 1976), claims have recently been made for the detection of SV40 in mesothelioma, ependymoma and other tumors (Butel and Lednicky 1999). However, in a blinded multi-center survey of mesothelioma biopsies, SV40 sequences were not evident, and this field remains controversial (International 2001). If SV40 detection in ependymoma is confirmed in infants born long after poliovirus vaccines were cleansed of SV40, either the vaccine was not the source of this simian virus being present in humans, or SV40 has become newly endemic in humans, and is vertically transmitted.

The other furore over polio vaccines is whether HIV-1 could have entered the human population through contaminated vaccines. Since HIV-1 appears to come from chimpanzees (Gao et al. 1999) this hypothesis demands that chimpanzee tissue was used to prepare oral polio vaccine (Hooper 1999). However, the vaccine pools from the 1950s which were under greatest suspicion of contamination have been found negative for HIV and SIV sequences and for chimpanzee DNA, while containing Rhesus macaque DNA as expected (Berry et al. 2001; Blancou et al. 2001; Weiss and Wain-Hobson 2001). Moreover, phylogenetic estimates of the time of cross-over of HIV-1 Group M from chimpanzee to human long predate the earliest polio vaccine trials (Korber et al. 2000; Rambaut et al. 2001). It thus appears that HIV-1 (and HIV-2) found their way into humans via other routes. As already remarked, cross-species infection by retroviruses has occurred repeatedly, and primate retroviruses are no exception. Examples are discussed by Heneine and by Allan in this volume, including those caused by animal bites and injection accidents.

Despite the probable natural transfer of lentiviruses such as HIV-1 and HIV-2 from nonhuman primates to humans, iatrogenic factors may well have played a crucial role in their early adaptation and spread in the new host. The growth in the use of syringes and needles together with the fall in unit cost of manufacture during the twentieth century has been analyzed (Marx et al. 2001). The period between the time at which HIV-1 Group M is thought to have first crossed into humans, and its emergence in epidemic form is consistent with the rapid growth in use and re-use of injecting and vaccination equipment in African countries that had few resources for sterilization. The rapid diversification of other parenterally transmitted viruses is also consistent with injection as a means of mass dispersion, e.g., HCV (Simmonds 2001). Just as the human act of building the Aswan Dam greatly increased the incidence of bilharzia in Egypt, so attempts to treat bilharzia by injection may have caused that country to become number one in HCV prevalence.

7.2 Xenotransplantation

"Animals have transmitted infections to humans throughout history. The additional risk of successful xenotransplantation might be minimal"

Paul Herrling, head of research and development at Novartis, has commented (Butler 1998). This is a more optimistic view than McNeill's (1976) quoted earlier that if there is a way to cross from one species to another, some microbe will find it. On the one hand, specific pathogen-free animals should be cleaner than 'free-range' human donors. On the other, three factors make the way to cross hosts rather easy in xenotransplantation. First, the physical barrier is removed so that the living tissues of the source species are engrafted into the human recipient; second, the recipient will be under immunosuppressive treatment; third, the source animal is likely to be genetically modified in a way that could aid zoonosis.

Transgenic or genetic knock-out pigs bred to ameliorate hyperacute and acute vascular rejection may release viruses that more readily infect humans (Weiss 1998). Pigs and humans are discordant in that only pigs express the carbohydrate antigen galactose α(1–3) galactose (known as αGal) on glycoproteins and glycolipids. As humans have high titer IgM antibodies to αGal, hyperacute rejection is effected through a complement-mediated lysis of cells expressing αGal (Rother and Squinto 1996). In addition, enveloped viruses such as PERV bear αGal antigens if the cells from which they bud express it. These viruses are then sensitive to complement-mediated inactivation whereas the same viruses grown in human cells are not (Patience et al. 1997; Takeuchi et al. 1996). If either the galactosyl transferase gene is knocked out of source animals, or human complement regulatory proteins are bred into them, enveloped viruses emanating from them are likely to be less sensitive to this natural immunity of humans to enveloped viruses of animals.

In addition, it is noteworthy that two of the human complement regulatory proteins bred into transgenic pigs can serve as virus receptors. CD46 is a measles receptor, and CD55/DAF can be utilized by the picornaviruses Echo 7, Coxsackie B3 and B5. Swine vesicular disease virus is related to Coxsackie B5 and can infect humans in a nontransmissible manner (Brown et al. 1976). Thus porcine viruses in transgenic pigs would have an opportunity to evolve by minor mutation to utilize human receptors, and would then be pre-adapted to infect and spread among humans (Weiss 1998).

8
Concluding Remarks

Cross-species infections occur frequently and widely. On rarer occasions they take off as pandemics in the new host species. The 1918/19 influenza pandemic, the appearance of canine parvovirus and the spread of HIV/AIDS are twentieth century examples. During the past 12,000 years humans have acquired and adopted as our own many infectious diseases originally of animal provenance, e.g., smallpox, measles, tuberculosis, trypanosomiasis. But humans have become so numerous that we now could be the source of 'anthroponoses' in animals. In particular, the infections that human primatologists and tourists bring into nature reserves harboring chimpanzees and gorillas pose a threat of infection to these already endangered species.

The history of zoonoses has surely not ended, and xenotransplantation provides one more route for potential transfer of pathogens. Does that mean that the infection hazards of xenotransplantation are so great that we should not proceed with clinical trials? Contrary to a decade ago when surgeons attempted clinical xenotransplantation with their 'eyes wide shut' (Groth et al. 1994; Starzl et al. 1993), there is now more responsible awareness of the infection hazards. Carefully monitored trials should go ahead, but source animals must be rigorously screened for viruses and other infections. If the physiological and immunological hurdles facing xenotransplantation are overcome, and its practice becomes routine, then the risk of zoonotic infection will increase. Even with the most stringent regulations and the most rigorous barrier containment of source animals, we must recognize that accidents and errors will occur. For those viruses that cannot readily be eliminated, means to control human infection if it were to take place should be established. For example, at least one anti-retroviral drug licensed for human use, zidovudine, appears to be effective against PERV (Qari et al. 2001).

Finally, we should give some thought to the quality of life of the xenotransplant recipients. They must not be 'imprisoned' for the safety of the community at large, but their life-style will be affected, for their own benefit too. In the UK, we have experienced three outbreaks of highly infectious porcine disease in as many years: swine vesicular disease, classical swine fever and foot and mouth disease. If such viruses gained access to the animal tissues in chimeric humans, they could destroy the transplant. I wonder if I were, say, a xenotransplant recipient with porcine lungs, whether I would be advised to give up a favorite pastime—hiking in the English countryside?

References

Allan GM, McNeilly F, McNair I, Curran MD, Walker I, Ellis J, Konoby C, Kennedy S, and Meehan B (2000) Absence of evidence for porcine circovirus type 2 in cattle and humans, and lack of seroconversion or lesions in experimentally infected sheep. Arch Virol. 145:853–857

Anderson RM, and May RM (1992) Infectious diseases of humans: dynamics and control, 2nd ed. Oxford University Press, Oxford

Barrett T, Visser IK, Mamaev L, Goatley L, van Bressem MF, and Osterhaus AD (1993) Dolphin and porpoise morbilliviruses are genetically distinct from phocine distemper virus. Virology 193:1010–1012

Benveniste RE, and Todaro GJ (1974) Evolution of C-type viral genes: inheritance of exogenously acquired viral genes. Nature 252:456–459

Berry N, Davis C, Jenkins A, Wood D, Minor P, Schild G, Bottiger M, Holmes H, and Almond N (2001) Vaccine safety. Analysis of oral polio vaccine CHAT stocks. Nature 410:1046–7

Blancou P, Vartanian JP, Christopherson C, Chenciner N, Basilico C, Kwok S, and Wain-Hobson S (2001) Polio vaccine samples not linked to AIDS. Nature 410:1045–1046

Boccaccio G (1995) The Decameron, Penguin Books, New York

Boeke JD, and Stoye JP. 1997. Retrotransposons, endogenous retroviruses, and the evolution of Retroelements, p. 343–435. *In* J. M. Coffin and S. H. Hughes and H. E. Varmus (ed.), *Retroviruses.* Cold Spring Harbor Laboratory Press, New York

Böni J, Stadler J, Reigel F, and Schupbach J (1996) Detection of reverse transcriptase activity in live attenuated virus vaccines. Clin. Diagn. Virol. 5:45–53

Brock TD (1975) *Milestones in microbiology.* American Society for Microbiology, Washington DC

Brown F, Goodridge D, and Burrows R (1976) Infection of man by swine vesicular disease virus. J Comp Pathol. 86:409–414

Budiansky S (1997) The covenant of the wild: why animals chose domestication. Phoenix, London

Burny A, Bruck C, Chantrenne H, Cleuter H, Cleuter Y, Dekegel D, Ghysdael J, Kettmann R, Leclercq M, Leunen J, Mammerick M, and Portatelle D. 1980. Bovine leukaemia virus: molecular biology and epidemiology, p. 231–289. *In* G. Klein (ed.), *Viral Oncology.* Raven Press, New York

Butel JS, and Lednicky JA (1999) Cell and molecular biology of simian virus 40: implications for human infections and disease. J Natl Cancer Inst. 91:119–134

Butler D (1998) Last chance to stop and think on risks of xenotransplants. Nature. 391:320–325

Carroll-Pankhurst C, Engels EA, Strickler HD, Goedert JJ, Wagner J, and Mortimer EA (2001) Thirty five year mortality following receipt of SV40-contaminated polio vaccine during the neonatal period. Brit J Cancer 85:In press

Clarke T (2001) Polio's last stand. Nature 409:278–280

Dalgleish AG, Marriott JB, Souberbielle B, Montesano C, Sheikh J, Sidebottom D, Westby M, and Austen B (1999) The role of HIV gp120 in the disruption of the immune system. Immunol Lett. 66:81–87

Darwin C (2001) The Voyage of the "Beagle". Modern Library, New York

Davidovici B, Karakis I, Bourboulia D, Ariad S, Zong J, Benharroch D, Dupin N, Weiss R, Hayward G, Sarov B, and Boshoff C (2001) Seroepidemiology and molecular epidemiology of Kaposi's sarcoma-associated herpesvirus among Jewish population groups in Israel. J Natl Cancer Inst. 93:194–202

Defoe D (1999) A journal of the plague year. Oxford University Press, Oxford

Desowitz RS (1997) Tropical Diseases from 50,000BC to 2,500AD. Harper Collins, London

Diamond J (1997) Guns, germs and steel: a short history of everybody for the last 13,000 years. Jonathan Cape, London

Domingo E, Webster R, and Holland J (1999) Origin and evolution of viruses. Academic Press, London

Ebert D, and Hamilton WD (1996) Sex against violence: the coevolution of parasitic diseases. Tree. 11:79–82

Ewald PW (1994) Evolution of infectious disease. Oxford University Press Inc, USA

Fenner F, and Fantoni B (1999) Biological control of vertebrate pests. Cabi Publishing, New York

Frank SA (1996) Models of parasite virulence. Q Rev Biol. 71:37–78

Frank SA, and Jeffrey JS (2001) The probability of severe disease in zoonotic and commensal infections. Proc R Soc Lond B. 268:53–60

Gao F, Bailes E, Robertson DL, Chen Y, Rodenburg CM, Michael SF, Cummins LB, Arthur LO, Peeters M, Shaw GM, Sharp PM, and Hahn BH (1999) Origin of HIV-1 in the chimpanzee Pan troglodytes troglodytes. Nature 397:436–441

Gao F, Yue L, White AT, Pappas PG, Barchue J, Hanson AP, Greene BM, Sharp PM, Shaw GM, and Hahn BH (1992) Human infection by genetically diverse SIVSM-related HIV-2 in west Africa. Nature. 358:495–499

Gibb HAR (1999) Ibn Battuta: Travels in Asia & Africa 1325–1354. Low Price Publications, New York

Groth CG, Korsgren O, Tibell A, Tollemar J, Moller E, Bolinder J, Ostman J, Reinholt FP, Hellerstrom C, and Andersson A (1994) Transplantation of porcine fetal pancreas to diabetic patients. Lancet 344:1402–1404

Hahn BH, Shaw GM, De Cock KM, and Sharp PM (2000) AIDS as a zoonosis: scientific and public health implications. Science 287:607–614

Harder TC, Kenter M, Appel MJ, Roelke-Parker ME, Barrett T, and Osterhaus AD (1995) Phylogenetic evidence of canine distemper virus in Serengeti's lions. Vaccine 13:521–523

Harris RJ, Dougherty RM, Biggs PM, Payne LN, Goffe AP, Churchill AE, and Mortimer R (1966) Contaminant viruses in two live virus vaccines produced in chick cells. J Hyg (Lond). 64:1–7

Hermon-Taylor J, Bull TJ, Sheridan JM, Cheng J, Stellakis ML, and Sumar N (2000) Causation of Crohn's disease by Mycobacterium avium subspecies paratuberculosis. Can J Gastroenterol. 14:521–539

Hooper E (1999) The River. *A journey back to the source of HIV and AIDS*. Penguin Books, London

Horimoto T, and Kawaoka Y (2001) Pandemic threat posed by avian influenza A viruses. Clin Microbiol Rev. 14:129–149

Huelsenbeck JP, Rannala B, and Yang Z (1997) Statistical tests of host-parasite cospeciation. Evolution 51:410–419

Hussain AI, Shanmugam V, Switzer WM, Tsang SX, Fadly A, Thea D, Helfand R, Bellini WJ, Folks TM, and Heneine W (2001) Lack of evidence of endogenous avian leukosis virus and endogenous avian retrovirus transmission to measles, mumps, and rubella vaccine recipients. Emerg Infect Dis. 7:66–72

International (2001) A multicenter evaluation of assays for detection of SV40 DNA and results in masked mesothelioma specimens. Cancer Epidemiology, Biomarkers & Prevention 10:523–532

Jacobs M (2000) Dengue: emergence as a global public health problem and prospects for control. Trans R Soc Trop Med Hyg. 94:7–8

Johnson JA, and Heneine W (2001) Characterization of endogenous avian leukosis viruses in chicken embryonic fibroblast substrates used in production of measles and mumps vaccines. J Virol. 75:3605–12

Korber B, Muldoon M, Theiler J, Gao F, Gupta R, Lapedes A, Hahn BH, Wolinsky S, and Bhattacharya T (2000) Timing the ancestor of the HIV-1 pandemic strains. Science. 288:1789–1796

Lanciotti RS, Roehrig JT, Deubel V, Smith J, Parker M, Steele K, Crise B, Volpe KE, Crabtree MB, Scherret JH, Hall RA, MacKenzie JS, Cropp CB, Panigrahy B, Ostlund E, Schmitt B, Malkinson M, Banet C, Weissman J, Komar N, Savage HM, Stone W, McNamara T, and Gubler DJ (1999) Origin of the West Nile virus responsible for an outbreak of encephalitis in the northeastern United States. Science 286:2333–2337

Laver WG, Bischofberger N, and Webster RG (2000) The origin and control of pandemic influenza. Perspect Biol Med. 43:173–192

Lederberg J (2000) Infectious history. Science 288:287–293

Levy JA (1998) HIV and the pathogensis of AIDS, 2nd ed. American Society of Microbiology, Washington DC

Lipsitch M, and Moxon ER (1997) Virulence and transmissibility of pathogens: what is the relationship? Trends Microbiol. 5:31–37

Mahy BWJ. 1998. Zoonoses and haemorrhagic fever, p. 31–36. *In* F. Brown and E. Griffiths and F. Horaud and J. C. Petricciani (ed.), Safety of biological products prepared from mammalian cell culture. Dev Biol Stand, vol. 93

Martin J, Herniou E, Cook J, O'Neill RW, and Tristem M (1999) Interclass transmission and phyletic host tracking in murine leukemia virus-related retroviruses. J Virol. 73:2442–2449

Martin J, Kabat P, and Tristem M. 2001. Cospeciation and horizontal transmission in the murine leukaemia-related retroviruses. *In* R. Page (ed.), Tangled trees: Phylogenies, cospeciation, and coevolution. University of Chicago Press, Chicago

Marx PA, Alcabes PG, and Drucker E (2001) Serial human passage of simian immunodeficiency virus by unsterile injections and the emergence of epidemic human immunodeficiency virus in Africa. Phil Trans R Soc Lond B. 356:911–920

McMichael AJ (2001) Human frontiers, environments and disease. Cambridge University Press, Cambridge

McNeill WH (1976) *Plagues and peoples.* Penguin, London

Morse SS (1994) Hantaviruses and the hantavirus outbreak in the United States. A case study in disease emergence. Ann N Y Acad Sci. 740:199–207

Nowak MA, and Bangham CR (1996) Population dynamics of immune responses to persistent viruses. Science 272:74–79

Oldstone MBA (1998) Viruses, plagues and history. Oxford University Press, Oxford

Osterhaus A (1989) A morbillivirus causing mass mortality in seals. Vaccine 7:483–484

Oxford JS (2000) Influenza A pandemics of the 20th century with special reference to 1918: virology, pathology and epidemiology. Rev Med Virol. 10:119–133

Palmer SR, Soulsby EJL, and Simpson DIH (eds) (1998) Zoonoses. Oxford University Press, Oxford

Parker JS, Murphy WJ, Wang D, O'Brien SJ, and Parrish CR (2001) Canine and feline parvoviruses can use human or feline transferrin receptors to bind, enter, and infect cells. J Virol. 75:3896–3902

Parrish CR (1999) Host range relationships and the evolution of canine parvovirus. Vet Microbiol. 69:29–40

Patience C, Switzer WM, Takeuchi Y, Griffiths DJ, Goward ME, Heneine W, Stoye JP, and Weiss RA (2001) Multiple groups of novel retroviral genomes in pigs and related species. J. Virol. 75:2771–2775

Patience C, Takeuchi Y, and Weiss RA (1997) Infection of human cells by an endogenous retrovirus of pigs. Nature Medicine 3:282–286

Pepys S (1995) The Diary of Samuel Pepys Vol 6:1665. HarperCollins, London

Perelson AS, Neumann AU, Markowitz M, Leonard JM, and Ho DD (1996) HIV-1 dynamics in vivo: virion clearance rate, infected cell life-span, and viral generation time. Science 271:1582–1586

Prato CM, Akers TG, and Smith AW (1974) Serological evidence of calcivirus transmission between marine and terrestrial mammals. Nature 249:255–256

Pybus OG, Rambaut A, and Harvey PH (2000) An integrated framework for the inference of viral population history from reconstructed genealogies. Genetics 155:1429–1437

Qari SH, Magre S, Garcia-Lerma JG, Hussain AI, Takeuchi Y, Patience C, Weiss RA, and Heneine W (2001) Susceptibility of the porcine endogenous retrovirus to reverse transcriptase and protease inhibitors. J Virol. 75:1048–1053

Quétel C (1990) History of syphilis. Blackwell, Oxford

Rambaut A, Robertson DL, Pybus OG, Peeters M, and Holmes EC (2001) Human immunodeficiency virus: Phylogeny and the origin of HIV-1. Nature. 410:1047–1048

Raoult D, Roux V, Ndihokubwayo JB, Bise G, Baudon D, Marté G, and Birtles R (1997) Jail fever (epidemic typhus) outbreak in Burundi. Emerg Infect Dis. 3:357–360

Rappole JH, Derrickson SR, and Hubalek Z (2000) Migratory birds and spread of West Nile virus in the Western Hemisphere. Emerg Infect Dis. 6:319–328

Richman LK, Montali RJ, Garber RL, Kennedy MA, Lehnhardt J, Hildebrandt T, Schmitt D, Hardy D, Alcendor DJ, and Hayward GS (1999) Novel endotheliotropic herpesviruses fatal for Asian and African elephants. Science 283:1171–1176

Rother RP, and Squinto SP (1996) The alpha-galactosyl epitope: a sugar coating that makes viruses and cells unpalatable. Cell 86:185–188
Sabin A, Hennessen WA, and Winser J (1954) Studies of variants of poliomyelitis virus. I. Experimental segregation and properties of avirulent variants of three immunological types. J. Exp. Med. 99:551–576
Shafer RW, and Sierra MF (1992) Mycobacterium xenopi, Mycobacterium fortuitum, Mycobacterium kansasii, and other nontuberculous mycobacteria in an area of endemicity for AIDS. Clin Infect Dis. 15:161–162
Shah K, and Nathanson N (1976) Human exposure to SV40: review and comment. Am J Epidemiol. 103:1–12
Simmonds P (2001) The origin and evolution of hepatitis viruses in humans. J Gen Virol. 82:693–712
Starzl TE, Fung J, Tzakis A, Todo S, Demetris AJ, Marino IR, Doyle H, Zeevi A, Warty V, Michaels M, Kusan S, Rudert WA, and Trucco M (1993) Baboon-to-human liver transplantation. Lancet 341:65–71
Sweet BH, and Hilleman MR (1960) The vacuolating virus, SV40. Proc. Soc. Exp. Biol. Med. 105:420–427
Takeuchi Y, Porter CD, Strahan KM, Preece AF, Gustafsson K, Cosset FL, Weiss RA, and Collins MK (1996) Sensitization of cells and retroviruses to human serum by (alpha 1–3) galactosyltransferase. Nature 379:85–88
Theiler M, and Smith HH (1937) The use of yellow fever virus modified by *in vitro* cultivation for human immunization. J. Exp. Med. 65:782–800
Truyen U, Geissler K, Parrish CR, Hermanns W, and Siegl G (1998) No evidence for a role of modified live virus vaccines in the emergence of canine parvovirus. J Gen Virol. 79:1153–1158
Webster R, Lin YP, Shaw M, Gregory V, Cameron K, Lim W, Klimov A, Subbarao K, Guan Y, Krauss S, Shortridge K, Cox N, and Hay A (2000) Avian-to-human transmission of H9N2 subtype influenza A viruses: relationship between H9N2 and H5N1 human isolates. Proc Natl Acad Sci USA. 97:9654–8
Weinstock GM (2000) Genomics and bacterial pathogenesis. Emerg Infect Dis. 6:496–504
Weiss RA (1982) Retroviruses produced by hybridomas. N Engl J Med. 307:1587
Weiss RA (1998) Transgenic pigs and virus adaptation. Nature 391:327–328
Weiss RA (2001) Gulliver's travels in HIVland. Nature. 410:963–967
Weiss RA, and Wain-Hobson S (eds) (2001) Origins of HIV and the AIDS epidemic. Phil Trans R Soc. B. 356:781–977
Wells RM, Sosa Estani S, Yadon ZE, Enria D, Padula P, Pini N, Mills JN, Peters CJ, and Segura EL (1997) An unusual hantavirus outbreak in southern Argentina: person-to-person transmission? Hantavirus Pulmonary Syndrome Study Group for Patagonia. Emerg Infect Dis. 3:171–174
White PJ, Norman RA, Trout RC, Gould EA, and Hudson PJ (2001) The emergence of rabbit haemorrhagic disease virus: will a non-pathogenic strain protect the UK? Phil Trans Roy Soc B. 356:1087–1096
Wren BW (2000) Microbial genome analysis: insights into virulence, host adaptation and evolution. Nat Rev Genet. 1:30–39
Ziegler P (1970) The black death, Penguin, London
Zinsser H (1934) Rats, lice & history. Macmillan, London

Nonhuman Primate Herpesviruses: Importance for Xenotransplantation

M. G. Michaels

Division of Allergy, Immunology and Infectious Diseases,
Children's Hospital of Pittsburgh, University of Pittsburgh School of Medicine,
3705 Fifth Avenue, Pittsburgh, PA 15213, USA
E-mail: marian.michaels@chp.edu
Supported by KOS AI01437

1 Introduction 73

2 Herpesviridae 74
2.1 Alpha-Herpesviruses of NHP 79
2.2 Beta-Herpesviruses of NHP 84
2.3 Gamma-Herpesviruses of NHP 90

3 Summary 95

References 95

Abstract Herpesviruses are found throughout the animal kingdom. Members of this family share properties including a highly orchestrated system of transcription, destruction of the host cell by active viral replication and an ability to persist in the host in a latent form. Human herpesviruses have all been implicated in causing substantial disease after allotransplantation. Often transmission of these viruses has been through the donor organ or blood products. Analogous species of herpesviruses exist in nonhuman primates. Accordingly, concern regarding the risk of their transmission and disease exists with xenotransplant procedures. This chapter reviews herpesviruses of nonhuman primates and their potential implication for causing disease after xenotransplantation.

1 Introduction

Xenotransplantation offers use of animal organs and tissues for human patients with a variety of diseases. Ultimately it holds the potential for use of organs for individuals who are not able to wait for allotransplantation because of the severity of their disease and/or the prolonged time on the waiting list for human organs. Xenotransplant procedures also include the use of animal derived cells for such diverse diseases as diabetes and Parkinson's syndrome, as well as extracellular circulation for individuals in hepatic coma (Taniguchi and Cooper 1997). While great hope has been given to these procedures to improve human health, concern has developed over the last decade regarding the potential of xenotransplantation to transmit new infections or xenozoonoses to the human population (Michaels and Simmons 1994). Herpesviruses are widespread throughout the animal kingdom. In addition, they are well known causes of serious disease after human-to-human allotransplantation. Accordingly, concern exists for whether this family of viruses will cause disease after xenotransplantation. This chapter reviews the herpesviruses of nonhuman primates (NHP) with particular emphasis on the potential for cross-species transmission and implications for xenotransplantation.

2
Herpesviridae

Viruses that fit into the family Herpesviridae are identified by their structure and contain a core with double-stranded DNA that is surrounded by an icosadeltahedral capsid with 162 capsomeres (Roizman and Pellett 2001). The capsid is separated from the surrounding viral envelope by an amorphous material called tegument. The envelope, a bilayered lipid membrane, is derived from the nuclear membrane and contains several different glycoprotein spikes. Herpesviruses vary in size from 120 to 300 nm and the length of genomic DNA ranges from approximately 120 to 230 kilobase pairs depending on the particular viral species. While the DNA sequence varies considerably between the different subfamilies, at the protein level there is good homology between a subset of core proteins that are shared by all herpesviruses.

While the herpesvirus family contains a variety of species with diverse natural hosts including humans, NHP, other vertebrate and invertebrate animals, they share four basic biologic properties (Roizman and Pellett 2001). First, transcription of viral genes occurs in a highly orchestrated, sequential fashion with the genes divided into three classes, immediate early, early, and late. Immediate early proteins, comprised primarily of regulatory proteins, are synthesized first and their production is essential for the subsequent synthesis of early proteins. The early proteins are largely responsible for viral nucleic acid metabolism and are followed by replication of viral DNA and the synthesis of late proteins. The late proteins form the structural components of the virions. Second, the synthesis of viral DNA and the assembly of the capsid occur in the nucleus of the host cell. Third, the host cell is destroyed by viral replication and the production of infectious viral progeny. Finally, herpesvirus infection of the host cell does not have to lead to viral production. Rather, the virus can be maintained in a latent or persistent state where only a subset of viral genes may be expressed and the host cell remains intact. Accordingly, herpesviruses are maintained in some of the host cells for the life span of the host. This ability to remain relatively quiescent within host cells while retaining the capacity to reactivate and produce infectious virus accounts for the herpesvirus' ability to be transmitted from one individual to another through transfusion or transplantation even if the host's original infection occurred years before.

Specific biologic properties vary between members of the herpesvirus family, including the host range, the cell range within a host species and the rapidity with which a productive infection destroys the infected cell. Herpesviridae are subdivided by their biologic properties into three subfamilies: alpha, beta and gamma. Examples of alphaherpesvirinae in humans are herpes simplex viruses 1 and 2, (HSV-1 and 2) and varicella-zoster virus (VZV). This group of viruses has a short reproductive span, a variable host range, efficient cell destruction, and the capacity to establish latency in sensory ganglion. Beta-herpesvirinae, typified by human cytomegalovirus (HCMV), have a more restricted host range and a long reproductive cycle. Latency is maintained in lymphoreticular cells and cells within secretory glands and kidneys. Human herpesvirus (HHV)-6 and HHV-7 are also classified as beta-herpesviruses. Gamma-herpesvirinae are lymphoid-associated viruses that are felt to be strongly host restricted. Examples of human gamma-herpesviruses include Epstein–Barr virus (EBV) and HHV-8. These viruses replicate and establish latency in the lymphoreticular cells of the host.

All of the human herpesviruses have been implicated in disease after human allotransplantation (Frances et al. 2000; Green and Michaels 1997; Mendez et al. 2001; Rubin 1990; Singh et al. 1988). Transmission of herpesviruses from the donor organ is most often associated with beta- and gamma-herpesviruses that establish latency in transplanted cells or tissues. In particular, HCMV and EBV have been proven to cause substantial disease after donor transmission (Cen et al.1991; Delmonico and

Table 1 Herpesviruses of NHP

Designated name	Vernacular names	Comments
Alphaherpesvirinae		
Cercopithecine herpesvirus 1	B virus, herpesvirus (HV) simiae	Similar to HSV in macaques; causes severe often fatal disease in humans
Cercopithecine herpesvirus 2	Simian agent (SA) 8	Similar to HSV in African green monkey
Cercopithecine herpesvirus 16	*H. papio* 2, baboon HV, SA8	Similar to HSV in baboons; has not been found to transmit to humans
Cercopithecine herpesvirus 6[a]	Liverpool vervet monkey virus (LVV, LVMV)	Similar clinical rash and disease to varicella in African green monkeys, high fatality rate
Cercopithecine herpesvirus 7[a]	Patas monkey HV (MMV or PHV) delta HV	Similar clinical rash to varicella in a group of imported Patas monkey, high fatality rate
Cercopithecine herpesvirus 9	Medical Lake macaque (MLM), simian varicella HV	Similar disease to varicella in macaques, low fatality rate
Ateline herpesvirus 1	Spider monkey HV	
Saimiriine herpesvirus 1	Marmoset HV, Herpes T, HV tamarinus, HV platyrrhinae type	Natural host is the Squirrel monkey virus; first recognized in marmosets and owl monkeys
Betaherpesvirinae		
Cercopithecine herpesvirus 3	SA 6	Isolated from African green monkeys
Cercopithecine herpesvirus 4	SA 15	Initially isolated from African green monkey kidney tissue culture, but subsequently isolated from healthy baboons
Cercopithecine herpesvirus 5	African green monkey cytomegalovirus	
Cercopithecine herpesvirus 8	Rhesus monkey cytomegalovirus	
Aotine herpesvirus 1	HV aotus type 1	Isolated from the kidney of an owl monkey
Aotine herpesvirus 3	HV aotus type 3	Isolated from the kidney of an owl monkey
Aotine herpesvirus 4	Owl monkey cytomegalovirus	

Table 1 (continued)

Designated name	Vernacular names	Comments
Callitrichine herpes-virus 2	SSG, marmoset cyto-megalovirus	CMV like organism isolated from the salivary glands of white-lipped marmosets (*Saguinus fuscicollis*)
Cebine herpesvirus 1	Capuchin HV (AL-5)	
Cebine herpesvirus 2	Capuchin HV (AP-15)	
	Baboon cytomegalo-virus	Isolated from baboons and from a patient who received a baboon liver transplant
	Squirrel monkey cyto-megalovirus	
Gammaherpesvirinae		
Cercopithecine herpesvirus 10	Rhesus leukocyte-associated HV strain 1	
Cercopithecine herpesvirus 11[a]	Rhesus leukocyte-associated HV strain 2	
Cercopithecine herpesvirus12	*H. papio*, baboon HV	Associated with lymphomas in baboons
Cercopithecine herpesvirus 14	African green monkey EBV-like HV	
Cercopithecine herpesvirus 15	Rhesus monkey EBV-like HV	
Aotine herpesvirus 2	HV aotus type 2	
Ateline herpesvirus 2	HV ateles	
Ateline herpesvirus 3	HV ateles strain 73	
Callitrichine herpes-virus 1	HV sanquinus	
Pongine herpesvirus 1	Chimpanzee HV, PtRV-1; Pan Rhadino HV 1a/1b	Two chimpanzee rhadi-noviruses have been identi-fied that are classed as RV-1 types (Greensill et al. 2000; Lacoste et al. 2000)
	Pan Rhadino-HV 2	A novel chimpanzee rhadi-novirus was identified that is more similar to RV-2 (Lacoste et al. 2001)
Pongine herpesvirus 2	Orangutan HV	
Pongine herpesvirus 3	Gorilla HV; GorRHV1	

Table 1 (continued)

Designated name	Vernacular names	Comments
Saimiriine herpesvirus 2	Squirrel monkey HV, *H. saimiri*, HVS	The first recognized rhadinovirus; natural host is the squirrel monkey (*Saimiri sciureus*); causes malignancies in marmosets and owl monkeys
	CalHV-3	Lymhocryptovirus isolated from lymphomas from common marmoset (*Callithrix jacchus*) (Cho et al. 2000)
	Retrofibromatosis herpesvirus *M. nemestrina* (RFHVMn)	Rhadinovirus type 1 isolated from a retrofibromatosis lesion of a pig-tailed macaque (*M. nemestrina*)
	Retrofibromatosis herpesvirus *M. mulatta* (RFHVMm)	Rhadinovirus type 1 isolated from a retrofibromatosis lesion of a rhesus macaque (*M. mulatta*)
	Rhesus Rhadinovirus (RRV)	Rhadinovirus type 2, Isolated from blood of *M. mulatta*

NHP, nonhuman primates.

[a] No longer included in viruses of the family Herpesviridae in Roizman and Pellett (2001).

Snydman 1998; Ho et al. 1985; Rubin 1990; Singh et al. 1988). These herpesviruses have stringent host restriction which implies that xenotransplantation may be less of a risk for transmission. However, some of the host restrictions classically found in nature are being challenged by experiments in xenotransplantation (Michaels et al. 2001).

Information on each of the three subfamilies of herpesviruses described below includes a brief description of the family in general, epidemiology in NHP, data on cross-species transmission if available and the potential importance for xenotransplantation. Finally a note on nomenclature is in order. The nomenclature for NHP herpesviruses remains somewhat controversial and has changed over time (Greensill et al. 2000; Kalter et al. 1980; Roizman and Pellett 2001; Roizman et al. 1981). Originally simian viruses from African monkeys were chronologically named simian agent (SA) and those from Asian monkeys, simian virus, without regard to their virus genera. Later researchers named viruses by their genera and disease finding or the species in which it was found. However, this too caused some complications as viruses were sometimes first identified in NHP species other than its natural host. For example, marmoset herpesvirus is actually the alpha-herpesvirus of the squirrel monkey. In 1981, the Herpesvirus Study Group attempted to reclassify all herpesviruses including those of NHP into a more uniform system (Roizman and Pellett 2001; Roizman et al. 1981). This system is listed in Table 1 along with the vernacular names that remain in more common use in the literature today.

2.1 Alpha-Herpesviruses of NHP

As noted above, this group of viruses has an adaptable host range, a short cycle of replication, and establishes latency in sensory ganglion. Alpha-herpesviruses have been identified in a number of NHP, including macaques, baboons, spider monkey, squirrel monkey and the great apes (Table 1; Eberle and Hilliard 1989; Hilliard and Soza 1996; Hilliard et al. 1989). Simian herpesviruses are biologically similar to HSV-1 and 2 in that they generally lead to self-limited lesions on mucocutaneous sites such as the oral mucosa, conjunctiva or genitals. In addition, these viruses establish latency in the sensory ganglia of the host and can have periodic recurrent lesions or asymptomatic shedding of virus.

Serological studies show variable seroprevalence rates to alpha-herpesviruses depending on the species, how they were reared and the antigen used (Table 2). Accordingly, great variations in seroprevalence may result from true differences in the prevalence of virus or be artifactual because of differences in methods or the antigens used. For example, a study of great apes in a zoo found seroprevalence to HSV-1 ranging from 7% in the orangutans to 65% in gorillas. Rather than reflecting true infection with a human virus, it is likely that the serological assay in this study cross-reacted with a related virus within each species. It is possible that this group of gorillas had a higher prevalence of alpha-herpesvirus infection. Alternatively it may be that the gorilla alpha-herpesvirus virus is more closely related antigenically to HSV-1 and therefore more accurately detected by the assay used (Eberle and Hilliard 1989). Despite these difficulties, seroprevalence studies do provide beneficial information, particularly when examining groups of primates within a study. Van der Reit and colleagues found a 70% positive rate for SA-8 in feral

Table 2 Seroprevalence of alpha-herpesviruses in different NHP

Virus	Species tested	Method reared	Result (%)	Comment	References
HSV-1	African green	Feral	7/10 (70)	Similar findings with SA-8 antigen	Van der Reit et al. 1987
	African green	NA	0/29 (0)	Higher incidence with SA-8 antigen	Kalter and Heberling 1990b
	Baboon	Feral	9/10 (90)		Van der Reit et al. 1987
	Macaque	NA	77/164 (47)	Dot-immunobinding assay	Heberling and Kalter 1986
	Macaque	NA	0/38	Higher prevalence with B virus antigen	Kalter and Heberling 1990b
	Chimpanzee and gorillas	NA	13/26 (50)		
	Chimpanzee	Zoo	7/38 (18)		Eberle and Hilliard 1984
	Gorilla	Zoo	53/81 (65)		
	Orangutan	Zoo	5/70 (7)	Low titers	
	Gibbon apes	Zoo	8/24 (33)		
B virus	Macaque	NA	415/1295 (32)		Kalter and Heberling 1990b
		NA	129/240 (54)	Dot-immunobinding assay	Heberling and Kalter 1986
		NA	4079/13000 (31)	Years 1987–1988	Kalter and Heberling 1990a
		Feral	164/204 (80)		Kessler et al. 1989
SA-8	African green	Captive	0/14 (0)	Significant difference feral versus captive animals	Van der Reit et al. 1987
	African green	Feral	7/10 (70)		
	African green	NA	28/58 (48)		Kalter and Heberling 1990b

Table 2 (continued)

Virus	Species tested	Method reared	Result (%)	Comment	References
SA-8 (IFA)	Baboon	Captive	18/26 (69)	Paired specimens	Michaels et al. 1994
SA-8 (DIA)	Baboon	Captive	30/31 (97)		
Herpes T virus	Squirrel monkey	NA	4/40 (10)	Dot-immunobinding assay	Heberling and Kalter 1986
VZV	African green	Captive	0/14 (0)		Van der Reit et al. 1987
	African green		2/111 (2)		Kalter and Heberling 1990b
	Baboon	Feral	7/10 (70)		Van der Reit et al. 1987
	Chimpanzee/gorilla	NA	19/26 (23)		Kalter and Heberling 1990b

NA, data not available.

African green monkeys while a captive group were negative showing that animals could be reared free of the virus (Van der Reit et al. 1987).

The most intensely reviewed herpesvirus of NHPs is *Cercopithecine herpesvirus* 1 as it is capable of causing virulent disease in humans. More commonly known as B virus, it was named by Sabin and Wright for the middle initial of a researcher who died with the infection and in whom the disease properties were first elucidated (Holmes et al. 1990). *C. herpesvirus* 1 is an alpha-herpesvirus of macaques, shed from mucocutaneous sites such as the oropharynx, conjunctiva and urogenital tract (Holmes et al. 1990; Weigler 1992). Similar to HSV-1 and 2, viral shedding can occur in the macaque with or without visible vesicular lesions. Acquisition in macaques increases with age and the onset of sexual maturity so that by adulthood, over 70% of captive macaques are infected (Weigler 1992). While the virus is found in most macaque species, strain differences have been hypothesized to correlate with different risks of infectivity to other hosts (Smith et al. 1998). To date, the majority of human disease has been associated with *C. herpesvirus* 1 of rhesus and cynomolgus monkeys. Whether this is due to true pathogenic strain differences or to significant differences in exposure rates of humans to these two monkeys compared with other monkeys is unproven at this time (Hilliard and Weigler 1999). Potential strain variations aside, it is clear that this virus is relatively benign in its natural host but leads to severe, usually fatal encephalitis in humans. *C. herpesvirus 1* infections of humans became increasingly evident in the 1950s as more intimate interactions with macaques developed during the course of biomedical research including the making of monkey cell lines for general virology and the development of poliomyelitis vaccines (Holmes et al. 1995). A resurgence of macaque work surrounding retrovirus research in the 1980s again led to increased occurrences of disease in humans and the development of public health guidelines for worker safety including protective clothing, wound care and potential treatment strategies (Holmes et al. 1995; Cohen et al. 2002).

Transmission of *C. herpesvirus 1* to humans occurs through contact of infectious material or exposure to infected monkey tissue with broken skin, such as from a bite or scratch (Holmes et al. 1995; Weigler 1992). However, a recent fatal infection of a young animal care worker occurred after a splash to the eye of unidentified material from a cage that housed a macaque (Anonymous 1998). Accordingly, regulations have been altered to include the use of protective eyewear in addition to previously recommended protective procedures. Secondary transmission of *C. herpesvirus* 1 to another person has also been documented (Holmes et al. 1990). This latter case was probably caused by self-inoculation of the virus when a spouse concurrently applied a topical steroid to her husband's *C. herpesvirus 1* infection and her own dermatitis. Although preventable, it demonstrates the capacity for human-to-human transmission.

While *C. herpesvirus 1* is highly pathogenic to humans, transmission appears to be relatively rare considering the number of potential exposures that occur yearly. Serologic studies of primate workers have not found evidence for asymptomatic infections (Freidfeld et al. 1995; Holmes et al. 1990). However, the extremely high case fatality rate of this infection led the National Institutes of Health to sponsor a multi-institutional program to establish macaque research colonies that would be negative for *C. herpesvirus 1* (Hilliard and Ward 1999).

C. herpesvirus 1 highlights several important concepts for xenotransplantation. It categorically proves that a herpesvirus of an NHP can be transmitted to humans. In addition, the resultant disease can be significantly more virulent than that found in the natural host. Further, once in the human the virus has the capacity for secondary transmission to close contacts. Finally, these risks can be eliminated through successful breeding plans that eliminate this virus from NHP colonies.

Other NHP species also have endogenous alpha-herpesviruses (Eberle and Hilliard 1989; Hilliard et al. 1989; Levin et al. 1988). *C. herpesvirus 2* of African green monkeys and *C. herpesvirus 16* of baboons are more commonly called SA8, (the latter is also called *H. papio 2*) and are the alpha-herpesviruses of their respective species (Eberle and Hilliard 1984; Levin et al. 1988; Michaels et al. 1994). Similar to HSV-1 and 2 in humans and *C. herpesvirus 1* in macaques, SA8 is neurotropic and can cause recurrent genital, oral mucosal and conjunctival lesions but is usually asymptomatic (Levin et al. 1988; Martino et al. 1998). Herpesviruses have been isolated from NHP species that had VZV-like vesicles (Blakely et al. 1973; McCarthy and Tosolini 1975; McCarthy et al. 1968). Similar to VZV disease in humans, macaque infection appeared to be a self-limited disease with few fatalities (Blakely et al. 1973). However, unlike humans and macaques disease outbreaks in patas monkeys and African green monkeys had a high fatality rate (Blakely et al. 1973; McCarthy and Tosolini 1975; McCarthy et al. 1968). Specific data regarding the host origin of these viruses is not available.

While SA8 has not been established as a cause of human infection or disease it's similarity to B virus raises the concern for potential transmission via xenotransplantation. To date, SA8 transmission was not found in the handful of baboon xenotransplant recipients studied (Michaels et al. 1996; Starzl et al. 1993). The development of specific enzyme linked immunosorbent assay and polymerase chain reaction assays (PCR) for SA8 that distinguish it from other alpha-herpesviruses will improve diagnostic abilities (Hilliard and Soza 1996). Should NHP be considered again for xenotransplantation trials, efforts should be made to raise them free of these viruses.

2.2 Beta-Herpesviruses of NHP

Beta-herpesviruses are abundant in mammals. A restrictive host range, long reproductive cycle and slow growth in tissue culture characterize this group of viruses (Roizman and Pellett 2001). Infected cells undergoing lytic viral replication are typically enlarged or cytomegalic. The viruses can maintain a latent infection in lymphoreticular cells, and cells of secretory glands, kidneys and possibly other tissues (Pass 2001). Cytomegalovirus (CMV), a ubiquitous virus, is the most well studied member of the beta-herpesvirus family. In humans, HCMV is usually a benign infection with either no symptoms or only mild disease. However, this is not always the case; recognition of HCMV and even its name was derived from the severe congenital infections that led to stillbirth fetuses characterized by enlarged cells with intranuclear inclusions in multiple organs (reviewed by Ho 1991 and Pass 2001). While the characteristic findings in stillbirths were initially wrongly ascribed to a parasitic infection, they were eventually recognized as being caused by a virus. Guinea pig experiments demonstrated a filterable agent to cause the same salivary gland pathology (Pass 2001). In addition, analogous pathologic findings in the salivary glands of children without systemic disease were noted along with a similarity to pathology caused by other herpesviruses. Tissue culture techniques of the 1950s permitted viral isolation allowing for the development of diagnostic studies such as antigen-based serologic assays. With these tools it became clear that HCMV was widespread in the adult population. Likewise it was recognized that blood transfusions, and transplantation of organs and bone marrow could transmit the virus (Delmonico and Snydman 1998; Ho 1991; Rubin 1990; Singh et al. 1988). Unlike the benign nature of infection in a healthy host, HCMV causes severe, even fatal, disease in immunosuppressed individuals (Green and Michaels 1997; Ho 1991; Rubin 1990; Singh et al. 1988).

NHP are also recognized as having infection with native CMV species and to shed intermittently, similar to humans (Brede and Murphy 1972; Kalter and Heberling 1990a, b; Swack et al. 1971; Vogel et al. 1994). A number of serologic surveys have been conducted showing 40%–100% of tested NHP to have antibody against CMV (Table 3). As noted above, serologic studies relying on antigens that cross-react with the herpesviruses of different species have been useful in starting to understand the epidemiology of herpesviruses in specific NHP populations but can cause difficulties in interpretation and underestimate the true prevalence of a virus. In part, this may explain some discrepancies in the seroprevalence found for specific NHP species. Direct comparisons of different assays on paired specimens can assist in evaluating this problem. Swack et al. (1971) found 91%–100% of African green monkeys to have neutralizing antibody against an African green monkey (AGM) CMV but none to have neutralizing antibodies against the human laboratory strain AD169. Likewise, Michaels et al. (1994) found a simian CMV antigen to yield a 97% seropositive rate in a captive group of baboons as opposed to only 76% seropositivity when a commercial HCMV antigen kit was used on the same sera.

A high seroprevalence to CMV was found in most NHP populations but differences existed depending on the species evaluated, their rearing conditions (feral versus captive bred), and the age of the animal tested. Animals raised in crowded, close quarters in captivity appeared to have higher rates of CMV seropositivity or acquisition of CMV infection over time (Kessler et al. 1989; Muchmore 1971; Swack et al. 1971; Vogel et al. 1994). Age of acquisition was addressed in a serial surveillance study of 142 captive macaques. Investigators found 100% of the animals over 1 year of age to be seropositive, while only 42% of the infant monkeys were seropositive (Vogel et al. 1994). Rather than reflecting a congenital infection it was felt that the eight seropositive infants had passive maternal antibody as evidenced by finding only IgG isotype antibody without the presence of IgM. All infants subsequently underwent seroreversion followed by new seroconversion or acquisition of IgM seropositivity by 18 months of age. This demonstrated a relatively early acquisition of CMV in this closed community. Risk factors such as sex, social dominance of the dam and birthing season did not affect the time of serocon-

Table 3 Seroprevalence of beta-herpesviruses in NHP

Virus	Species tested	Method reared	Result (%)	Comment	References
HCMV	African green	Feral	6/10 (60)	Minimal difference feral vs. captive	Van der Reit et al. 1987
	African green	Captive	6/14 (43)		
	Baboon	Feral	10/10 (100)		
	Baboon	Captive	19/25 (76)	Lower prevalence compared to simian CMV antigen	Michaels and Simmons 1994
African green CMV	African green	Feral	33/175 (19)		Kalter and Heberling 1990b
	African green	NA	52/57 (91)		Swack et al. 1971
	African green	NA	61/61 (100)		
	African green	Feral	42/47 (89)	Serial testing over time	Muchmore 1971
		Captive 1–3 months	46/47 (98)		
	Rhesus monkey	Captive 1–3 months	27/59 (46)	Serial testing over time	
		Captive >1 year	10/13 (77)		
	Rhesus monkey	NA	27/59 (46)		Swack et al. 1971
	Baboon	NA	6/15 (40)		Swack et al. 1971
	Baboon	Captive 1–3 months	6/15 (40)	Serial testing over time	Muchmore 1971
		Captive >1 year	36/41 (88)		

Table 3 (continued)

Virus	Species tested	Method reared	Result (%)	Comment	References
Baboon CMV	Baboon	Captive, caged	66/66 (100)	Both with 100% prevalence	Neubauer et al. 1979
Captive, free range	30/30 (100)				
'Simian' CMV	Baboon	Captive	30/31 (97)	Higher prevalence compared to HCMV antigen	Michaels and Simmons 1994

version. The high prevalence rates in adult animals and easy transmission to other animals in close quarters are important points if considering the use of NHP for xenotransplant research. If animals free of CMV are required for study or xenotransplantation then specific pathogen free rearing conditions must be maintained using very young animals.

Studies comparing proteins from fibroblasts infected by different species of simian CMV found most isolates to have counterparts of the principal structural and nonstructural proteins of HCMV (Gibson 1983; Weiner and Gibson 1981). A 145-KDa protein that represents the predominant structural protein of the viral icosahedral capsid appeared to be well conserved over NHP species including CMV from Old World monkeys (baboon, African green and rhesus) and New World monkeys *Cebus* and *Aotus* (Weiner and Gibson 1981). Interestingly, this and other proteins of Rhesus CMV (RhCMV) and AGM CMV strains were more similar to each other than to HCMV (Gibson 1983). Sequence comparison of the promoter regions of the immediate early genes of AGM CMV, RhCMV and HCMV likewise found more homology between the two simian strains than with HCMV (70% homology between RhCMV and AGM CMV versus only 48% homology between RhCMV and HCMV (Alcendor et al. 1993). Diagnostic assays for xenotransplant research can take advantage of some of these differences. Restriction endonuclease cleavage of CMV genomes shows differences in the DNA of simian and human CMV but is not readily applicable for rapid diagnostic studies (Kilpatrick et al. 1976; Michaels et al. 1997). However, the development of species-specific CMV PCR assays based on differences in the major immediate early genes have proven to be useful tools for xenotransplant research (Hilliard et al. 1996; Michaels et al. 1997).

Most healthy NHP do not exhibit signs or symptoms from CMV infection, but similar to humans, disease can occur in states of immunosuppression. RhCMV caused disseminated disease in 14 macaques (13 rhesus monkeys and one cynomologous monkey) that were infected with simian immunodeficiency virus (SIV) (Baskin 1987). Pathologic abnormalities with characteristic CMV inclusions were identified in the lungs of 11 animals and in the lymph nodes of eight. Less frequent involvement was found in nerves, arteries, intestines, liver, and brain. Likewise, Ohtaki and colleagues (1986) found disseminated CMV infection in cynomologous monkeys that were immunosuppressed with a combination of steroids, anti-thymocyte globulin and cyclosporin. The lungs and lymph nodes were particularly affected. Unlike humans, congenital

CMV infection has not been recognized in the surveillance studies of NHP. However, experimental in utero inoculation of rhesus monkeys either intracerebrally or intra-amniotically led to brain disease in 50% and placental abnormalities in 81% (London et al. 1986). Therefore simian CMV can lead to disease in NHP that are congenitally infected or immunosuppressed, similar to HCMV in humans.

As noted above, while the alpha-herpesviruses, such as B virus, are transmissible across species lines, they are less likely be donor associated in a xenotransplant setting because their site of latency is not within most tissues or lymphoreticular cells. Beta- and gamma-herpesviruses on the other hand are classic donor transmitted infections after allotransplantation (Cen et al. 1991; Ho et al. 1985; Rubin 1990; Singh et al. 1988). Accordingly, the ability of these viruses to traverse species barriers is of substantial concern for xenotransplantation. Several findings suggest that transmission of CMV between species is possible both in vivo and in vitro. The laboratory Towne strain of HCMV replicates in cultures of chimpanzee skin fibroblasts (Perot et al. 1992). Likewise baboon CMV (BCMV) replicates well in human foreskin fibroblast and MRC-5 cell lines (Michaels et al. 1997). Growth characteristics of BCMV in these cell lines are similar to those of HCMV.

Simian CMV has been implicated as the cause of neurologic disease in several humans. A brain biopsy from an encephalopathic boy led to the isolation of CMV, strain Colburn which has substantial homology with AGM CMV (strain GR2757) (Gibson 1983; Huang et al. 1978). In separate cases, Martin and colleagues isolated an AGM-like CMV from a woman suffering from chronic fatigue syndrome (Martin et al. 1994; Martin et al. 1995) and from the cerebrospinal fluid of a patient with encephalopathy (Martin 1996). While these findings suggest the possibility of simian CMV crossing over to humans the sources of these potential simian infections were not ascertained.

Replication competent BCMV was isolated from a patient who received a baboon liver xenotransplant 29 days after transplantation (Michaels et al. 2001). The virus was isolated from a blood sample obtained 10 days after the cessation of ganciclovir, but was not isolated again after the reinstitution of ganciclovir. Sequence analysis of the PCR product from the isolated virus was identical to that of the donor baboon's BCMV. Susceptibility assays showed it to be more sensitive to ganciclovir than the patient's native HCMV giving a biologically plausible explanation for not finding it in the patient when ganciclovir was administered. While disease association was not proven, the finding of replication competent BCMV in the blood of a xenotransplant recipient 1 month after transplantation highlights the importance of CMV transmission across species lines.

2.3 Gamma-Herpesviruses of NHP

Gamma-herpesviruses are divided into two genera, gamma-1 also called *Lymphocryptoviruses* (LCV) and gamma-2 or *Rhadinoviruses.* The two genera are represented in humans by EBV and HHV-8 respectively (Roizman and Pellett 2001). Both genera are associated with the development of tumors.

The biologic characteristic of EBV and its NHP homologues is their ability to latently infect B lymphocytes and transform them in vitro into lymphoblastoid cell lines (LCL) (Rickinson and Kieff 2001). In humans, EBV is usually an asymptomatic infection when acquired early in life or causes a mononucleosis syndrome when acquired during adolescence or young adulthood. More than 90% of people are seropositive for EBV by adulthood (Rickinson and Kieff 2001). EBV has been associated with several tumors including Burkitt's lymphoma, T-cell lymphoma, gastric carcinoma, nasopharyngeal carcinoma and fatal proliferative disorders in boys with X-linked aggamaglobulinemia (reviewed by Rickinson and Kieff 2001). Immunosuppressed individuals are at particular risk for EBV-associated lymphoproliferative disorders and leiomyosarcoma (Cen et al. 1991; Green and Michaels 1997; Ho et al. 1985). The need for chronic immunosuppressive drugs for xenotransplantation raises substantial concern for transmission of NHP gamma-herpesviruses viruses and their malignant potential (Michaels and Simmons 1994).

Serologic studies have found the presence of cross-reacting antibodies to EBV viral capsid antigen (VCA) in most Old World monkeys suggesting that homologous viruses exist in these species (Falk et al. 1976; Kalter and Heberling 1990a, b; Michaels et al. 1994; Table 4). However, similar to serologic studies with alpha- and beta-herpesviruses, reliance on cross-reacting antigens can give variable results. For example cross-reacting antibody to EBV nuclear antigen (EBNA) appears to be less common in NHP. In one study only 4% of paired baboon sera tested positive to EBV EBNA compared with 97% seropositivity to EBV VCA (Michaels et al. 1994). Accordingly, some serologic studies grossly underestimate

Table 4 Seroprevalence of gamma-herpesviruses in NHP

Virus	Species tested	Method reared	Result (%)	Comment	References
EBV VCA	Baboon	Captive	30/31 (97)	Paired samples found VCA more sensitive than EBNA in this population	Michaels et al. 1994
EBV EBNA		Captive	1/26 (4)		
H. papio	Baboons, juveniles	Captive	19/52 (37)	Serial evaluation over time juveniles	Jenson et al. 2000
			39/52 (75)		
	Baboons, adults	Captive	88/92 (96)		
H. papio VCA	Baboons with lymphoma	Caged	31/31 (100)	High titer	Neubauer et al. 1979
	Baboons, healthy	Free range forest	26/30 (87)	Low titer	
H. papio EA	Baboons with lymphoma	Caged	21/31 (70)	More commonly found in caged animals with lymphoma	
	Baboons healthy	Free range forest	2/30 (6)		
H. papio EBNA	Baboons with lymphoma	Caged	10/31 (32)	More commonly found in caged animals with lymphoma	
	Baboons, healthy	Free range forest	0/30 (0)		

Table 4 (continued)

Virus	Species tested	Method reared	Result (%)	Comment	References
H. saimiri	Squirrel monkeys	Colony-born <1 year	6/16 (38)	Early acquisition without evidence of disease	Deinhardt et al. 1973
		>2 years	19/19 (100)		
		>3 years	67/67 (100)		
		NA	45/98 (46)	Dot-immunobinding assay	Heberling and Kalter 1986
KSHV (HHV-8)	Chimpanzee	NA	20/25 (80)	1:40 dilutions	Reviewed by Lacoste et al. 2001
	Gorilla	NA	2/5 (40)		

NA, data not available.

the presence of LCVs in NHP. The definitive recognition of the existence of NHP LCVs came with the establishment of LCLs from splenic lymphocytes of a lymphomatous baboon and was termed *Herpesvirus papio* (Falk et al. 1976). Subsequently, simian LCVs have been characterized in most other Old World monkeys and more recently in New World monkeys (Cho et al. 2001; Moghaddam et al. 1998).

In primates, similar to humans, LCV infections are often asymptomatic and tend to be acquired at a young age. A large seroepidemiologic study on baboons found *H. papio* to be ubiquitous in adults and to be most often acquired within the first year of life (Jenson et al. 2000). Simian LCVs have been implicated in the pathogenesis of lymphomas and squamous epithelial proliferative disease in immunosuppressed primates (Baskin et al. 1995; Li et al. 1993).

The LCVs share many properties but their ability to immortalize B cells of other species is variable (Moghaddam et al. 1998). While human EBV and baboon *H. papio* can immortalize marmoset lymphocytes (Falk et al. 1976) in general, immortalization only occurs between closely related NHP. Moghaddam and colleagues (1998) found that human EBV could not transform B cells of rhesus monkeys. Likewise neither baboon nor rhesus LCVs could transform human B cells. However, *H. papio* efficiently immortalized B cells of rhesus monkeys. This demonstrated that infection could occur between related Old World primates.

A number of studies were carried out to attempt to elucidate why LCVs of distant NHP species could not immortalize human peripheral B cells. The rhesus monkey LCV major membrane glycoprotein was characterized with the hypothesis that the problem with immortalization was at the site of binding and entry. However, the investigators found the binding epitope of this glycoprotein to be highly conserved and that simian LCVs could actually infect human B cells and express CD23 (Moghaddam et al. 1998). Thus the blocking of immortalization in disparate species had to be after virus penetration. Other investigators found that the EBNA 2 of *H. papio* differs significantly from EBNA-2 of human EBV (Franken et al. 1995; Ling et al. 1993). Because EBNA-2 is a critical component leading to B cell immortalization it is possible that this genetic variability plays a role in host susceptibility to LCVs of different species. Of interest, baboon LCV could persistently co-infect human B cells that were already immortalized by EBV (Moghaddam et al. 1998). This may be of consequence in xenotransplant studies. While NHP LCVs might be able to attach to and enter human B cells they may not be able immortalize directly them. However, superinfection might be possible in the setting of xenotransplantation if EBV-associated post-transplant lymphoproliferative disorder developed coincidentally in a recipient. Species-specific PCR assays, developed by taking advantage of the differences in EBNA-2 sequences could be helpful to better explore these possibilities in a xenotransplant setting (Hayashi et al. 2001).

H. saimiri was the first gamma-2 herpesvirus recognized and led to the name rhadinovirus describing the 'slender' or 'fragile' appearance of the viral DNA when visualized by electron microscopy (Greensill et al. 2000). A virus isolated from the leukocytes of rhesus monkeys (rhesus leukocyte-associated herpesvirus) likewise fits into this class of viruses (Frank et al. 1973).

The human rhadinovirus, HHV-8, was discovered in 1993 in a Kaposi's sarcoma lesion of an AIDS patient using representational difference analysis (Chang et al. 1994). Unlike other herpesviruses that appear to be ubiquitous in the human population, HHV-8 is encountered less frequently . Certain parts of the world, such as Africa, have high endemic seroprevalence, whereas the Mediterranean area and Middle East have a moderate seroprevalence, and North America, Asia and Northern Europe have a low seroprevalence (Moore and Chang 2001). Disease manifestation of HHV-8 was first proven for Kaposi's sarcoma. Subsequently it has been associated with body cavity based lymphomas, and multicentric Castleman's disease. Most often the tumors are associated with immunosuppressed states. After the discovery of HHV-8 in humans a number of related rhadinoviruses have been found in NHPs including macaques (rhesus, cynomologous and pig-tailed monkeys), African green monkeys, gorillas, chimpanzees and orangutans (Desrosiers et al. 1997; Holmes et al. 1990; Moore and Chang 2001; Schultz et al. 2000).

H. saimiri of the squirrel monkey appears to be benign in its natural host but causes rapidly progressive tumors when transmitted across species lines to other NHP (Del Prete et al. 1994). Similarly the spider monkey (*Ateles sp.*) is not affected adversely by infection with *H. ateles* but tumors can be induced in other primates (Greensill and Schultz 2000). *H. saimiri* and *H. ateles* can transform in vitro the CD4 cells of a number of other primate species including humans (Del Prete et al. 1994; Greensill and Schultz 2000). Cross-reacting antibody to *H. saimiri* in colonies of rhesus monkeys suggested widespread infection of a related virus in these colonies. In 1997 Desrosiers and colleagues isolated rhesus monkey rhadinovirus but did not show a specific disease. Earlier that same year Rose and colleagues also identified homologs to HHV-8 in retroperitoneal fibromatosis tumors of both rhesus and pig-tailed macaques (Rose et al. 1997). These tumors, which were similar to Kaposi's sarcoma, occurred in an outbreak in the Washington and Oregon Primate colonies in 1976 through the mid 1980s and appeared to be associated with animals having simian AIDS (Rose et al. 1997). In addition, a related rhadinovirus was isolated from a multicentric lymphoproliferation (similar to multicentric Castleman's disease) of an SIV infected rhesus macaque (Wong et al. 1999). This virus caused similar disease when injected into other SIV infected rhesus monkeys (Wong et al. 1999). Therefore, analogous to humans, immunosuppressed states appear to allow these viruses to have greater oncogenic potential. More recently two disparate lineages of rhadinoviruses have been recognized in macaques and African green monkeys (Schultz et al. 2000). While the range of disease potential of rhadinoviruses after transplantation is not known their presence in B cells and oncogenic potential particularly in immunosuppressed states is a concern for xenotransplantation.

3 Summary

Herpesviruses are widespread in the NHP world. Some such as *C. herpesvirus 1* are known to cross species lines into humans with significant effect. Others may be benign or unable to cross into different species. Lessons learned from allotransplantation and early primate-to-human xenotransplantation suggest that some of these classes of herpesviruses are capable of being transmitted with xenotransplant procedures. Accordingly, caution should be exercised when pursuing these procedures. Molecular diagnostic tools should be used whenever possible.

References

Alcendor DJ, Barry PA, Pratt-Lowe E, Luciw PA (1993) Analysis of the rhesus cytomegalovirus immediate-early gene promoter. Virology 194:815–821

Anonymous. (1998) Fatal Cercopithecine herpesvirus 1 (B virus) infection following a mucocutaneous exposure and interim recommendations for worker protection. MMWR 47:1073–1076, 1083

Baskin GB (1987) Disseminated cytomegalovirus infection in immunodeficient rhesus monkeys. Am J Pathol 129:345–352

Baskin GB, Roberts ED, Kuebler D, Martin LN, Blauw B, Heeney J, Zurcher C (1995) Squamous Epithelial proliferative lesions associated with rhesus Epstein-Barr virus in simian immunodeficiency virus-infected rhesus monkeys. J Infect Dis 172:535–539

Blakely GA, Lourie B, Morton WG, Evans HH, Kaufmann AF (1973) A varicella-like disease in macaque monkeys. J Infect Dis 127:617–625

Brede HD, Murphy GP. (1972) Bacteriologic and virologic considerations in primate transplants. Primate Med 7:18–28

Cen H, Breinig MC, Atchinson RW, Ho M, McKnight JLC (1991) Epstein-Barr virus transmission via the donor organs in solid organ transplantation: polymerase chain reaction and restriction fragment length polymorphism analysis of IR2, IR3 and IR4. J Virol 65:976

Chang Y, Cesarman E, Pessin MS et al (1994) Identification of herpesvirus-like DNA sequences in AIDS-associated Kaposi's sarcoma. Science 265:1865–1869

Cho Y, Ramer J, Rivailler P, Quink C, Garber RL, Beier DR, Wang F (2001) An Epstein-Barr-related herpesvirus from marmoset lymphomas. Proc Natl Acad Sci USA 98(3):1224–1229

Cohen JI, Davenport DS, StewartJA, Deitchman S, Hilliard JK, Chapman LE and the B Virus Workring Group (2002) Recommendations for Prevention of and therapy for exposure to B virus (Cercopithecine Herpesvirus 1). Clin Infect Dis 35:1191–1203

Deinhardt F, Falk LA, Wolfe LG. (1973) Simian herpesviruses Cancer Research 33:1424–26

Del Prete G, De Carli M, D'Elios MM, Fleckenstein IM, Fickenscher H, Fleckenstein B, Almerigogna F, Romagnani S (1994) Polyclonal B cell activation induced by herpesvirus saimiri-transformed human CD^4+ T cell clones: Roll for membrane TNF-α/TNF-α receptors and CD2/CD58 interactions. J Immun; pp 4872–4879

Delmonico FL, Snydman DR (1998) Organ donor screening for infectious diseases. Transplantation 65:603–610

Desrosiers RC, Sasseville VG, Czajak SC, Zhang X, Mansfield KG, Kaur A, Johnson RP, Lackner AA, Jung JU (1997) A herpesvirus of rhesus monkeys related to the human Kaposi's sarcoma-associated herpesvirus. J Virol 71(12):9764–9769

Eberle R, Hilliard JK (1984) Replication of simian herpesvirus SA8 and identification of viral polypeptides in infected cells. J Virol 50:316–324

Eberle R, Hilliard JK (1989) Serological evidence for variation in the incidence of herpesvirus infections in different species of apes. J Clin Microbiol 27:1357–1366

Eberle R, Black DH, Lehenbauer TW, White GL (1998) Shedding and transmission of baboon herpesvirus papio 2 (HPV2) in a breeding colony. Lab Anim Sci 48:23–28

Falk L, Deinhardt F, Nonoyama M, Wolfe LG, Bergholf C (1976) Properties of a baboon lymphotropic herpesvirus related to Epstein–Barr virus. Int J Cancer 18:798–807

Frances C, Mouquet C, Marcelin AG, et al (2000) Outcome of kidney transplant recipients with previous human herpesvirus-8 infection. Transplantation 69:1776–1779

Frank AL, Bissell JA, Rowe DS, Dunnick NR, Mayner RE, Hopps HE, Parkman PD, Meyer HM Jr. (1973) Rhesus leukocyte associated herpesvirus. I. Isolation and characterization of a new herpesvirus recovered from rhesus monkey leukocytes. J Infect Dis 128:618–628

Franken M, Annis B, Ali AN, Wang F (1995) 5' coding and regulatory region sequence divergence with conserved function of the Epstein–Barr Virus LMP2A homolog in herpesvirus papio. J Virol 69:8011–8019

Freidfeld AG, Hilliard J, Southers J, Murray M, Savarese B, Schmitt JM, Straus SE (1995) A controlled seroprevalence survey of primate handlers for evidence of asymptomatic herpes B virus infection. J Infect Dis 171:1031–1034

Gibson W (1983) Protein counterparts of human and simian cytomegaloviruses. Virology 128:391–406

Green M, Michaels MG (1997) Infections in solid organ transplant recipients. Principles and Practice of Pediatric Infectious Diseases Eds: Long SS, Pickering L, Prober C, Churchill Livingstone Inc. New York

Greensill J, Schultz TF (2000) Rhadinoviruses (gamma-herpesviruses) of Old World primates: models for KSHV/HHV8-associated disease? AIDS 14 (Suppl 3):S11-S19

Greensill J, Sheldon JA, Murthy KK, Bessonette JS, Beer BE, Schulz TF (2000) A chimpanzee rhadinovirus sequence related to Kaposi's sarcoma-associated herpesvirus/human herpesvirus 8: increased detection after HIV-1 infection in the absence of disease. AIDS 14(17):F129-F135

Hayashi K, Ohara N, Teramoto N, Onoda S, Chen HL, Oka T, Kondo E, Yoshino T, Takahashi K, Yates J, Akagi T (2001) An animal model for human EBV-associated hemphagocytic syndrome: Herpesvirus papio frequently induces fatal lymphoproliferative disorders with hemophagocytic syndrome in rabbits. Am J Pathol 158:1533–1542

Heberling RL, Kalter SS 1986 Rapid dot-immunobinding assay on nitrocellulose for viral antibodies. J Clin Micro 23:109–113

Hilliard JK, Soza I (1996) Rapid identification and differentiation of baboon alphaherpesvirus SA8 from closely related HSV-1 and HSV-2 in xenograft transplant recipients. Molecular Diagnosis 1:261–265

Hilliard JK, Ward JA (1999) B-virus specific-pathogen-free breeding colonies of macaques (Macaca mulatta): retrospective study of seven years of testing. Lab Anim Sci 49:144–148

Hilliard JK Weigler BJ (1999) Commentary on Smith AL, Black DH, Eberle R. The existence of differing monkey B virus genotypes with possible implications for degree of virulence in humans. J Virol 72:9224–32 Lab Anim Sci 49:10–11

Hilliard JK, Black D, Eberle R (1989). Simian alphaherpesviruses and their relation to the human herpes simplex virus. Arch Virol 109:83–102

Hilliard J, Lachmi B, Soza I, Brasky K, Mirkovic R (1996) PCR identification and differentiation of baboon cytomegalovirus from other human and nonhuman primate cytomegaloviruses. Molecular Diagnosis 1:267–273

Ho M (1991) Cytomegalovirus: biology and infection. 2nd edn New York: Plenum Medical Book.

Ho M, Miller G, Atchinson RW, et al (1985) Epstein-Barr virus infections and DNA hybridization studies in post-transplantation lymphoma and lymphoproliferative lesions: the role of primary infection. J Infect Dis 152(5):876–886

Holmes GP, Hilliard JK, Klontz KC, et al (1990) B virus (herpesvirus simiae) infection in humans: Epidemiological investigation of a cluster. Ann Intern Med 112:833–839

Holmes GP, Chapman LE, Stewart JA, et al (1995) Guidelines for the prevention and treatment of B-virus infections in exposed persons. Clin Infect Dis 20:421–439

Huang E, Kilpatrick B, Lakeman A, Alford CA (1978) Genetic analysis of a cytomegalovirus-like agent isolated from human brain. J Virol 26:718–723

Jenson HB, Ench Y, Gao S-J, Rice K, Carey D, Kennedy RC, Arrand JR, Mackett M (2000) Epidemiology of Herpesvirus Papio infection in a large captive baboon colony: Similarities to Epstein-Barr virus infections in humans. J Infect Dis 181:1462–1466

Kalter SS, Heberling RL (1990a) Primate viral diseases in perspective. J Med Primatol 19:519–535

Kalter SS, Heberling RL (1990b) Viral battery testing in nonhuman primate colony management. Lab Anim Sci 40:21–23

Kalter SS, Heberling RL, Ratner JJ (1972) EBV antibody in sera of non-human primates. Nature 238:353–354

Kalter SS, Ablashi D, Espana C, Heberling RL, Hull RN, Lennette EH, Malherbe, McConnell S, Yohn DS (1980). Simian virus nomenclature, 1980 Intervirology 13:317–330

Kessler MJ, London WT, Madden DL, Dambrosia JM, Hilliard JK, Soike KF, Rawlins RG (1989) Serological survey for viral diseases in the Cayo Santiago rhesus macaque population. Puerto Rican Health Sci J 8:95–97

Kilpatrick BA, Huang E, Pagano JS (1976) Analysis of cytomegalovirus genomes with restriction endonucleases HinD III and EcoR-1. J Virology 18:1095–1105

Lacoste V, Mauclere P, Dubreuil G, Lewis J, Georges-Courbot MC, Gessain A (2000) Virology: KSHV-like herpesviruses in chimps and gorillas. Nature 407:151–152

Lacoste V, Mauclere P, Dubreuil G, Lewis J, Georges-Courbot MC, Gessain A (2001) A novel gamma 2-herpesvirus of the Rhadinovirus 2 lineage in chimpanzees. Genome Research 11(9):1511–1519

Levin JL, Hilliard JK, Lipper SL, Butler TM, Goodwin WJ (1988) A naturally occurring epizootic of Simian Agent 8 in the baboon. Lab Anim Sci 38:394–397

Li SL, Feichtinger H, Kaaya E, Migliorini P, Putkonen P, Biberfeld G, Middeldorp JM, Biberfeld P, Ernberg I (1993) Expression of Epstein-Barr-virus-related nuclear antigens and B-cell markers in lymphomas of SIV-immunosuppressed monkeys. Int J Cancer 55(4):609–615

Ling PD, Ryon JJ, Hayward SD (1993) EBNA-2 of herpesvirus papio diverges significantly from the type A and type B EBNA-2 proteins of Epstein-Barr Virus but retains an efficient transactivation domain with a conserved hydrophobic motif. J Virol 67:2990–3003

London WT, Marinez AJ, Houff SA, Wallen WC, Curfman BL, Traub RB, Sever JL (1986) Experimental congenital disease with simian cytomegaloviruses in rhesus monkeys. Teratology 33:323–331

Martin WJ (1996) Simian cytomegalovirus-related stealth virus isolated from the cerebrospinal fluid of a patient with bipolar psychosis and acute encephalopathy. Pathobiology 64:64–66

Martin WJ, Zen LC, Ahmed K, Roy M (1994) Cytomegalovirus-related sequence in an atypical cytopathic virus repeatedly isolated from a patient with chronic fatigue syndrome. Am J Pathol 145(2):440–451

Martin WJ, Ahmed K, Zeng LC, Olsen JC, Seward JG, Seehrai JS (1995) African green monkey origin of the atypical cytopathic 'stealth virus' isolated from a patient with chronic fatigue syndrome. Clin and Diag Virol 4:93–103

Martino MA, Hubbard GB, Butler TM, Hilliard JK (1998) Clinical disease associated with simian agent 8 infection in the baboon. Lab Anim Sci 48:18–22

McCarthy K, Tosolini FA (1975) A review of primate herpes virus. Proc Roy Soc Med 68:145–149

McCarthy K, Thorpe E, Laursen AC, Heymann CS, Beale AJ (1968) Examatous disease in patas monkeys caused by a herpesvirus. Lancet 856–857

Mendez JC, Dockrell DH, Espy MJ, et al (2001) Human beta herpesvirus interactions in solid organ transplant recipients. J Infect Dis 183:179–184

Michaels MG, Simmons RL (1994) Xenotransplant associated zoonoses: strategies for prevention. Transplantation, 57:1–7

Michaels MG, McMichael J, Brasky K, et al (1994) Screening donors for xenotransplantation: the potential for xenozoonoses. Transplantation 57:1462–1465

Michaels MG, Hilliard J, Deeks S, et al (1996) Baboon bone marrow xenotransplant in a patient with advanced HIV: A model for the evaluation of potential xenozoonoses. Institute of Human Virology Annual Meeting, Baltimore, MD. Acquired Immune Deficiency Syndromes and Human Retrovirology, Abstract #11, p 3

Michaels MG, Alcendor DJ, St George K, et al (1997) Distinguishing baboon cytomegalovirus from human cytomegalovirus: importance for xenotransplantation. J Infect Dis 176:1476–1483

Michaels MG, Jenkins FJ, St George K, Nalesnik MA, Starzl TE, Rinaldo CR Jr (2001) Detection of infectious baboon cytomegalovirus after baboon-to-human liver xenotransplantation. J Virol 75:2825–2828

Moghaddam A, Koch J, Annis B, Wang F (1998) Infection of human B lymphocytes with lymphocryptoviruses related to Epstein-Barr virus. J Virol 72:3205–3212

Moore PS, Chang Y (2001) Kaposi's Sarcoma – Associated Herpesvirus. In Fields Virology, 4th edn Knipe DM, Howley PM. eds Lippincott Williams &Wilkins Philadelphia. Chapter 82 pp 2835

Muchmore E (1971) Possible cytomegalovirus infection in man following chimpanzee bite. Lab Anim Sci 21(6 II):1080–1081

Neubauer RH, Rabin H, Strnad BC, Lapin BA, Yakovleva LA, Indzie E (1979) Antibody responses to herpesvirus papio antigens in baboons with lymphoma. Int J Cancer 23:186–192

Ohtaki S, Kodama H, Hondo R, Kurata T (1986) Activation of cytomegalovirus infection in immunosuppressed cynomologous monkeys inoculated with varicella-zoster virus. Acta Pathol Jpn 36:1537–1552

Pass RF (2001) Cytomegalovirus. In Fields Virology, 4th edn Knipe DM, Howley PM. Eds Lippincott Williams &Wilkins Philadelphia. Chapter 77, pp 2675–2706

Perot K, Walker CM, Spaete RR (1992) Primary chimpanzee skin fibroblast cells are fully permissive for human cytomegalovirus replication. J Gen Virol 73:3281–3284

Rickinson AB, Kieff E (2001) Epstein-Barr virus. In Fields Virology, 4th Edition. Knipe DM, Howley PM. Eds. Lippincott Williams &Wilkins Philadelphia. Chapter 75 pp 2575–2628

Roizman B, Pellett PE (2001) The family Herpesviridae: A brief introduction. In Fields Virology, 4th Edition. Knipe DM, Howley PM. Eds. Lippincott Williams &Wilkins Philadelphia. Chapter 71 pp 2381–2397

Roizman B, Carmichael LE, Deinhardt F, de-The G, Nahmias AJ, Plowright W, Rapp F, Sheldrick P, Takahashi M, Wolf K (1981) Herpesviridae: Definition, provisional nomenclature and taxonomy. Intervirology 16:201–217

Rose TM, Strand KB, Schultz ER, Schaefer G, Rankin GW, Thouless ME, Tsai CC, Bosch ML (1997) Identification of two homologs of the Kaposi's sarcoma-associated herpesvirus (human herpesvirus 8) in retroperitoneal fibromatosis of different macaque species. J Virol 71(5):4138–4144

Rubin RH (1990) Impact of cytomegalovirus infection on organ transplant recipients. Rev Infect Dis 12(suppl 7):S754-S766

Schultz ER, Rankin GW Jr, Blanc MP, Raden BW, Tsai CC, Rose TM (2000) Characterization of two divergent lineages of macaque rhadinoviruses related to Kaposi's sarcoma-associated herpesvirus. J Virol 74(10):4919–4928

Singh N, Dummer JS, Kusne S, Breinig MK, Armstrong JA, Makowka L, Starzl TE, Ho M (1988) Infections with cytomegalovirus and other herpesviruses in 121 liver transplant recipients: transmission by donated organ and the effect of OKT3. J Infect Dis 158:124–131

Smith AL, Black DH, Eberle R (1998) Molecular evidence for distinct genotypes of monkey B virus (Herpesvirus simiae) which are related to macaque host species. J Virol 72:9224–9232

Starzl TE, Fung J, Tzakis A, Todo S, Demetris AJ, Marino IR, Doyle H, Zeevi A, Warty V, Michaels M, Kusne S, Rudert WA, Trucco M (1993) Baboon-to-human liver transplantation. Lancet 341:65–71

Swack NS, Liu OC, Hsiung GD (1971) Cytomegalovirus infections of monkeys and baboons. Am J Epidemiol 94:397–402

Taniguchi S, Cooper DKC (1997) Clinical xenotransplantation – a brief review of the world experience. In: Cooper DKC, et al, eds. Xenotransplantation 2nd Ed. Heidelberg, Germany: Springer, 776

Van der Reit F de St J, Human PA, Cooper DKC, et al (1987) Virological consideration of the use of primates in xenotransplantation. Transplant Proc 19:4068–4069

Vogel P, Weigler BJ, Kerr H, Hendrickx AG, Barry PA (1994) Seroepidemiologic studies of cytomegalovirus infection in a breeding population of rhesus macaques. Lab Anim Sci 44(1):25–30

Weigler BJ (1992) Biology of B virus in macaque and human hosts: a review. Clin Infect Dis 14:555–567

Weiner D, Gibson W (1981) Identification of a primate cytomegalovirus group-common protein antigen. Virology115:182–191

Wong SW, Bergquam EP, Swanson RM, Lee FW, Shiigi SM, Avery NA, Fanton JW, Axthelm MK (1999) Induction of B cell hyperplasia in simian immunodeficiency virus-infected Rhesus Macaques with the simian homologue of Kaposi's Sarcoma-associated herpesvirus. J Exp Med 190(6):827–840

Understanding Xenotransplantation Risks from Nonhuman Primate Retroviruses

J. S. Allan
Department of Virology and Immunology,
Southwest Foundation for Biomedical Research,
7620 N.W. Loop 410 at Military Drive, San Antonio, TX 78227, USA
E-mail: Jallan@icarus.sfbr.org

1 Introduction 102

2 Exogenous Retroviruses 104
2.1 Simian Immunodeficiency Viruses 104
2.2 Simian T Cell Lymphotropic Viruses 106
2.3 Simian Foamy Viruses 108
2.4 Simian Retrovirus (Type D) 111

3 Endogenous Retroviruses 112
3.1 Baboon Endogenous Retrovirus 114
3.2 Simian Endogenous Retrovirus 115
3.3 *Papio cynocephalus* Endogenous Retrovirus 115

4 Conclusions 116

References 118

Abstract Significant progress in making animal-to-human transplantation a viable adjunct to human organ donation will require a greater understanding of the intricacies of immunologic rejection. Recent success in generating cloned knockout piglets increases the possibility that xenotransplantation may find its way into the clinics. Nonhuman primates' organs have been used for human transplants in the past and there is reason to believe that if ethical considerations and inherent problems with supply were overcome, their close genetic proximity to humans would lessen complications of rejection. Unfortunately, nonhuman primates harbor several pathogens known to be infectious in humans and the potential of other viral infections has precluded further use of monkeys in this setting. Baboons are generally considered the nonhuman primate species of choice yet this species carries several retroviruses considered a threat to humans in transplantation. Both known and potentially undiscovered retroviruses pose an important risk that is the focus of this review.

1 Introduction

Retroviruses are insidious by nature due of their lifelong persistence in the host. The machinery used by retroviruses for replication requires reverse transcription of viral RNA into a double-stranded DNA copy followed by its integration into the host chromosome establishing a persistent infection. From a disease perspective, there is an assortment of retrovirus types: some are highly cytopathic, cause no disease in the natural host yet induce profound immunodeficiency in an unnatural host (e.g., AIDS); some are highly cytopathic but cause no apparent disease in either host; others are weakly oncogenic in both natural and unnatural host; and some are simply fossil records of bygone infections. The situation in which previously unknown 'apathogenic' animal retroviruses are introduced into humans is of immediate concern in xenotransplantation.

Among the modes for retroviral persistence used by these different retroviruses is the resilience of chronicity—the ability to persist in spite of potent immune responses. Retroviruses use diverse strategies in their replication and persistence. The complex retroviruses have any number of accessory genes, in addition to conventional *gag*, *pol*, and *env* genes, which allow for replication in cells that are not undergoing cell division as is the case with the primate lentiviruses in targeting macrophages. Other complex retroviruses such as the human T cell lymphotropic viruses (HTLVs) produce almost no cell-free virus yet persist primarily by accelerating cell division of infected T cells (clonal expansion). Still other genes downregulate host cellular receptors in order to subvert host immune response. While many retroviruses are considered exogenous in origin—they are transmitted horizontally and are seen by the host as foreign invaders—the endogenous retroviruses represent an important risk in the transplant setting because they are considered part of the germ line of the host. Every cell contains multiple copies of retroviral elements that are inherited in a Mendelian fashion. Providing retrovirus-free source animals becomes a daunting task and may require further technological breakthroughs to eliminate or disentangle the host from its resident passengers. Recently, it has been estimated that as much as 8% of the human genome represents retroviral sequences (Hughes and Coffin 2001). These buried freeloaders are infrequently expressed in the host but given the right circumstances, i.e., development of the embryo, or transplanting an organ into another species, may yield infectious virus.

Nonhuman primates have had a long and sometimes dubious history in xenotransplantation. From transplanted chimpanzee kidneys and hearts in the early 1960s, a baboon heart into a pediatric patient in 1986, to baboon livers and a bone marrow in the 1990s, either the patients did not survive or in the case of the bone marrow transplant patient, the cells failed to survive implantation (Traeger 1969; Giles et al. 1970; Deodhar 1986; Starzl et al. 1993; Fricker 1996). Successful primate-to-human transplants could introduce both known and unknown viral infections that could have long-term public health consequences (Allan 1994, 1996a, 1996b, 1998). Due to this perceived heightened risk from nonhuman primates, and to problems in resource supply, the Food and Drug Administration published a *Guide to Industry* in 1999 advising against the use of nonhuman primate tissues in human clinical trials thus directing industry towards porcine tissues (Bloom 2001). This should not be construed as the final word on the availability and use of primates as source donors for human transplantation and these guides may change as there is no absolute ban on their use. Novel cell therapies and the possibility of rogue transplanters introducing simian organs and viruses into the human population must be considered a serious threat to the public health. One can imagine an evolving transplant industry providing organ replacement on request in a foreign country to any individual willing to pay for such a procedure. This 'Xenotourism' trade could prompt a surgeon in a foreign country with few regulations on xenotransplantation to use baboon, macaque or chimpanzee organs or cell therapies.

Of all of the nonhuman primate donors, the baboon has been most commonly used as a source animal for xenotransplantation. The focus of this review is limited to the presentation of primate retroviruses in the context of infectious disease risks in xenotransplantation with special emphasis on those harbored by baboons because of their historical status as 'best choice' source animals. A more comprehensive discussion of simian viruses and their risk in xenotransplantation can be found elsewhere (Allan 1996a, 1996b, 1998).

2
Exogenous Retroviruses

Exogenous nonhuman primate retroviruses represent a continuous threat to the blood supply and are prominent sexually transmitted agents. While some retroviruses can be transmitted by saliva, most are blood borne or sexually transmitted infections limiting transmission to close contacts. Important questions for determining risk from nonhuman primate retroviruses, whether exogenous or endogenous in nature, are: Can the virus infect human cells? Can it replicate and produce cell-free virus for further rounds of replication in human cells and tissues? What cell types are targeted? Is the virus cytopathic/tumorigenic in human cells? Can infection lead to clinical disease in humans? and importantly, Can the virus be transmitted from the recipient to contacts? (Allan 1998) For some of these retroviruses, we have more detailed knowledge of their biology and replication while others remain poorly studied. As with endogenous retroviruses, these exogenous viruses retain the capacity to integrate a DNA version (provirus) into the host genome. Chance integration near a cellular proto-oncogene may lead to the expression of cellular growth factors that along with some later event might result in cancer. Regardless of the strategy used by these different retroviral types, all maintain this capacity for the lifetime of the infected host. Repeated rounds of infection and proviral insertion increase the odds for such an event. Beyond this possibility other exogenous retroviruses may induce anemia, lymphopenia, neurologic disease and opportunistic infections (Coffin et al. 1997). The viruses are described in the context of both their previous and new classification schemas.

2.1
Simian Immunodeficiency Viruses

Simian immunodeficiency viruses (SIV) presumably do not pose a significant threat in the xenotransplant setting. This family of viruses, while persistent residents in most African primates, has apparently spared baboons although cross-species infections of baboons from African green monkeys have been reported (Jin et al. 1994). In addition, baboons have been experimentally infected with SIVmac, HIV-2, and a recombinant virus containing the HIV-1 *env* gene on a SIVmac backbone (Cranage et al. 1992; Castro et al. 1991; Letvin et al. 1987; Allan et al. 1995). As a general rule, naturally infected African nonhuman primates do not develop any signs of AIDS and depletion of SIV target cells ($CD4^+$) is not seen in these species (Chakrabarti et al. 2000; Kaur et al. 1998). In contrast, Asian macaques display most of the hallmarks of AIDS after experimental infection with SIV and due to their smaller size and as carriers of herpes B virus, which is usually fatal to humans, have not been a primary choice for source organs.

Having resided in African primates for thousands of years means that SIV may have evolved with its natural host altering its virulence (Allan et al. 1991). Only when SIV infects non-African primates are immunologic deficits commonly seen. It is this natural host dichotomy that creates concern in xenotransplantation. What if baboons harbor a 'nonpathogenic' lentivirus that has yet to be discovered? The lessons of the AIDS epidemic have taught us that infectious agents may be present in an animal species without causing disease and thus below the radar for discovery. Only when escape from the natural host through butchering as is believed the case for HIV-1 from chimpanzees or through contaminated needle sticks are humans at risk (Gao et al. 1999). The best possible avenue for a novel primate zoonosis would be the transplantation of a whole organ from a primate to a human in the presence of immunosuppressive agents. Baboons may still harbor an SIV strain that is distantly related from the known SIVs making the job of isolation and characterization problematic. Studies have detected antibodies to SIV and type D retroviruses in approximately 35% of wild caught baboons (Benveniste et al. 1993). In particular, antibodies reactive to the Gag protein of HIV/SIV are commonly recognized; however, isolation and other methods of detection have failed. The question remains whether this diminished reactivity denotes actual infection or merely a cross-reactive heterophilic antibody profile.

The threat of lentiviral transmission from nonhuman primates also stems from the fact that cellular receptors required for viral entry are most conserved between apes, monkeys and humans. The primary receptor CD4 and a series of coreceptors including CCR5 and CXCR4 (chemokine receptors) are required for SIV to gain entry (Doms 2001). The binding sites on these molecules are highly conserved between nonhuman primates and humans whereas this conservation is diminished the farther down the phylogenetic tree one proceeds (Fomsgaard et al. 1997; Marx and Chen 1998). In addition, cellular factors necessary for completion of the virus life cycle also limit viral replication to primates (Cohen

2001). Major research efforts are directed toward developing transgenic mice capable of being infected with HIV (Cohen 2001). These mice have been engineered to express several human genes necessary for HIV replication yet these models still have not allowed for the completion of the HIV life cycle due to other yet undefined cellular genes. These results clearly demonstrate that the infectious disease risk from retroviral infections in most cases correlates with the genetic proximity of donor and recipient in the transplant setting.

2.2 Simian T Cell Lymphotropic Viruses

The first human exogenous retrovirus was isolated in 1981 after epidemiologic studies revealed a cluster of lymphoid cancers in humans of Japanese ancestry (Uchiyama et al. 1977). HTLV was linked to a clinical syndrome called adult T cell leukemia and lymphoma (ATLL) whose incidence paralleled infection (Hinuma et al. 1981; Poiesz et al. 1981). Unlike previously characterized retroviruses that have simple genomes comprised of long terminal repeats (LTRs) which drive viral replication, and the structural genes, *gag*, *pol* and *env* , HTLV also carries at the 3′ end of its genome several multiply spliced genes (pX region), one of which (*tax*) has been shown to disrupt normal cell growth by promoting the activation of a variety of cellular genes involved in T cell activation including interleukin-2 and interleukin-2Rα (Seiki et al. 1983; Franchini 1995). Furthermore, transformation of $CD4^+$ T cells through clonal expansion of lymphocytes leads to leukemia and lymphoid tumors.

As was the case for HIV, studies have revealed that Old World primates harbor a virus closely related to HTLV and are natural reservoirs for infection of humans. This simian counterpart, STLV, is highly related to HTLV (as much as 95% homology) and phylogenetic analyses point to several cross-species transmissions from African nonhuman primates including baboons to humans in the distant past (Seiki et al. 1984; Gessain and De The 1996; Van Dooren et al. 2001; for a comprehensive review see Allan et al. 2001) Furthermore, STLV can be propagated in human T cell lines suggesting no barrier for STLV infection in humans. The receptor for HTLV/STLV has not been identified but the primary targets for this group of retroviruses are $CD4^+$ T cells. Lymphocytes are a major source of viral infections especially in transfusion situations and most allotransplants contain a high number of lymphocytes that can harbor such viruses.

In order to assess the relative risk from STLV, epidemiologic studies have been performed on many Old World primate species including baboons. In the transplant setting, STLV represents a significant pathogen. Introduction of new STLV-related infections at the least may duplicate HTLV infection; however, it is impossible to predict the pathogenic outcome of new STLV infections in humans; perhaps more acute disease involving the lymphoid system may evolve. Screening of species for known STLV infections may significantly reduce the risk of infection. However, in a study of macaques experimentally infected with HTLV, evidence of seroconversion was delayed for more than a year and a half (Liska et al. 1997). Sophisticated molecular diagnostic testing is therefore required to detect virus positive, antibody negative suspect animals.

In order to understand the routes of transmission of STLV between baboons and to determine overall seroprevalence, we developed a sensitive PCR-based method for detecting STLV. The baboon breeding colony from which source animals have been used for previous transplantation to humans, is by no means a specific pathogen free colony. Initial studies indicated a high prevalence of STLV in captive baboons with infection rates approaching 80% in adult animals (Mone et al. 1992). Furthermore, spontaneously arising non-Hodgkin's lymphomas and leukemias indistinguishable from ATLL in humans have been seen in baboons (Hubbard et al. 1993). The life-time incidence of cancer in the infected animals approaches 4% which is similar to cancer rates seen in HTLV infected humans. There is also high variability between baboons in the number of STLV infected lymphocytes present in asymptomatic animals ranging from 9 to 12,332 DNA copies/10^6 cells assessed by quantitative DNA Real-Time PCR (J. S. Allan, unpublished results). Theoretically, those animals with higher viral burdens may be more prone to development of cancer and may be more infectious in the transplant setting.

Molecular and serologic diagnostic methods developed for screening the human blood supply are also effective for testing nonhuman primates. Commercially available enzyme-linked immunoabsorbent assays, Western blotting and PCR-based diagnostics are generally satisfactory for identifying infected animals. Transmission of STLV amongst baboons occurs primarily at sexual maturity; however, mother-to-infant transmission through milk has been detected (J. S. Allan, unpublished results). The fact that we have adequate means of detecting and thus eliminating STLV from potential donors would certainly lessen the risk for transmission to humans in xenotransplantation. Nevertheless, the rates of natural infection and the lack of pathogen free breeding colonies would necessitate a tremendous commitment of time and resources to develop such a colony.

2.3 Simian Foamy Viruses

Foamy viruses (FV) remain an enigma in the retroviral field. In tissue culture, these viruses are highly cytopathic and their name belies this observation as large ballooning syncytia are present in cells infected with FV. Curiously, there has been no clear association between FV infection and naturally occurring disease. Surveys of nonhuman primates demonstrate extremely high rates of infection in wild-caught populations of monkeys and apes and within captive breeding colonies (Schweizer et al. 1995; Broussard et al. 1997; Blewett et al. 2000). Recent phylogenetic analyses of simian FV (SFV) have revealed a close relationship between host and its virus strain suggesting SFV has co-evolved with its host (Schweizer and Neumann-Haefelin 1995; Broussard et al. 1997). These species-specific SFVs are nonetheless infectious for a wide range of other hosts including humans, rabbits, and mice (Brown et al. 1982; Santillana-Hayat et al. 1993; Saib et al. 1997; Hooks and Detrick-Hooks 1979). Of the primate family, only humans seem to have been spared a resident FV (Ali et al. 1996). A 'human' FV isolated from a case of nasopharyngeal carcinoma was later found to represent a tissue culture contaminant and most likely had its origins in chimpanzees (Achong et al. 1971; Herchenroder et al. 1994). Nevertheless, SFV grows well in a variety of human cell types including lymphocytes (B and T), macrophages, fibroblasts, endothelial cells, kidney cells as well as canine thymus cells and rodent cells and invariably induces cell killing (Mergia et al. 1996). There are few cell types resistant to infection with SFV. The receptor for SFV has not been identified but is presumably a common cell surface molecule with a great degree of conservation between species as SFV replicates in most animal cells.

Baboons harbor SFV at high rates. Our studies indicate that virtually all adult baboons harbor SFV and 95% of adult baboons were found to be infected with SFV in another study (Broussard et al. 1997; Blewett et al. 2000). Like other SFV, baboon SFV replicates to high levels in human cell lines and primary cells and is cytolytic. The source animals for two baboon liver transplants performed in 1992–1993 were found to harbor SFV (Allan et al. 1998). Examination of the human recipients revealed that many tissues including liver, lymph node, gastrointestinal tract and kidney had SFV DNA present. Anti-SFV antibodies were not detected in these patients; however, they lived only 26 and 70 days after xenotransplantation. In addition, potent immunosuppressive drugs may have impeded B cell responses. We do not know if SFV replicated in the human host or if SFV resided in any human cell types. Evidence of baboon endogenous retrovirus (ERV) sequences were also present in the recipients' tissues, and baboon mitochondrial DNA was detected, strongly suggesting the migration of baboon lymphocytes throughout the patients' tissues (Allan et al. 1998). Known as *microchimerism*, donor passenger cells present in the transplanted organ spread to other sites in the body (Starzl et al. 1996). If these patients had survived, would persistent infection with SFV become a reality?

Studies of primate workers, zoo workers and laboratory personnel exposed to bites of captive primates and to needle sticks demonstrated active and persistent infection in approximately 4% of the individuals which seemed to correlate with type and length of exposure to primates (Schweizer et al. 1995, 1997; Heneine et al. 1998; Sandstrom et al. 2000). Genetic analyses of SFV performed on several infected humans revealed cross-species infection from chimpanzees, baboons and African green monkeys (Schweizer et al. 1997; Heneine et al. 1998). In one such study, antibodies to SFV were detected in four of 231 primate workers and viral DNA could be amplified by PCR from peripheral blood cells of two of these humans. These studies support the notion that tissue recipients of SFV infected animals would probably become persistent carriers of SFV infection. There has been no apparent disease associated with infection in any of these humans nor were their close contacts infected, providing some measure of assurance that perhaps, even if humans became infected via xenografts, SFV infection might be a dead-end opportunist. On the other hand, there is a variety of SFV strains present in nonhuman primates and there could be profound differences among isolates in their transmissibility from human to human as well in their potential to cause clinical disease.

FVs have been variously associated with disease in experimental models. For example, transgenic mice harboring an SFV genome developed a severe neurologic disease linked to the expression of FV transactivating gene, *bel-1* (Tschopp et al. 1996; Aguzzi et al. 1993). Experimental infection of rabbits with SFV led to transient immunosuppression although these animals remained persistently infected and asymptomatic for more than 5 years (Saib et al. 1997; Hooks and Detrick-Hooks 1979; Santillana-Hayat et al. 1993). Experimental inoculation of SFV into mice also led to persistent infection without associated pathology (Brown et al. 1982). Furthermore, the lack of disease in the natural host does not alleviate the possible risk of FV-induced diseases in humans. For example, SIV causes no disease in African nonhuman primates but transfer to humans or Asian macaques has resulted in severe immunodeficiency and a global AIDS pandemic. We cannot predict what persistent SFV infection in the human population may lead to in terms of transmission and disease. The fact that SFV is infectious for exposed humans means that every effort must be made to reduce exposure in occupations that involve contact with animals or tissues and fluids from these animals in order to safeguard individual and public health.

Reliable research tools have been developed to determine whether individual primates are infected which can be used to screen for SFV-free animals. We have recently performed a survey of infants, juveniles and adult baboons in a large breeding colony to determine when and how SFV is transmitted amongst baboons (J. S. Allan, unpublished results). While virtually all adult baboons are infected with SFV, suggesting ease of transmission, SFV is not transmitted from mother to infant. However, we found that infection rates began to rise after the first 6 months when maternal antibodies wane, suggesting a nonsexual route of infection. Furthermore, the rates steadily rose in juvenile baboons (0.8–2.6 years of age) reaching 25% positivity by PCR. By contrast, only 5% of these same animals were infected with STLV. In general, SFV remains in a latent nonreplicative state that is apparently controlled both by neutralizing antibody responses and by inactivation of the provirus through methylation, although active replication is seen in the oral mucosa and virus can be isolated from infected animals via oral swabs (Von Laer et al. 1996; Schweizer et al. 1993). Based on these findings, the most reasonable mode of transmission is through biting and introduction of virus from the saliva through breaks in the skin. Because of fundamental differences in behaviors (no biting) between humans we have fortunately been spared the establishment of SFV infection in the human population.

SFV is also being investigated as a possible vector for gene therapy and vaccine delivery (Mergia et al. 2001). The advantages of SFV include its wide cell and host tropism, its ability to replicate in nondividing cells, and its apparent lack of pathogenicity. Questions will remain as to the risk of SFV in humans. Since SFVs from several Old World primates have persistently infected humans in the past, public health prevention would justify eliminating SFV from transplant donors.

2.4 Simian Retrovirus (Type D)

Simian retroviruses (SRV) are members of the beta-retrovirus group and were initially linked to simian AIDS outbreaks at several National Institute of Health (NIH) primate centers. SRV induces immunosuppressive disease in macaques in addition to retroperitoneal fibromatosis (Marx et al. 1984). SRV infects both B and T cells and elicits strong neutralizing antibody responses (Maul et al. 1988). Vaccines against SRV have been tested successfully in macaques. Formalin inactivated SRV protected six monkeys from intravenous challenge with SRV-1 and in another study, an Env-expressing vaccinia vector was effective in preventing infection after an SRV challenge (Marx et al. 1986; Hu et al. 1989). Recently, two groups identified the receptor for type D retroviruses including SRV, and a related cat virus RD-114 as a sodium-dependent neutral-amino acid transporter. This receptor is highly conserved amongst animals and explains the wide tropism for type D retroviruses (Tailor et al. 1999; Rasko et al. 1999).

Exogenous SRV infections appear to be limited primarily to Asian nonhuman primates with disease manifestations common in macaques (Lowenstine et al. 1986). A highly related endogenous SRV was reported in langurs and it has been speculated that cross-species infection of macaques may have occurred (Nandi et al. 2000; Bryant et al. 1978). African nonhuman primates are not generally considered natural carriers for exogenous type D infections, however antibodies have been detected to SRV in African Talapoin monkeys (Ilyinskii et al. 1991). Anti-SRV antibodies were also found in 5% of captive baboons although baboons are more likely to harbor endogenous forms (Grant et al. 1995; see "Baboon Endogenous Retroviruses").

SRVs represent a potential threat to humans both from primate xenografts and possibly via other avenues. A recent study confirms the presence of antibodies to SRV in primate workers implying zoonotic infection; however, attempts to isolate a bona fide SRV from these individuals have failed (Lerche et al. 2001). Whether further adaptation to humans is necessary to establish the infection in the population remains to be determined.

An SRV-like virus has also been reported in an HIV-1 infected AIDS patient (Ford et al. 1992). Virus isolation confirmed infection in this patient but a link to disease could not be estimated due to ongoing immunodeficiency caused by HIV. An epidemiologic investigation found no link between the SRV infection in this case and exposure to any primates so it is uncertain how this individual became infected. Besides infection with herpes B virus, a fatal zoonotic infection in primate workers, another important reason for the exclusion of macaques in xenotransplantation is common infection by SRV in these monkeys and the immunosuppressive properties of the virus. Most strains of SRV replicate well in human cell lines and certainly pose a threat in the transplant arena. Further studies are necessary to sort out the relationship between endogenous Type D viral infections in baboons and possible exogenous infections to ascertain the risk from baboon SRV-like viruses. Molecular diagnostic techniques are available to screen for SRV in monkeys and to assist in developing SRV-free breeding colonies (Lerche et al. 1994; 1997; Liska et al. 1997).

3
Endogenous Retroviruses

ERVs have become a major infectious disease risk in xenotransplantation because a porcine endogenous retroviruses (PERV) was originally shown to replicate in human cells and has thus become a major focus of investigation to determine whether PERV represents a serious risk in porcine xenografts (see chapter by Niebert and Tönjes, this volume). Simian endogenous retroviruses are present in nonhuman primates and are scattered throughout their genomes. Although ERVs were described early in the history of retroviruses, research into the breadth of infectious ERVs in nonhuman primates has been scarce. Most of the ERV-like elements are commonly defective. Indeed, ERVs probably represent a fossil record of exogenous retroviruses that have long since become part of the host genome (Hughes and Coffin 2001). Genes have been deleted or silenced through mutations and most ERVs are only nonreplicated pieces of prior infections. However, all animals contain ERVs that are littered throughout their genomes; some of which may be replication competent. Some are ERVs in one species but are exogenous pathogenic infections in other species. Some can reinitiate infection in the same host (ecotropic), some are only able to infect cells from other species (xenotropic) while others can infect cells from the same species and disparate species (polytropic). The host range of a few retroviruses, for example the murine leukemia viruses (MuLVs), has even been exploited in designing vectors to deliver genes currently being used in gene therapy.

In one study, a MuLV vector was used for gene delivery and expression in macaque bone marrow cells (Donahue et al. 1992). Reinfusion of these modified cells into macaques led to T cell lymphomas in three of ten animals. Examination of the tumors indicated that the MuLV vector had recombined within the packaging cell line used to generate MuLV and had become infectious. Further studies revealed high viral loads in these macaques without the generation of immunologic responses to infection (Vanin et al. 1994). In addition, MuLV was found to be monoclonally integrated into the tumor cells implicating MuLV as the cause of these cancers (Purcell et al. 1996). Two important conclusions can be drawn from these studies. First, animal retroviruses are potent cancer agents and must be carefully evaluated to ensure that replication competent vectors do not arise. Second, the introduction of retroviruses into bone marrow cells may indirectly tolerize the host to infection. MuLV expression in bone marrow cells may undermine immune surveillance. Despite high viral loads in the blood of these monkeys, there were no antibody responses to MuLV indicating a lack of recognition by the host. These studies illustrate potential problems in xenotransplantation if donor bone marrow is used in an attempt to tolerize the human recipient to the animal organ. Inadvertently, tolerizing protocols involving bone marrow cells may also have the unintended effect of hiding resident retroviruses associated with the xenograft from the host.

ERVs have been implicated in autoimmune diseases and in some cases have been proposed as necessary for normal biologic function in the host through altering cellular gene regulation. A comprehensive review of the role of ERVs in normal biologic processes and in pathology can be found elsewhere (Larsson and Andersson 1998). Via promoter insertion, the LTRs of these ERVs function as promoters and enhancers to regulate gene expression in areas of insertion. One such example is the transcriptional regulation of salivary amylase by human ERVs (HERVs) in humans (Ting et al. 1992). Recent studies based on new information from the human genome project have estimated that there are as many as 23 copies of HERV-K in the human genome and certain HERV genes may be expressed at any given time (Hughes and Coffin 2001). ERVs in nonhuman primates are slowly being described but what is apparent is that baboons carry several different types of ERV that have relevance to xenotransplantation.

3.1 Baboon Endogenous Retrovirus

Baboon endogenous retrovirus (BaEV) was the first primate retrovirus discovered in 1973 from placental tissue (Benveniste et al. 1974). Until that time it was thought that humans and monkeys were spared from retroviral infections. Interestingly, BaEV is a recombinant endogenous retrovirus comprised of a 5′ *gag–pol* region derived from a type C retrovirus and a 3′ portion, including *env*, from a type D retrovirus. BaEV thus shares a high degree of similarity with the murine retrovirus type C group yet the envelope is most closely related to other SRV of the type D group. BaEV replicates well in human cells and since it is replication competent represents an important risk in transplantation (Huang et al. 1989). Old World monkeys and humans lack the expression of a specific type of α-gal sugar on their cell surfaces. Therefore, both have natural antibodies to this α-gal sugar that will be expressed on nonprimate enveloped viruses and infected cells and can neutralize infection (Takeuchi et al. 1996). In contrast, transplantation of baboon or other nonhuman primate cells into humans would avoid the α-gal immunity for retroviral infection.

We do not know if BaEV would actually be infectious in humans. As mentioned earlier, BaEV was detected in tissues from two humans who received baboon livers in 1992 but later died (Allan et al. 1998). Besides evidence of BaEV in tissues of these patients, baboon genomic sequence (mitochondrial DNA) and SFV DNA were also present most likely a result of baboon lymphocytes populating several human tissues. Human donor lymphocytes are commonly detected in allotransplant recipients long after transplantation suggesting that xenotransplantation may lead to the establishment of xenogeneic lymphocytes in human recipients (Starzl et al. 1996). We failed to detect antibodies to BaEV or SFV in archived serum samples from both liver recipients. The immunosuppressed patients survived for only 27 and 70 days which may not have been sufficient time for significant infection and replication in human cells.

3.2 Simian Endogenous Retrovirus

Further examination of the baboon genome for evidence of ERV-like sequences led to the discovery of a new simian endogenous type D retrovirus (SERV) (Van Der Kuyl et al. 1997). Full-length proviruses were detected in multiple copies but direct sequence analysis of two of these clones revealed several internal stop codons suggesting that at least some SERVs may not be replication competent. Further studies will be necessary to determine whether every copy present in the genome is defective. Of interest, the envelope of SERV was found to be highly related to the *env* gene of BaEV supporting the notion that BaEV arose via recombination between SERV and an endogenous type C ERV (see "Baboon Endogenous Retrovirus"). In parallel with these studies, investigators at the University of Washington detected antibodies to type D retroviruses in captive baboons (Grant et al. 1995). Five percent of 236 baboons examined were SRV positive. Virus was successfully isolated from the peripheral blood from three seropositive baboons and sequence analysis revealed homology with other SRVs. While it was theorized at the time that baboons were infected while in captivity with an exogenous type D retrovirus possibly from macaques, sequence similarity with the more recently discovered SERV suggests these antibodies may have been directed toward SERV. These data illustrate the difficulty in determining whether a given retrovirus is strictly exogenous or endogenous and significantly how to address the infectious disease risks from these seemingly harmless travelers. Further studies are needed to define the extent of type D infections in baboons and if these SERVs are infectious and transmissible among primates.

3.3 *Papio cynocephalus* Endogenous Retrovirus

In addition to the aforementioned baboon ERVs, a more recent study has revealed a full-length endogenous retrovirus present in the baboon genome that helps to solve the mystery about the origins of BaEV (Mang et al. 1999). This newly discovered ERV, *Papio cynocephalus* endogenous retrovirus (PcEV), is a type C retrovirus closely related to other type C species including the prototypic murine MuLV and porcine PERV. The proviral copy number of PcEV is greater than BaEV at 38–59 copies/genome compared with 10–30 copies/genome, therefore PcEV is considered older than BaEV. Based on PcEV sequence comparisons with BaEV, the 5′ *gag-pol* portion of BaEV originated from PcEV while the 3′ provirus originated from type D SERV. The proviral clones of PcEV represent an entire type C genome yet like SERV, both clones analyzed had multiple mutations that would disrupt some gene expression and LTR function. These findings are thus consistent with a recombination event among defective ERVs leading to intact, replication competent BaEV. Implanting animal ERVs along with either nonhuman primate or porcine cells and tissues into humans might lead to recombination with any number of human ERVs resulting in unexpected recombinants. Whether or not these hypothetical zoonotic ERVs (ZERVs) could then infect and induce disease or be transmitted to other humans remains speculative but will require close scrutiny in future clinical trials.

4 Conclusions

Retroviral infections in nonhuman primates are common and diverse, covering many if not all of the various retroviral groups. Some of these viruses are capable of inducing disease in monkeys while others appear to be innocent passengers. There is compelling evidence that retroviruses in nonhuman primates carry a greater risk in the transplant setting than nonprimates. STLV and SIV, which have both crossed into humans and established significant infectious diseases, use cellular receptors present in monkeys, apes and humans with little or no infectivity of other lower primates or mammals. Not only would receptors more likely be shared between related primates, but the cellular machinery in human cells necessary for viral replication would be more easily appropriated by simian viruses. From a historical perspective, there have been at least three simian retroviral zoonotic infections from apes and monkeys to humans which have in some cases led to the establishment of new emerging human infections leading to illness and death from such simian infections (HIV, HTLV and SFV). From AIDS to lymphoid cancers, heightened awareness of the possible zoonotic spread of retroviruses and other viral infections (herpesviruses) to humans is the foremost consideration in prohibiting the use of primate cells and tissues in xenotransplantation. Phylogenetic proximity of humans to other primates increases the probability of cross-species viral infections, thus the use of primates for xenografting raises higher concerns to human public health.

Sexual and blood transmission coupled with, in some instances, an extremely long clinical latency makes it exceedingly difficult to determine whether introduction of a new infectious agent would gain a foothold in the population and whether we might expect a new infectious disease. Such long clinical latencies might mask a new emerging infection; its discovery coming only after several hundred or a thousand transplants have been completed and after decades have passed. State-of-the-art molecular diagnostics are available to significantly reduce the risk for transmission of the known retroviral infections and the use of specific pathogen free animals would further lower this risk. Many of these potential pathogens are not transmitted vertically between mother and infant so that strategies to develop 'clean' animals would significantly reduce both known and unknown infections in humans. Other as yet undiscovered retroviruses, for which we have no reliable assays for detection, are undoubtedly present in these primate populations. On the other hand, there are presently no *known* exogenous retroviruses in swine and the replication competent endogenous versions like PERV replicate relatively poorly in human cell cultures compared with viruses of nonhuman primates. For these reasons, swine must be viewed as a relatively safer alternative to primates as source animals for xenotransplantation yet vigilance will still be necessary to circumvent the spread of novel porcine viruses into human populations. Predictions about the pathogenic potential of an animal retrovirus in humans are exceedingly difficult to make based on what happens in the natural host. Responsible public health policy may mean that if a porcine virus is found to replicate in a human transplant patient one must assume pathogenicity. Animal models such as pig-to-monkey experimental transplantation can help to resolve some of these risks, but monkeys and their viral risk profiles are clearly not the same as those of humans.

The need for organ replacement must be balanced with the possible introduction of new viral infections that could have disastrous consequences. In this light, public health officials have had to find common ground in allowing small well-controlled clinical trials involving porcine cells to move forward while at the same time, prohibiting nonhuman primate tissues. It must be remembered that safeguarding the public from new viral epidemics should remain our first priority when developing new technologies that include the use of animal cells or tissues to treat human disease.

References

Achong BG, Mansell PW, Epstein MA and Clifford P (1971) An unusual virus in cultures from a human nasopharyngeal carcinoma. J Natl Cancer Inst 46:299–307

Aguzzi A, Wagner EF, Netzer KO, Bothe K, Anhauser I and Rethwilm A (1993) Human foamy virus proteins accumulate in neurons and induce multinucleated giant cells in the brain of transgenic mice. Am J Pathol 142:1061–1071

Ali M, Taylor GP, Pitman RJ, Parker D, Rethwilm A, Cheingsong-Popov R, Weber JN, Bieniasz PD, Bradley J and McClure MO (1996) No evidence of antibody to human foamy virus in widespread human populations. AIDS Res Hum Retroviruses 12:1473–1483

Allan JS (1994) Primates and new viruses. Science 265:1345–1346

Allan JS (1996a) Xenotransplantation and Possible Emerging Infectious Diseases. Mol Diagn 1:209–217

Allan JS (1996b) Xenotransplantation at a crossroads: prevention versus progress. Nat Med 2:18–21

Allan JS (1998) The risk of using baboons as transplant donors. Exogenous and endogenous viruses. Ann N Y Acad Sci 862:87–99

Allan JS, Broussard SR, Michaels MG, Starzl TE, Leighton KL, Whitehead EM, Comuzzie AG, Lanford RE, Leland MM, Switzer WM and Heneine W (1998) Amplification of simian retroviral sequences from human recipients of baboon liver transplants. AIDS Res Hum Retroviruses 14:821–824

Allan JS, Leland M, Broussard S, Mone J and Hubbard G (2001) Simian T-cell lymphotropic Viruses (STLVs) and lymphomas in African nonhuman primates. Cancer Invest 19:383–395

Allan JS, Ray P, Broussard S, Whitehead E, Hubbard G, Butler T, Brasky K, Luciw P, Cheng-Mayer C, Levy JA, Steimer K, Li J, Sodroski J and Garcia-Moll M (1995) Infection of baboons with simian/human immunodeficiency viruses. J Acquir Immune Defic Syndr Hum Retrovirol 9:429–441

Allan JS, Short M, Taylor ME, Su S, Hirsch VM, Johnson PR, Shaw GM and Hahn BH (1991) Species-specific diversity among simian immunodeficiency viruses from African green monkeys. J Virol 65:2816–2828

Benveniste RE, Hill RW, Knott WB, Tsai CC, Kuller L and Morton WR (1993) Detection of serum antibodies in Ethiopian baboons that cross-react with SIV, HTLV-I, and type D retroviral antigens. J Med Primatol 22:124–128

Benveniste RE, Lieber MM, Livingston DM, Sherr CJ, Todaro GJ and Kalter SS (1974) Infectious C-type virus isolated from a baboon placenta. Nature 248:17–20

Blewett EL, Black DH, Lerche NW, White G and Eberle R (2000) Simian foamy virus infections in a baboon breeding colony. Virology 278:183–193

Bloom ET (2001) Xenotransplantation: regulatory challenges. Curr Opin Biotechnol 12:312–316

Broussard SR, Comuzzie AG, Leighton KL, Leland MM, Whitehead EM and Allan JS (1997) Characterization of new simian foamy viruses from African nonhuman primates. Virology 237:349–359

Brown P, Moreau-Dubois MC and Gajdusek DC (1982) Persistent asymptomatic infection of the laboratory mouse by simian foamy virus type 6: a new model of retrovirus latency. Arch Virol 71:229–234

Bryant ML, Sherr CJ, Sen A and Todaro GJ (1978) Molecular diversity among five different endogenous primate retroviruses. J Virol 28:300–313

Castro BA, Nepomuceno M, Lerche NW, Eichberg JW and Levy JA (1991) Persistent infection of baboons and rhesus monkeys with different strains of HIV-2. Virology 184:219–226

Chakrabarti LA, Lewin SR, Zhang L, Gettie A, Luckay A, Martin LN, Skulsky E, Ho DD, Cheng-Mayer C and Marx PA (2000) Normal T-cell turnover in sooty mangabeys harboring active simian immunodeficiency virus infection. J Virol 74:1209–1223

Coffin JM, Hughes, SH, and Varmus HE (eds) (1997) Retroviruses. Cold Spring Harbor Laboratory Press, Cold Spring Harbor, NY.

Cohen J (2001) Building a small-animal model for AIDS, block by block. Science 293:1034–1036

Cranage MP, Cook N, Stott EJ, Cook R, Baskerville A and Greenaway PJ (1992) Transmission studies with simian immunodeficiency virus of macaques; persistent infection of baboons. Intervirology 34:53–61

Deodhar SD (1986) Review of xenografts in organ transplantation. Transplant Proc 18:83–87

Doms RW (2001) Chemokine receptors and HIV entry. Aids 15 Suppl 1:S34–35

Donahue RE, Kessler SW, Bodine D, McDonagh K, Dunbar C, Goodman S, Agricola B, Byrne E, Raffeld M, Moen R and et al. (1992) Helper virus induced T cell lymphoma in nonhuman primates after retroviral mediated gene transfer. J Exp Med 176:1125–1135

Fomsgaard A, Muller-Trutwin MC, Diop O, Hansen J, Mathiot C, Corbet S, Barre-Sinoussi F and Allan JS (1997) Relation between phylogeny of African green monkey CD4 genes and their respective simian immunodeficiency virus genes. J Med Primatol 26:120–128

Ford RJ, Donehower LA and Bohannon RC (1992) Studies on a type D retrovirus isolated from an AIDS patient lymphoma. AIDS Res Hum Retroviruses 8:742–751

Franchini G (1995) Molecular mechanisms of human T-cell leukemia/lymphotropic virus type I infection. Blood 86:3619–3639

Fricker J (1996) Baboon xenotransplant fails but patient improves. Lancet 347:457

Gao F, Bailes E, Robertson DL, Chen Y, Rodenburg CM, Michael SF, Cummins LB, Arthur LO, Peeters M, Shaw GM, Sharp PM and Hahn BH (1999) Origin of HIV-1 in the chimpanzee Pan troglodytes troglodytes. Nature 397:436–441

Gessain A and de The G (1996) Geographic and molecular epidemiology of primate T lymphotropic retroviruses: HTLV-I, HTLV-II, STLV-I, STLV-PP, and PTLV-L. Adv Virus Res 47:377–426

Giles GR, Boehmig HJ, Amemiya H, Halgrimson CG and Starzl TE (1970) Clinical heterotransplantation of the liver. Transplant Proc 2:506–512

Grant RF, Windsor SK, Malinak CJ, Bartz CR, Sabo A, Benveniste RE and Tsai CC (1995) Characterization of infectious type D retrovirus from baboons. Virology 207:292–296

Heneine W, Switzer WM, Sandstrom P, Brown J, Vedapuri S, Schable CA, Khan AS, Lerche NW, Schweizer M, Neumann-Haefelin D, Chapman LE and Folks TM (1998) Identification of a human population infected with simian foamy viruses. Nat Med 4:403–407

Herchenroder O, Renne R, Loncar D, Cobb EK, Murthy KK, Schneider J, Mergia A and Luciw PA (1994) Isolation, cloning, and sequencing of simian foamy viruses from chimpanzees (SFVcpz): high homology to human foamy virus (HFV). Virology 201:187–199

Hinuma Y, Nagata K, Hanaoka M, Nakai M, Matsumoto T, Kinoshita KI, Shirakawa S and Miyoshi I (1981) Adult T-cell leukemia: antigen in an ATL cell line and detection of antibodies to the antigen in human sera. Proc Natl Acad Sci U S A 78:6476–6480

Hooks JJ and Detrick-Hooks B (1979) Simian foamy virus-induced immunosuppression in rabbits. J Gen Virol 44:383–390

Hu SL, Zarling JM, Chinn J, Travis BM, Moran PA, Sias J, Kuller L, Morton WR, Heidecker G and Benveniste RE (1989) Protection of macaques against simian AIDS by immunization with a recombinant vaccinia virus expressing the envelope glycoproteins of simian type D retrovirus. Proc Natl Acad Sci U S A 86:7213–7217

Huang LH, Silberman J, Rothschild H and Cohen JC (1989) Replication of baboon endogenous virus in human cells. Kinetics of DNA synthesis and integration. J Biol Chem 264:8811–8814

Hubbard GB, Mone JP, Allan JS, Davis KJ, 3rd, Leland MM, Banks PM and Smir B (1993) Spontaneously generated non-Hodgkin's lymphoma in twenty-seven simian T-cell leukemia virus type 1 antibody-positive baboons (Papio species). Lab Anim Sci 43:301–309

Hughes JF and Coffin JM (2001) Evidence for genomic rearrangements mediated by human endogenous retroviruses during primate evolution. Nat Genet 29:487–489

Ilyinskii P, Daniel M, Lerche N and Desrosiers R (1991) Antibodies to type D retrovirus in talapoin monkeys. J Gen Virol 72 (Pt 2):453–456

Jin MJ, Rogers J, Phillips-Conroy JE, Allan JS, Desrosiers RC, Shaw GM, Sharp PM and Hahn BH (1994) Infection of a yellow baboon with simian immunodeficiency virus from African green monkeys: evidence for cross-species transmission in the wild. J Virol 68:8454–8460

Kaur A, Grant RM, Means RE, McClure H, Feinberg M and Johnson RP (1998) Diverse host responses and outcomes following simian immunodeficiency virus SIVmac239 infection in sooty mangabeys and rhesus macaques. J Virol 72:9597–9611

Larsson E and Andersson G (1998) Beneficial role of human endogenous retroviruses: facts and hypotheses. Scand J Immunol 48:329–338

Lerche NW, Cotterman RF, Dobson MD, Yee JL, Rosenthal AN and Heneine WM (1997) Screening for simian type-D retrovirus infection in macaques, using nested polymerase chain reaction. Lab Anim Sci 47:263–268

Lerche NW, Switzer WM, Yee JL, Shanmugam V, Rosenthal AN, Chapman LE, Folks TM and Heneine W (2001) Evidence of infection with simian type D retrovirus in persons occupationally exposed to nonhuman primates. J Virol 75:1783–1789

Lerche NW, Yee JL and Jennings MB (1994) Establishing specific retrovirus-free breeding colonies of macaques: an approach to primary screening and surveillance. Lab Anim Sci 44:217–221

Letvin NL, Daniel MD, Sehgal PK, Yetz JM, Solomon KR, Kannagi M, Schmidt DK, Silva DP, Montagnier L and Desrosiers RC (1987) Infection of baboons with human immunodeficiency virus-2 (HIV-2). J Infect Dis 156:406–407

Liska V, Fultz PN, Su L and Ruprecht RM (1997) Detection of simian T cell leukemia virus type I infection in seronegative macaques. AIDS Res Hum Retroviruses 13:1147–1153

Liska V, Lerche NW and Ruprecht RM (1997) Simultaneous detection of simian retrovirus type D serotypes 1, 2, and 3 by polymerase chain reaction. AIDS Res Hum Retroviruses 13:433–437

Lowenstine LJ, Pedersen NC, Higgins J, Pallis KC, Uyeda A, Marx P, Lerche NW, Munn RJ and Gardner MB (1986) Seroepidemiologic survey of captive Old-World primates for antibodies to human and simian retroviruses, and isolation of a lentivirus from sooty mangabeys (Cercocebus atys). Int J Cancer 38:563–574

Mang R, Goudsmit J and van der Kuyl AC (1999) Novel endogenous type C retrovirus in baboons: complete sequence, providing evidence for baboon endogenous virus gag-pol ancestry. J Virol 73:7021–7026

Marx PA and Chen Z (1998) The function of simian chemokine receptors in the replication of SIV. Semin Immunol 10:215–223

Marx PA, Maul DH, Osborn KG, Lerche NW, Moody P, Lowenstine LJ, Henrickson RV, Arthur LO, Gilden RV, Gravell M and et al. (1984) Simian AIDS: isolation of a type D retrovirus and transmission of the disease. Science 223:1083–1086

Marx PA, Pedersen NC, Lerche NW, Osborn KG, Lowenstine LJ, Lackner AA, Maul DH, Kwang HS, Kluge JD, Zaiss CP and et al. (1986) Prevention of simian acquired immune deficiency syndrome with a formalin-inactivated type D retrovirus vaccine. J Virol 60:431–435

Maul DH, Zaiss CP, MacKenzie MR, Shiigi SM, Marx PA and Gardner MB (1988) Simian retrovirus D serogroup 1 has a broad cellular tropism for lymphoid and nonlymphoid cells. J Virol 62:1768–1773

Mergia A, Chari S, Kolson DL, Goodenow MM and Ciccarone T (2001) The efficiency of simian foamy virus vector type-1 (SFV-1) in nondividing cells and in human PBLs. Virology 280:243–252

Mergia A, Leung NJ and Blackwell J (1996) Cell tropism of the simian foamy virus type 1 (SFV-1). J Med Primatol 25:2–7

Mone J, Whitehead E, Leland M, Hubbard G and Allan JS (1992) Simian T-cell leukemia virus type I infection in captive baboons. AIDS Res Hum Retroviruses 8:1653–1661

Nandi JS, Bhavalkar-Potdar V, Tikute S and Raut CG (2000) A novel type D simian retrovirus naturally infecting the Indian Hanuman langur (Semnopithecus entellus). Virology 277:6–13

Poiesz BJ, Ruscetti FW, Reitz MS, Kalyanaraman VS and Gallo RC (1981) Isolation of a new type C retrovirus (HTLV) in primary uncultured cells of a patient with Sezary T-cell leukaemia. Nature 294:268–271

Purcell DF, Broscius CM, Vanin EF, Buckler CE, Nienhuis AW and Martin MA (1996) An array of murine leukemia virus-related elements is transmitted and expressed in a primate recipient of retroviral gene transfer. J Virol 70:887–897

Rasko JE, Battini JL, Gottschalk RJ, Mazo I and Miller AD (1999) The RD114/simian type D retrovirus receptor is a neutral amino acid transporter. Proc Natl Acad Sci U S A 96:2129–2134

Saib A, Neves M, Giron ML, Guillemin MC, Valla J, Peries J and Canivet M (1997) Long-term persistent infection of domestic rabbits by the human foamy virus. Virology 228:263–268

Sandstrom PA, Phan KO, Switzer WM, Fredeking T, Chapman L, Heneine W and Folks TM (2000) Simian foamy virus infection among zoo keepers. Lancet 355:551–552

Santillana-Hayat M, Rozain F, Bittoun P, Chopin-Robert C, Lasneret J, Peries J and Canivet M (1993) Transient immunosuppressive effect induced in rabbits and mice by the human spumaretrovirus prototype HFV (human foamy virus). Res Virol 144:389–396

Schweizer M, Falcone V, Gange J, Turek R and Neumann-Haefelin D (1997) Simian foamy virus isolated from an accidentally infected human individual. J Virol 71:4821–4824

Schweizer M, Fleps U, Jackle A, Renne R, Turek R and Neumann-Haefelin D (1993) Simian foamy virus type 3 (SFV-3) in latently infected Vero cells: reactivation by demethylation of proviral DNA. Virology 192:663–666

Schweizer M and Neumann-Haefelin D (1995) Phylogenetic analysis of primate foamy viruses by comparison of pol sequences. Virology 207:577–582

Schweizer M, Turek R, Hahn H, Schliephake A, Netzer KO, Eder G, Reinhardt M, Rethwilm A and Neumann-Haefelin D (1995) Markers of foamy virus infections in monkeys, apes, and accidentally infected humans: appropriate testing fails to confirm suspected foamy virus prevalence in humans. AIDS Res Hum Retroviruses 11:161–170

Seiki M, Hattori S, Hirayama Y and Yoshida M (1983) Human adult T-cell leukemia virus: complete nucleotide sequence of the provirus genome integrated in leukemia cell DNA. Proc Natl Acad Sci U S A 80:3618–3622

Seiki M, Watanabe T, Komuro A, Miyoshi I, Hayami M and Yoshida M (1984) Characterization of simian retrovirus genome related to human T-cell leukemia virus type I. Princess Takamatsu Symp 15:241–249

Starzl TE, Demetris AJ, Murase N, Trucco M, Thomson AW and Rao AS (1996) The lost chord: microchimerism and allograft survival. Immunol Today 17:577–584; discussion 588

Starzl TE, Fung J, Tzakis A, Todo S, Demetris AJ, Marino IR, Doyle H, Zeevi A, Warty V, Michaels M and et al. (1993) Baboon-to-human liver transplantation. Lancet 341:65–71

Tailor CS, Nouri A, Zhao Y, Takeuchi Y and Kabat D (1999) A sodium-dependent neutral-amino-acid transporter mediates infections of feline and baboon endogenous retroviruses and simian type D retroviruses. J Virol 73:4470–4474

Takeuchi Y, Porter CD, Strahan KM, Preece AF, Gustafsson K, Cosset FL, Weiss RA and Collins MK (1996) Sensitization of cells and retroviruses to human serum by (alpha 1-3) galactosyltransferase. Nature 379:85–88

Ting CN, Rosenberg MP, Snow CM, Samuelson LC and Meisler MH (1992) Endogenous retroviral sequences are required for tissue-specific expression of a human salivary amylase gene. Genes Dev 6:1457–1465

Traeger J (1969) Transplantations of kidneys from chimpanzees to man. Primates Med 3:52–54

Tschopp RR, Brandner S, Marino S, Bothe K, Horak I, Rethwilm A and Aguzzi A (1996) Analysis of the determinants of neurotropism and neurotoxicity of HFV in transgenic mice. Virology 216:338–346

Uchiyama T, Yodoi J, Sagawa K, Takatsuki K and Uchino H (1977) Adult T-cell leukemia: clinical and hematologic features of 16 cases. Blood 50:481–492

van der Kuyl AC, Mang R, Dekker JT and Goudsmit J (1997) Complete nucleotide sequence of simian endogenous type D retrovirus with intact genome organization: evidence for ancestry to simian retrovirus and baboon endogenous virus. J Virol 71:3666–3676

Van Dooren S, Salemi M and Vandamme AM (2001) Dating the origin of the African human T-cell lymphotropic virus type-i (HTLV-I) subtypes. Mol Biol Evol 18:661–671

Vanin EF, Kaloss M, Broscius C and Nienhuis AW (1994) Characterization of replication-competent retroviruses from nonhuman primates with virus-induced T-cell lymphomas and observations regarding the mechanism of oncogenesis. J Virol 68:4241–4250

von Laer D, Neumann-Haefelin D, Heeney JL and Schweizer M (1996) Lymphocytes are the major reservoir for foamy viruses in peripheral blood. Virology 221:240–244

Exogenous Porcine Viruses

P. S. Paul[1] · P. Halbur[2] · B. Janke[2] · H. Joo[3] · P. Nawagitgul[4] · J. Singh[2] · S. Sorden[2]

[1] Department of Veterinary and Biomedical Sciences, University of Nebraska-Lincoln, Lincoln, NE 68588, USA
E-mail: ppaul2@unl.edu

[2] College of Veterinary Medicine, Iowa State University, Ames, IA 50011, USA

[3] College of Veterinary Medicine, University of Minnesota, Saint Paul, MN 55108, USA

[4] Faculty of Veterinary Medicine, Kasetsart University, Kasetsart, Thailand

1 Introduction . . . 127

2 Orthomyxoviruses . . . 129
2.1 Swine Influenza Virus . . . 129
2.1.1 Virus Characteristics . . . 129
2.1.2 Pathogenesis . . . 129
2.1.3 Diagnosis . . . 132
2.1.4 Control and Eradication . . . 133
2.1.5 Xenozoonoses . . . 134

3 Paramyxovirus . . . 134
3.1 Nipah Virus Infection in Swine . . . 135
3.1.1 Viral Characteristics . . . 135
3.1.2 Pathogenesis . . . 136
3.1.3 Diagnosis . . . 137
3.1.4 Control and Eradication . . . 137
3.1.5 Xenozoonoses . . . 137
3.2 Menangle Virus . . . 138
3.3 Le Piedad Paramyxovirus . . . 138
3.4 Porcine Paramyxovirus . . . 139

4 Arteriviruses . . . 141
4.1 Porcine Reproductive and Respiratory Syndrome Virus . . . 141
4.1.1 Virus Characteristics . . . 141
4.1.2 Pathogenesis . . . 142
4.1.3 Diagnosis . . . 144
4.1.4 Control and Eradication . . . 145
4.1.5 Xenozoonoses . . . 145

5 Japanese Encephalomyelitis Virus . . . 146
5.1 Virus Characteristics . . . 146
5.2 Pathogenesis . . . 146
5.3 Diagnosis . . . 148
5.4 Control and Eradication . . . 148

5.5 Xenozoonoses 149

6 Encephalomyocarditis Virus 150
6.1 Virus Characteristics 150
6.2 Pathogenesis 151
6.3 Diagnosis 152
6.4 Control and Eradication 152
6.5 Xenozoonoses 153

7 Porcine Circovirus 153
7.1 Viral Characteristics 153
7.2 Pathogenesis 154
7.3 Diagnosis 158
7.4 Control and Eradication 159
7.5 Xenozoonoses 159

8 Herpesviruses 160
8.1 Pseudorabies Virus 160
8.1.1 Virus Characteristics 160
8.1.2 Pathogenesis 160
8.1.3 Diagnosis 161
8.1.4 Eradication and Control 161
8.1.5 Xenozoonoses 162
8.2 Porcine Lymphotropic Herpesvirus 162
8.3 Porcine Cytomegalovirus 164
8.3.1 Xenozoonoses 166

9 Porcine Parvovirus 166
9.1 Virus Characteristics 166
9.2 Pathogenesis 167
9.3 Diagnosis 167
9.4 Control and Eradication 168
9.5 Xenozoonoses 169

10 Coronaviruses 169

11 Adenoviruses 171

12 Conclusion 172

References 173

Abstract Porcine organs, cells and tissues provide a viable source of transplants in humans, though there is some concern of public health risk from adaptation of swine infectious agents in humans. Limited information is available on the public health risk of many exogenous swine viruses, and reliable and rapid diagnostic tests are available for only a few of these. The ability of several porcine viruses to cause transplacental fetal infection (parvoviruses, circoviruses, and arteriviruses), emergence or recognition of several new porcine viruses during the last two decades (porcine circovirus, arterivirus, paramyxoviruses, herpesviruses, and porcine respiratory coronavirus) and the immunosuppressed state of the transplant recipients increases the xenozoonoses risk of humans to porcine viruses through transplantation. Much of this risk can be eliminated with vigilance and sustained monitoring along with a better understanding of pathogenesis and development of better diagnostic tests. In this review we present information on selected exogenous viruses, highlighting their characteristics, pathogenesis of viral infections in swine, methods for their detection, and the potential xenozoonoses risk they present. Emphasis has been given in this review to swine influenza virus, paramyxovirus (Nipah virus, Menagle virus, LaPiedad paramyxovirus, porcine paramyxovirus), arterivirus (porcine reproductive and respiratory syndrome virus) and circovirus as either they represent new swine viruses or present the greatest risk. We have also presented information on porcine parvovirus, Japanese encephalitis virus, encephalomyocarditis virus, herpesviruses (pseudorabies virus, porcine lymphotropic herpesvirus, porcine cytomegalovirus), coronaviruses (TGEV, PRCV, HEV, PEDV) and adenovirus. The potential of swine viruses to infect humans needs to be assessed in vitro and in vivo and rapid and more reliable diagnostic methods need to be developed to assure safe supply of porcine tissues and cells for xenotransplantation.

1
Introduction

Recent interest in the use of porcine organs, cells, and tissues for transplantation in humans (xenotransplantation) to alleviate the critical shortage of human organs has initiated a debate on the possible public health risk from swine infectious agents. Of concern are both the potential adaptation of swine infectious agents to humans and the emergence of new human pathogens (xenozoonoses) (Chapman et al. 1995; Fishman 1994; Weiss 1998; Bach et al. 1998; Gunzburg and Salmons 2000).

The major initial focus of concern has been porcine endogenous retrovirus, because of its potential to integrate into the host genome, its demonstrated ability to infect human cells (Patience et al. 1997; Weiss 1998), and its potential to recombine with human retroviruses. In contrast, limited information is known about the risk to humans of many exogenous swine viruses, and reliable diagnostic tests are available for only a few of the swine infectious agents that are xenozoonotic risks. It is generally believed that swine can easily be raised free of infectious agents in a sterile environment, and therefore do not pose a significant public health threat. Practical experience has shown this to be a false security, as transplacental infection of fetuses has been demonstrated with a number of viruses, e.g., parvoviruses, circoviruses, and arteriviruses, and contamination of specific pathogen-free (SPF) herds with swine pathogens occurs periodically. Furthermore, a number of new swine viruses, such as porcine circovirus, arterivirus, paramyxoviruses, herpesviruses, and coronaviruses, whose origins are not fully understood, have emerged in the last 20 years. Xenotransplant recipients also are potentially more susceptible hosts for adoption of porcine exogenous viruses as they are immunosuppressed over a long period of time. The greatest risk is from those viruses that have a high mutation rate and/or produce latent or persistent infections. New viruses can also emerge from recombination with human viruses such as herpesviruses and coronaviruses, and reassortment of genes between porcine and human viruses, as demonstrated for influenza viruses.

Exogenous porcine viruses that present the greatest xenozoonoses risk are those that have already been shown to be zoonotic or that infect humans, e.g., orthomyxoviruses, paramyxoviruses, encephalitis viruses, and picornaviruses. Many of these viruses have been extensively studied. Viruses that present unknown yet important potential risk are those that cause persistent and/or latent infections; cross the transplacental barrier and infect swine fetuses; have high recombination or mutation rates; infect cells, organs and tissues used for human transplantation; infect multiple species; infect human or nonhuman primate cells; or cross species barriers. Much of this risk can be eliminated with vigilance and sustained monitoring along with a better understanding of pathogenesis and development of better diagnostic tests.

In this review we present information on selected exogenous viruses, highlighting their characteristics, pathogenesis of viral infections in swine, methods for their detection, and the potential xenozoonoses risk they present. Emphasis has been given in this review to swine influenza virus, paramyxovirus, arterivirus and circovirus as either they represent new swine viruses or present the greatest risk.

2 Orthomyxoviruses

2.1 Swine Influenza Virus

There has been longstanding interest in swine influenza virus (SIV) as a public health risk. The 1918 pandemic of influenza that resulted in 20 million human deaths worldwide has been suspected to be caused by SIV. There has been renewed interest in swine influenza as new strains and types have appeared in swine in the last decade.

2.1.1 Virus Characteristics

Influenza viruses are enveloped, single-stranded RNA viruses belonging to the Family *Orthomyxoviridae*. The viral genome is segmented, with eight segments. Major structural viral proteins are ribonucleoprotein (NP), matrix proteins (M1, M2), hemagglutinin (HA) and neuraminidase (NA). The NP and M proteins are type-specific antigens that are used to identify virus isolates as influenza and to classify influenza viruses as type A, B, or C. Influenza viruses that infect animals are almost exclusively type A viruses, as are most of the influenza viruses of significance in humans. In contrast to the type A viruses, influenza B and C viruses are human viruses and have occasionally been isolated from pigs, probably as limited incidental infections from contact with humans. The more variable HA and NA proteins are used to classify influenza viruses into subtypes. Fifteen HA and nine NA subtypes have been established among type A viruses. Influenza viruses have extensive heterogeneity as a result of reassortment between two viruses, a process known as antigenic shift. They also go through random mutations in the HA and NA, known as antigenic drift, which results in new variants.

2.1.2 Pathogenesis

Swine are quite susceptible to infection with viruses from humans and birds; however, many of the infections are subclinical or result in only mild disease. Serological studies indicate that many such strains remain in swine populations for only a short time. Occasionally, a human strain will continue to circulate in swine populations long after it had disappeared from human populations (Brown 2000). Until recently, H1N1 and H3N2 had been identified as the predominant subtypes pathogenic for swine. An H1N2 subtype virus, first identified in England in 1995, has become the predominant subtype responsible for clinical disease in England (Brown et al. 1995). H1N2 isolates also have been reported in France (Gourreau et al. 1994), Japan (Ouchi et al. 1996), Belgium (Van Reeth et al. 2000), and the United States (Karasin et al. 2000a). A recent report of H4N6 subtype infection in a single herd in Canada possibly was the first description of this subtype in swine (Karasin et al. 2000b).

The course of influenza virus infection in swine is quite rapid (Easterday and van Reeth 1999). The virus attaches via HA to sialic acid receptors on the surface of epithelial cells lining the airways of the respiratory tract. Virus is internalized and multiplication occurs within the cytoplasm and nucleus with assembly of virions at the plasma membrane. Within 5 h post infection, virus has been observed by electron microscopy budding from the surface of infected cells. Virus initially infects epithelial cells on nasal turbinates and in medium-sized bronchioles in the lung. Infection results in depression and high fever by 24–36 h post infection that lasts for 24–48 h. At 24 h after infection, the bronchiolar epithelium is filled with virus but little damage has occurred. During the next 24–48 h, epithelial cells become necrotic and slough into bronchiolar lumens. Infected cells can be detected at this time in airways of all sizes and in alveoli. The damage to bronchioles stimulates irritation that results in the harsh barking cough characteristic of the disease. Restricted airflow from bronchiolar damage and interference with oxygen transfer due to interstitial pneumonia result in hyperpnea/dyspnea. By 96–120 h after infection, the amount of virus in the lung has dropped considerably, body temperatures have returned to normal, and clinical signs of respiratory distress have abated.

Because of the airborne route of entry and the initial infection of the airways, the gross lesions induced by SIV resemble the bronchopneumonia of bacterial origin. By 48 h post infection, irregularly distributed coalescing gray to red foci of lobular consolidation are evident grossly in the cranial and middle lobes and in hilar areas of the lung (Fig. 1). In severe infections, the entire lung may be edematous and noncollapsed because of interstitial pneumonia. Focal ecchymotic hemorrhages or interlobular bullae may occasionally be present. The consolidated areas

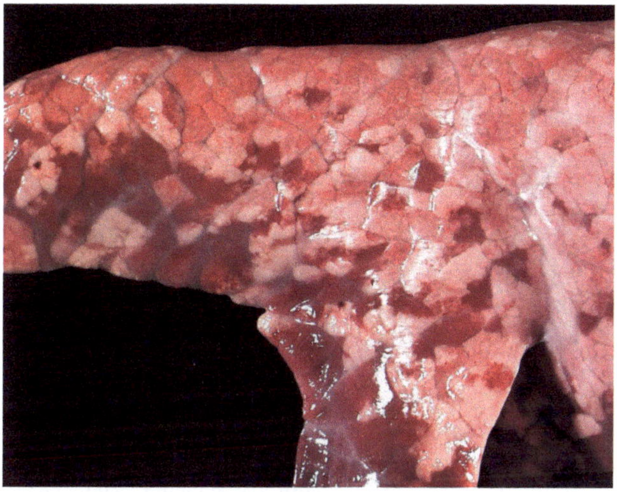

Fig. 1 Lung from a pig infected with SIV. Note *gray* to *red* foci of lobular consolidation

become darker red and depressed below the surface of the surrounding lung as the affected lung tissue contracts during resolution. Gross lesions may remain visible, though shrinking in size, for 2–3 weeks.

Microscopically, the hallmark lesion of influenza virus infection is necrotizing bronchiolitis. By 48 h after infection, necrotic infected epithelial cells are sloughing into bronchiolar lumens and a light loose infiltration of lymphocytes is present around affected airways (Fig. 2). Alveolar walls are thickened by infiltration of mononuclear leukocytes and by pneumocyte swelling. In severe infections, bronchioles and partially collapsed alveoli may contain necrotic cellular debris in which virus can be demonstrated. Alveolar hemorrhage and edema are variable. At 72–96 h after infection, many bronchioles will be lined by attenuated to proliferative epithelium as the airways begin to repair. By 120 h after infection, epithelial proliferation is prominent and little active necrosis is present. Peribronchiolar and perivascular lymphocytic cuffing may be extensive by this time. Lesions vary considerably in severity from lobule to lobule.

Swine influenza is a highly contagious disease. Pigs inoculated experimentally via the intranasal route develop fever and begin shedding virus in nasal secretions within 24 h. Shedding routinely continues for 5–6 days. The primary mode of transmission is through aerosolization of virus in droplets disseminated by the cough induced by virus damage to

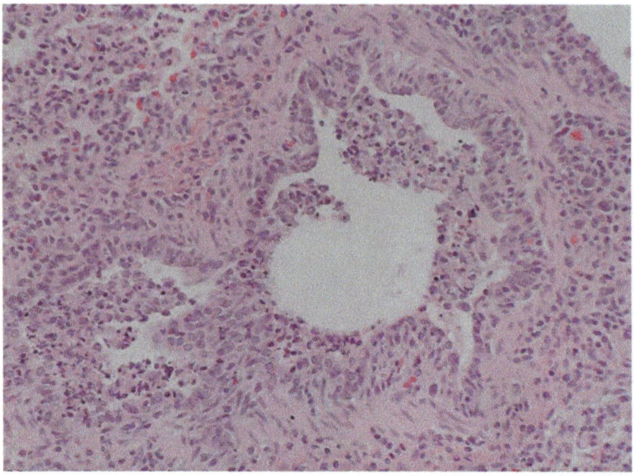

Fig. 2 Photomicrograph of lung from pig infected with SIV showing lesions characterized by necrotizing bronchiolitis, sloughing of necrotic infected epithelial cells into bronchiolar lumens and a loose infiltration of lymphocytes around affected airways

airways in the lung. Infection also can be acquired through direct contact with nasal and oral secretions from infected pigs.

At 24 h after infection, many epithelial cells lining medium-sized bronchioles will contain virus. By 48 h, virus will be present in airways of all sizes as well as in pneumocytes in alveoli. Virus also can be found in epithelial cells lining the nasal passages, but very little virus is present in tracheal epithelium. The tonsil also does not appear to be directly infected. Although a few research studies have reported transient viremia (Brown et al. 1993), in most pigs the virus does not invade beyond the respiratory tract to any great extent.

2.1.3 Diagnosis

A variety of diagnostic tests are available to detect SIV infections (Janke 2000). An antigen-capture enzyme linked immunosorbent assay (ELISA) for type A influenza viruses (Directogen by Becton-Dickinson) developed for use in humans has been used successfully to detect SIV in nasal or bronchiolar swabs. Application of fluorescein-conjugated antibody to frozen sections of lung, and immunohistochemical methods to sections

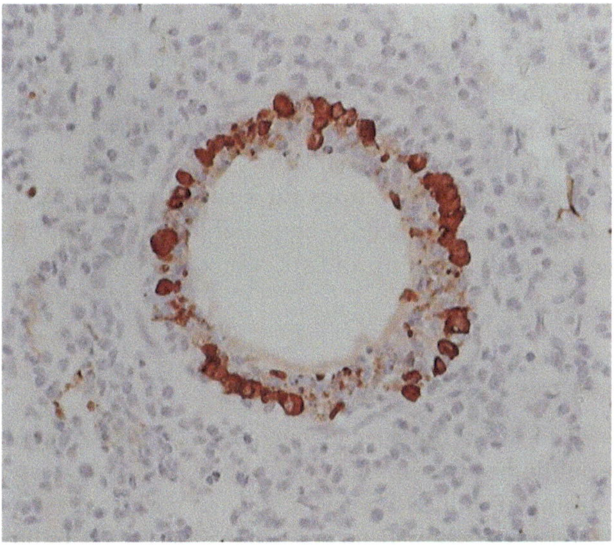

Fig. 3 SIV antigen in lung of a pig infected with SIV detected by immunohistochemistry using monoclonal antibody

of formalin-fixed lung are used routinely to detect SIV in tissues from pigs submitted for necropsy (Vincent et al. 1997; Fig. 3). Virus isolation techniques routinely use embryonated chicken eggs or Madin–Darby Canine kidney cells. Isolates that exhibit hemagglutinating activity are identified as influenza viruses through reaction with hyperimmune typing serum or with polymerase chain reaction (PCR)-based assays. PCR techniques also are used for direct detection of SIV in homogenized lung tissue or on nasal swabs and to determine virus subtype. Hemagglutination inhibition (HI) tests have been the standard serologic test for swine influenza. Recently, a commercially developed ELISA for antibody against H1N1 SIV has become available.

2.1.4 Control and Eradication

SIVs are ubiquitous and very few herds are free of infection. Researchers seeking virus- and antibody-free pigs for experimental purposes have great difficulty locating such herds. Because of this ubiquity and the recurrence of disease each fall in many herds, even without the introduction of additional pigs that could serve as a source of infection, a carrier state has been proposed. However, no evidence of prolonged infection of individual pigs has been found. Virus probably survives within a herd at a low level by transmission to susceptible individuals within the group. Immune pigs that do not develop clinical illness after challenge have been shown to shed virus in nasal secretions for a short period post infection. Elimination of infection is likely to be possible only by repopulation through segregated early weaning and strict biosecurity measures.

2.1.5 Xenozoonoses

SIVs have been shown to cross the species barrier and infect humans, posing a significant public health risk. Pigs also serve as mixing vessels for generating new strains of influenza viruses through genetic reassortment. SIV subtype H1N1 is suspected to be responsible for 20 million human deaths in the 1918 influenza pandemic. However, the first SIV infection from humans was not demonstrated until 1976 when SIV was isolated from US military recruits (Goldfield et al. 1977). Since then H1N1 has been shown to cross the species barrier and infect humans as SIV was isolated from pigs and caretakers from a farm in Wisconsin (Hinshaw et al. 1978) and from a boy who lived on a farm and spread the virus to classmates. Patriarca et al. (1984) isolated SIV from an animal caretaker who died of pneumonia in Maryland (Wentworth et al. 1994). The latter virus was similar to that circulating in the pig population. Wentworth et al. (1997) reported on infection and mild disease in two individuals conducting experiments in pigs with H1N1 virus. H3N2 of possible swine origin has also been isolated from young children in the Netherlands (Claas et al. 1994).

3 **Paramyxovirus**

Paramyxoviruses are a diverse group of viruses, some of which present a public health risk. A number of paramyxoviruses of animal origin have clearly crossed the species barrier and have become established as human pathogens; others appear to be narrow in host range. Paramyxoviruses belong to the family *Paramyxoviridae* with four genera: *Paramyxovirus*, *Rubulavirus*, *Morbillivirus*, and *Pneumovirus*. All members have a single-stranded negative-sense RNA genome and share affinity for the respiratory tract. In some host species, paramyxoviruses also infect the central nervous system. Members of the genus *Paramyxovirus* include human parainfluenza virus types 1 and 3, and bovine parainfluenza virus type 3. *Rubulavirus* genus includes Newcastle disease virus of birds, Simian virus 5, canine parainfluenza virus type 2, mumps virus, human parainfluenza virus types 2, 4a, and 4b, and Le Piedad paramyxovirus (LPMV) of swine associated with blue eye disease in Mexico. Members of *Morbillivirus* genus include canine distemper virus, measles virus, phocine morbillivirus and rinderpest virus. *Pneumovirus* genus includes human respiratory syncytial virus, bovine respiratory syncytial virus, and turkey rhinotracheitis virus of turkeys. A new genus, *Henipavirus*, to accommodate Hendra virus and Nipah virus, has been proposed. Here we discuss Nipah virus and briefly LPMV and porcine paramyxovirus (PPMV).

3.1 Nipah Virus Infection in Swine

The Nipah virus outbreak was detected in Malaysia in 1999, and resulted in 265 cases of encephalitis in humans, 100 deaths in swine farm workers, and an economic loss of millions of dollars to the swine industry (Tchoyoson-Lim et al. 2000; Parashar et al. 2000). Nipah virus infection was also observed in abattoir workers in Singapore that processed pigs imported from Malaysia (Chew et al. 2000). The disease is characterized by pronounced respiratory and neurologic signs with low morbidity and mortality in pigs. The disease in pigs was closely associated with an epidemic of viral encephalitis in pig farm workers. A viral agent with the morphology of paramyxovirus was isolated and later confirmed to be the agent responsible for the human and swine diseases (Chua et al. 2000a; 2000b). Late presentation of encephalitis was also seen in patients, even months after being exposed to the virus (Wong et al. 2001).

3.1.1 Viral Characteristics

The Nipah virus is an RNA virus with morphology typical of viruses belonging to the family *Paramyxoviridae*. Nipah virus is closely related to Hendra virus of horses (Chua et al. 2000a), formally designated as equine morbillivirus. Hendra virus was associated with an outbreak of respiratory disease in horses in Hendra, Queensland, Australia, in which 14 horses and one human died (Murray et al. 1995). Comparison of nucleotide sequence of Nipah with other paramyxoviruses shows that Nipah virus is closely related to Hendra Virus but is distinct from members of other genera of the family *Paramyxoviridae* and should be considered a new genus (Harcourt et al. 2000; McCormack 2000). Wang et al. (2000) have suggested *Henipa* as a name for this new genus. Nipah and Hendra viruses have a broad host range that includes humans. The virus replicates in the African green monkey kidney cell line Vero and the baby hamster kidney cell line producing syncytial cells typical of those produced by other paramyxoviruses. Electron microscopy reveals a 'herring bone' appearance of its nucleocapsid, typical of paramyxoviruses.

3.1.2 Pathogenesis

Limited information is available on its pathogenesis and is mostly based on field observations. Clinical disease varies with the age of affected animals and a large number of infected animals have subclinical infection. Adult swine primarily show neurologic signs, but respiratory disease is commonly observed. Mortality was higher in younger pigs of up to 6 months of age. The incubation period is 7–14 days.

The major lesions in lungs include consolidation, emphysema, and petechial to ecchymotic hemorrhages. Mild to severe interstitial pneumonia with widespread hemorrhages and syncytial cells in the endothelial cells of the lung blood vessels are the common histological lesions observed (Hooper et al. 2001). Congestion and edema are common lesions in the brain. Histological lesions in lungs, kidney, and brain tissues include vasculitis with fibrinoid necrosis, hemorrhages, and infiltration of mononuclear cells. Nonsuppurative meningitis with gliosis is common in the brain. High concentrations of viral antigens have been detected by immunohistochemistry in the endothelium of the blood vessels, especially in the lung (Daniels 1999).

3.1.3
Diagnosis

Because of its public health significance, public health officials and the United States Department of Agriculture should be contacted immediately if Nipah virus infection is suspected. All samples should be handled under biosafety level 4 (BL-4) conditions. ELISA and virus neutralization tests are the serological tests currently available. Currently, the viral antigen used in ELISA is gamma-irradiated virus. Before testing, sera are treated with sodium dodecyl sulphate (SDS) and Triton X-100 and by heating at 56 C for 1 h to inactivate virus. Virus can be isolated in Vero cells, which should only be attempted under strict biosecurity conditions.

3.1.4
Control and Eradication

Nipah virus infections have been detected in swine, horses, dogs, and humans. Infections of cats and goats exposed to infected pigs have also been observed. Serological surveys have detected neutralizing antibodies in fruit bats of the genus *Pteropus*, which have been incriminated as a potential reservoir for Nipah virus. Possible modes of transmission between farms within farming communities include movement of infected swine, contaminated boar semen, and dogs and cats. Because of the public health significance of Nipah virus infection, eradication of the disease is the best method of control. In Malaysia, Nipah virus was eliminated by culling all swine from herds affected in Nipah virus outbreaks. Once ELISA became available, swine were tested for serological evidence of Nipah virus infection. Fifteen sows from each of 889 farms were tested of which 50 were found positive. All pigs on these farms were destroyed. This strategy was successful in eradicating Nipah virus infections in Malaysia.

3.1.5
Xenozoonoses

Nipah virus has clearly been shown to infect humans, causing encephalitis with high mortality and hence it is of public health importance. Epidemiologic investigations suggest that pigs are the major source of virus transmission to humans through direct contact with pigs or their secretions (urine) and excretions (feces) (Goh et al. 2000). Many of the infections occurred amongst pig farmers and abattoir workers (Chew et al. 2000; Goh et al. 2000). Virus may be transmitted by respiratory droplets as persons that did not have direct contact with pigs developed Nipah virus infection (Goh et al. 2000). However, it should be noted that there have been no documented cases of human-to-human transmission of Nipah virus (chan et al. 2002). The main clinical signs in humans include fever, headache, vomiting, reduced level of consciousness, and prominent brain stem dysfunction (Chua et al. 2000a). Fortunately, the virus infection has been eliminated from domestic swine. Fruit bats and other as yet unidentified reservoirs present potential risk for reintroduction of Nipah virus in swine, so constant vigilance is required. Additional studies are needed to determine the reservoirs of Nipah virus and to understand the pathogenesis of Nipah viral infection.

3.2 Menangle Virus

Menangle virus is another porcine paramyxovirus isolated from pigs in Australia (Chant et al. 1998). This virus has been associated with stillbirths in swine (Philbey et al. 1998). Human infections with Menangle virus have been reported. Two workers from a pig farm infected with this new paramyxovirus suffered a respiratory illness and developed high convalescent-phase antibody titers of 128 and 512 to the new virus. Both workers with antibodies had suffered a sudden onset of fever, chills, severe headaches and myalgia. Other personnel with no to low occupational hazard remained seronegative to this new virus. Limited available information suggests that Menangle virus presents a public health and xenozoonoses risk. Information on its epidemiology is limited and additional studies are justified.

3.3 Le Piedad Paramyxovirus

LPMV is a causative agent of blue eye disease first observed in Le Piedad, Mexico (Stephano et al. 1988; Stephano 1999). The virus has not been detected in the USA. LPMV is a member of *Rubulavirus* genus of *Paramyxovirinae* subfamily of *Paramyxoviridae* family. Virus characteristics as to the morphology, size, and physicochemical properties are typical of other paramyxoviruses; however, LPMV is distinguishable antigenically. LPMV is associated with respiratory, reproductive, and neurological disease in pigs. Clinical signs include fever, arched back, nervous signs of ataxia, weakness, muscle tremor, and abnormal posture. Pigs are hyperexcitable and squeal with paddling movements. Conjunctivitis and corneal opacity are common. Reproductive failure is characterized by return of females to estrus, stillbirths and mummified fetuses.

Mild pneumonia is a common gross lesion observed with microscopic evidence of interstitial pneumonia. Microscopic lesions are also observed in brain and spinal cord. LPMV infection should be suspected in countries where this virus is prevalent when encephalitis, corneal opacity and reproductive failure in sows or orchitis in boars are observed. LPMV can be easily isolated in pig kidney (PK-15) cell line as it induces syncytium characteristic of paramyxoviruses. Viral antigen can be detected in cells by fluorescent antibody tests. Antibodies can be detected by HI, virus neutralization and ELISA.

3.4 Porcine Paramyxovirus

We have reported a neurological and respiratory disease in a swine herd in the northern USA associated with PPMV (Janke et al. 2001). A swine unit with 400 pigs suffered an outbreak of neurological and respiratory disease. Disease spread to second unit within a few days. The clinical respiratory and neurological disease was similar to that observed with PPMV (Nipah virus) infection except the disease was milder. Clinical signs included dyspnea, harsh barking cough, central nervous system (CNS) disturbance, persistent squealing, and whole body tremors, rear end ataxia, and intermittent episodes of head pressing. Gross lesions included congestion of the lungs with consolidation of the ventral tips of the lung lobes. Two pigs were submitted to the veterinary diagnostic laboratory at Iowa State University. Both pigs were in good condition but did exhibit CNS signs as previously described. Clinical signs of respiratory disease were not evident. At necropsy, lungs in both pigs had bilateral pale gray consolidation of the ventral half of the cranial and middle lobes. The rest of the lung tissue was only slightly firmer than normal. No gross lesions were observed in the brain or other internal organs. Mi-

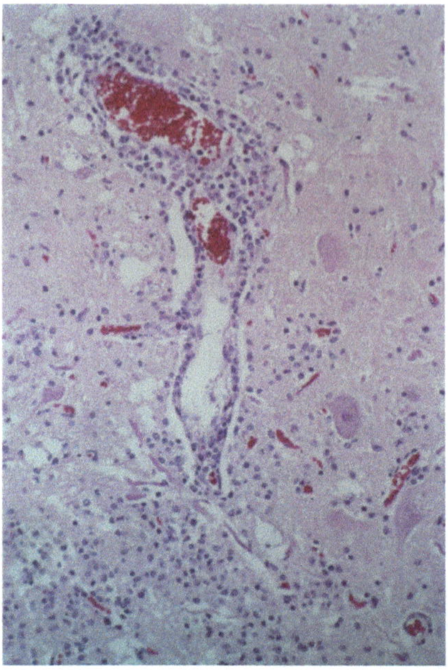

Fig. 4 Lymphocytic perivasculitis in the midbrain of a pig naturally infected with PPMV. Macrophages and lymphocytes surround small vessels. H&E

croscopically, lungs had moderate to severe bronchointerstitial pneumonia characterized by thickening of alveolar septa with infiltrating macrophages and swollen pneumocytes and endothelial cells. Alveolar capillaries were congested. Alveolar lumens were partially collapsed and contained proteinaceous fluid, fibrin, and variable numbers of macrophages, lymphocytes, sloughed pneumocytes, and neutrophils. Epithelium lining of some bronchioles was attenuated and focally disrupted; other bronchioles had intact hyperplastic epithelium. Bronchiolar lumens were filled with neutrophils. Peribronchiolar and perivascular lymphocytic cuffing was prominent. The brain from both pigs had mild but widespread perivasculitis and mild diffuse gliosis (Fig. 4).

Virus was isolated in Vero cells and characterized. PPMV was serologically and genetically related to bovine paramyxovirus 1. The origin of virus has not been identified but based on high sequence homology it is believed to have originated from cattle. There is no evidence as to its public health risk. However, the virus has been shown to replicate in HEp-2 human cell line producing syncytia and can possibly complicate differential diagnosis of Nipah virus infections as there is similarity in many of the gross and microscopic lesions induced by PPMV and Nipah virus.

Several other paramyxoviruses have been isolated from pigs around the world. These include paramyxovirus isolated from pigs with encephalomyelitis in Japan (Sasahara et al. 1954) and Canada (Greig et al. 1971). Lipkind et al. (1986) isolated paramyxovirus from nasal swabs of swine in Israel. PPMV related to Newcastle disease virus of chickens has been isolated from pigs in Germany (Groschup et al. 1993), and a parainfluenza virus type 2 has been isolated from a sow showing respiratory and reproductive syndrome-like symptoms in Netherlands (Heinen et al. 1998).

4 Arteriviruses

4.1 Porcine Reproductive and Respiratory Syndrome Virus

A new reproductive and respiratory disease characterized by stillborn, mummified and weak-born piglets and pneumonia in neonatal pigs appeared in 1987 in the USA (Hill 1990). The disease was shown to be caused by a new virus designated as porcine reproductive and respiratory syndrome virus (PRRSV) in the USA (Collins et al. 1992) and Lelystad virus (LV) in Europe (Wensvoort et al. 1991). The disease has now become one of the most important viral diseases in swine herds around the world. Salient features of PRRSV infection are persistent infections in swine, in utero infections, and transmission of virus through semen. A high mutation rate leading to high variability and recombination among PRRSV isolates has been reported. Although, no known public health risk has been presented, PRRSV presents a potential xenozoonoses risk due to its high mutation rate, the ability to recombine and the ability to cause persistent infections.

4.1.1 Virus Characteristics

PRRSV is a member of the genus *Arterivirus* under family *Arteriviridae* of the order *Nidovirales*. Other members of this virus family include lactate dehydrogenase-elevating virus of mice, equine arteritis virus, and simian hemorrhagic fever virus (Plagemann and Moenning 1992). The virions are enveloped and 40–65 nm in diameter, with spikes of 8–12 nm. Six structural proteins have been identified for LV prototype European strain of PRRSV, of which four are glycoproteins. The viral genome is a single-stranded genome of 15 kb with eight open reading frames (ORFs). ORF 1a and 1b code for RNA polymerase and proteases involved in replication, and ORFs 2–7 code for structural proteins. ORF 2–6 products are membrane proteins and the ORF 7 product is a nucleocapsid protein. ORFs 2, 3, and 4 of LV are of 30, 45–50, and 31–35 kDa, respectively. The ORF4 product is believed to contain an important immunogen as monoclonal antibodies to ORF4 have been shown to possess neutralizing activity. ORF7 codes for a nucleoprotein of ~12–15 kDa.

There is extensive antigenic, biological and genetic variability among PRRSV isolates. PRRSV isolates vary in virulence and their ability to cause respiratory disease (Halbur et al. 1995). There also is an extensive variability amongst PRRSV isolates in their ability to cause reproductive failure (Mengeling et al. 1996). Antigenic differences have also been detected between European LV and North American isolates. The American and European strains represent two separate serotypes as amino acid sequence homology in ORFs 2–7 among the US strains is over 90% where it is less than 60% with European strains (Meng et al. 1995). ORF 5 is most variable as amino acid homology amongst PRRSV isolates is 89–92% whereas it is 51–55% between US and European isolates (Meng et al. 1995).

4.1.2 Pathogenesis

The primary route of viral infection is oronasal; however, sexual transmission through semen has been reported. The primary site for PRRSV replication is in macrophages and dendritic cells in tonsils, upper respiratory tract and lungs. Virus replication has been detected in lymph nodes, spleen, thymus, bone marrow, heart and lungs. Viremia is detected 6–12 h after infection and persists for several weeks even in the presence of antibodies.

Clinical disease varies from subclinical infections in pigs on many farms to severe reproductive and respiratory disease on other farms. Virus strain, challenge dosage, and the age and breed of pigs influence the severity of the disease. Clinical disease can vary from subclinical infec-

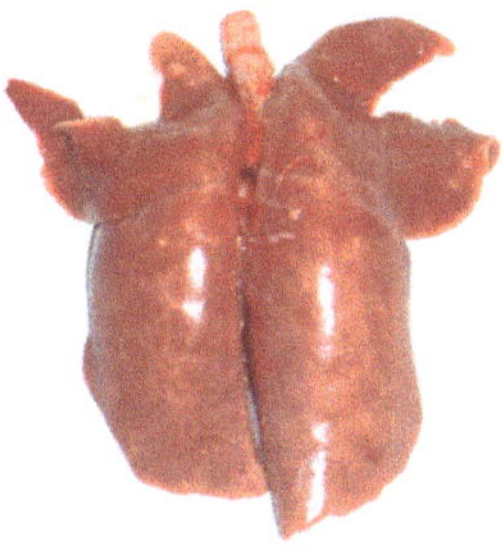

Fig. 5 Lung of a pig infected with highly virulent strain of PRRSV. Note severe consolidation of the lung giving it a rubbery appearance

tion to mild pneumonia for low virulence strains to severe pneumonia for virulent strains. Clinical signs in growing pigs include pyrexia, lethargy, anorexia, dyspnea, tachypnea, chemosis, conjunctivitis, and patchy dermal cyanosis.

Gross lesions can vary from none to pneumonia depending upon the virus strain and the age and genetic strain of the pigs (Halbur et al. 1995). Lungs have mild to severe multifocal involvement and with rubbery appearance and fail to collapse (Fig. 5). Evidence of pneumonia can be seen as early as 3 days after infection and are most severe by 7–10 days and are resolved by 14–28 days. Lymph node enlargement is a consistent gross lesion observed after 10 days of infection. However, microscopic lesions of interstitial pneumonia are common in infected pigs and are characterized by alveolar septal infiltration with mononuclear cells, type 2 pneumocyte hypertrophy and hyperplasia, and alveolar exudates consisting of mixed mononuclear cells and necrotic debris. Lymphohistiocytic encephalitis, myocarditis, and rhinitis may be observed with some strains.

PRRSV replicates in cells of the immune lineage and is believed to cause immunosuppression or at least immune modulation: infected animals are more susceptible to secondary infections. PRRSV infects and destroys pulmonary alveolar macrophages and pulmonary intravascular macrophages and causes decreased function of antigen presenting cells, dendritic cells and macrophages. Reduction in number of alveolar macrophages and circulating monocytes is postulated to be as a direct result of PRRSV-induced apoptosis, which has been detected in mononuclear cells and in the lung and lymphoid tissues of PRRSV-infected cells (Sirinarumitr et al. 1998). PRRSV has also been shown to be immunosuppressive as in utero PRRSV-infected pigs that are born viremic have been

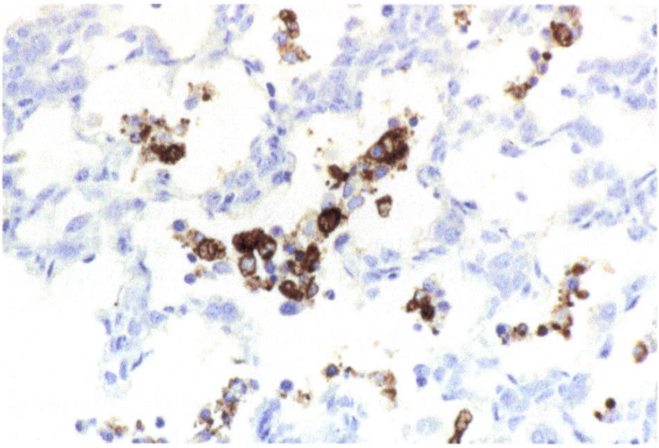

Fig. 6 Immunohistochemical stain of lung from a pig infected with PRRSV. Antigen is seen as a *brown color* within the mononuclear cells

shown to be more susceptible to *Streptococcus suis* infection (Feng et al. 2001).

Antibodies have been shown to be both beneficial and deleterious. Passively acquired antibodies are protective against PRRSV infection. However, antibody dependent enhancement of virus replication has been demonstrated in vitro and is postulated to play a role in PRRSV pathogenesis (Yoon et al. 1996).

4.1.3
Diagnosis

PRRSV can be isolated in primary alveolar macrophage cultures, MA-104 cell lines, and several other proprietary cell lines (Benfield et al. 1992; Meng et al. 1996). Virus is cytolytic for primary alveolar macrophage cultures and macrophage cultures are most susceptible for virus isolation. Viral antigens in cell cultures and tissues can be detected by immunofluorescence (Yoon et al. 1992) and immunohistochemistry (Fig. 6; Halbur et al. 1994). Monoclonal antibodies SDOW 12 and 17 detect a conserved epitope on nucleoprotein of PRRSV and LV (Nelson et al. 1993). These monoclonal antibodies have been very useful in the detection of PRRSV in tissues of infected animals using immunohistochemistry (Halbur et al. 1994). Viral nucleic acid can be detected by in situ hybridization (Haynes et al. 1997) and PCR (Christopher-Hennings et al. 1995). Virus strains can be differentiated by restriction endonuclease fingerprinting (Wesley et al. 1996). Fluorescent antibody, immunoperoxidase, virus neutralization tests and ELISA are available to detect antibodies. Detectable serum antibodies appear 6–10 days after infection, peak by 4–10 weeks and persist for 5–10 months.

4.1.4 Control and Eradication

PRRSV infections are widespread in swine herds around the world. The source of the virus into the herd is usually new genetic stock. PRRSV is spread either via sexual transmission through semen causing in utero infection of fetuses or through direct contact with pigs that are shedding virus. PRRSV persists in pigs for as long as 157 days (Wills et al. 1997). Virus is shed in feces for over 35 days, urine for 14 days, and saliva for 42 days. Infectious PRRSV has also been detected in semen for 43 days after infection and viral nucleic acid has been detected by PCR in semen for as long as 92 days. A number of management practices such as partial depopulation, segregated early weaning, and multi-site production strategies have been attempted to limit the spread of virus. These methods minimize the duration and severity of the PRRSV-associated disease. However, the best way to control PRRS is to keep PRRSV out of negative herds. This can be accomplished by strict biosecurity practices and assuring that the incoming seed stock is of known PRRSV-free status. PRRSV-free pigs can also be derived by Cesarean section as long as sows are immune to minimize in utero infection of fetuses.

4.1.5 Xenozoonoses

There is no evidence to date of public health risk from PRRSV. Furthermore, we have attempted to infect a large number of human cell lines in vitro with PRRSV but have been unable to show replication. However, additional studies are warranted as PRRSV has been shown to replicate in vitro in nonhuman primate cells. Furthermore, an arterivirus-associated disease, simian hemorrhagic fever, has been observed in monkeys. PRRSV genome is also fairly unstable with a high mutation rate and a vaccine strain has been suspected to have reverted to the wild-type pathogenic strain in Denmark (Botner et al. 1997; Nielsen et al. 2001).

Recombination among PRRSV (van-Vugt-Joke et al. 2001) has also been demonstrated and there is a concern that new strains of PRRSV may emerge through recombination that may adapt in humans through xenotransplantation. Because of these concerns additional studies are warranted to assess xenozoonoses risk of PRRSV.

5 Japanese Encephalomyelitis Virus

Japanese encephalitis (JE) is a mosquito-borne viral disease of animals and humans. In swine, the virus causes lesions in the CNS in young pigs and various forms of reproductive failures in pregnant sows. In other animals, infection is usually subclinical. Geographic distribution of the disease is restricted to Southeast Asia.

5.1 Virus Characteristics

JE virus (JEV) is classified in the genus *Flavivirus* of the family *Flaviviridae*. The virus is spherical, about 40 nm in diameter, enveloped, and it contains single-stranded RNA with an icosahedral capsid. There are three structural and several nonstructural proteins. The structural proteins are envelope glycoprotein E (54 kDa), nonglycosylated envelope protein M (8 kDa), capsid protein C (14 kDa). The oligonucleotide fingerprinting technique (Hori et al. 1986) reveals that mutations of JEV are present in strains that were isolated years apart in Japan and Thailand. JEV is unstable in the environment and easily inactivated by disinfectants. The virus is sensitive to ether, chloroform, and sodium desoxycholate, and also to proteolytic or lipolytic enzymes. It is readily inactivated at 56°C after 30 min and has an optimal pH stability of 8.5. JEV replicates well and produces a cytopathic effect in a wide range of host cell culture systems. Cells originating from mosquitoes also are susceptible.

5.2 Pathogenesis

Pigs become infected with JEV via the bites of mosquitoes carrying the virus. Infected pigs develop viremia that persists for 1–6 days. After the initial viremia, the virus disseminates to vascular tissues such as the liver, spleen and muscle. The virus enters the CNS via cerebrospinal fluid, endothelial cells, macrophage, lymphocyte infection, or a hematogenous route. In humans and mice, JEV infects and destroys neurons selectively, mostly in areas of the brain stem, thalamus, basal ganglion, and lower layer of cortex. In mosquitoes, JEV infection is noncytopathic.

Transplacental infection of JEV has been reported in pigs (Shimizu et al. 1954). In pregnant pigs, fetuses may become infected during the viremic period. Experimentally, after intravenous infection of pregnant sows with JEV, virus could be recovered from fetuses as early as 7 days post infection. In some pigs, the virus fails to cross the placenta. Successful transplacental infection may depend on the time of gestation at which the dam was infected or on the strain of virus. When infection of pregnant dams takes place in the mid-third of gestation, transplacental infection and pathogenic effects are more obvious. Field observations show that fetal death and mummification have been associated with JEV infection of dams between 40 and 60 days of gestation; fetuses from gilts infected after 85 days gestation were little affected.

No major gross lesions have been found in pigs infected with JEV. However, various abnormalities have been observed in litters from sows infected with the virus during pregnancy. Stillborn or weak neonatal piglets may show hydrocephalus, subcutaneous edema, hydrothorax, ascites, petechial hemorrhages on serous membranes, congestion of lymph nodes, necrotic foci in liver and spleen, and congested meninges or spinal cord. Cerebellar hypoplasia and spinal hypomyelinogenesis have also been described (Morimoto 1969).

Significant microscopic lesions in affected piglets or stillborn pigs have been restricted to the CNS. Most CNS lesions, mainly involving the cortex, basal ganglion, brain stem, and spinal cord, occur in young pigs. Perivascular cuffing and scattered neuronal degeneration and necrosis are found in the cerebrum and cerebellum in pigs. Neuronal degeneration is prominent in the gray matter and Purkinje layers.

Pathologic changes in the testes in association with JEV infection were described (Ogasa et al. 1977). In naturally affected boars, a large amount of mucous fluid was observed in the cavity tunica vaginalis, as well as fibrous thickening along the edge of the epididymis and the visceral layer of the tunica vaginalis. Microscopically, such testicles showed edema and inflammatory changes, with cellular infiltrations in the interstitial tissue of the epididymis and tunica vaginalis. Cell infiltration and hemorrhage were also evident in the interstitial tissue of the testes.

5.3 Diagnosis

Diagnosis of JEV infection has been based on isolation of the virus from fetuses and infected pigs. Isolation of the virus can be performed by intracerebral inoculation of brain extracts into suckling mice between 1 and 5 days of age. Signs of CNS disturbance or death follow between 4 and 14 days post inoculation, and virus in mouse brain tissue can readily be identified by in vivo neutralization tests in suckling mice or in cell culture. The commonly used cell cultures are derived from hamster, pig kidney, and mosquito, in all of which the virus causes a cytopathic effect. Detection of viral antigen in infected tissues such as brains, placenta and mummified fetuses has also been diagnostically important. Methods such as avidin-biotin staining and fluorescent antibody staining have been used to detect JE viral antigen in formalin-fixed tissues. Several serologic tests are available that detect antibody titers of JEV infection in pig serum such as the HI test, ELISA, antigen biotin-labeled ELISA, single radial hemolysin, and serum neutralization technique. An ELISA to detect IgM antibodies to JEV has been developed (Burke et al. 1985). Detection of cerebral spinal fluid IgM using ELISA diagnostic kits has been used in humans. However, in an area where vaccination is routine, paired serum samples should be considered in the serology. The presence of the antibody in fetuses is of diagnostic value.

5.4 Control and Eradication

Infection with JEV in nature is maintained cyclically, involving vector mosquitoes (*Culex tritaeniorhynchus*), birds, and mammals. A correlation between infection in pigs and infection in humans is apparent, with evidence indicating that swine play an important role in the build-up of the virus within a population. In enzootic zones, pigs are favored feeding sources for mosquitoes. Consistent development of viremia in susceptible pigs ensures a continued supply of infected mosquitoes. However, epidemiologic patterns could differ among areas of Southeast Asia, as activity for the vector mosquito was modified by differing climatic conditions (Takashima et al. 1988). Other animals and different mosquito species could alter infection cycles and have been factors involved in the transmission of JEV. Chickens and wild birds, especially herons and egrets, have been able to maintain the virus.

Population density of susceptible animals for JEV is the most important predisposing factor. In countries within the temperate zone, the mosquito season starts in late spring and the pig–mosquito cycle becomes evident shortly afterward. During this time the pig population contains a high proportion of susceptible breeding pigs, whose passive immunity has waned during the winter. Given these conditions, high concentration of the virus can be built up and maintained in the pig population. This buildup will not be as prevalent in the tropical countries of Southeast Asia, where the mosquito–pig cycle may continue throughout the year.

The treatment of JE in humans with human recombinant interferon-α has shown some satisfactory results. For swine, breaking the infectious cycle in this mosquito-borne disease is an important step. However, because insect control is impractical, immunizing breeding pigs with JEV vaccine is widely applied as a control and preventive measure. Live-attenuated vaccines have been developed for the prevention of JE in pigs and are being used successfully in the field (Hsu et al. 1972; Fujisaki et al. 1975). Inactivated vaccines have proved to be less efficient. It is recommended that attenuated vaccines be given to young gilts or boars twice at an interval of 2–3 weeks before the start of the mosquito season. The live virus vaccines are not recommended for use in pregnant pigs.

5.5 Xenozoonoses

JE is one of the common mosquito-borne diseases of the human CNS, with epidemics having been recorded in several Southeast Asian countries. Pigs are considered the most important natural amplifying animal for the virus. Episodes of human infection occur annually during the mosquito season. Disease due to JEV in most people is subclinical or mild, but fatal encephalitis develops in some children. It should be recognized that tissue suspected of being infected with JEV must be handled with care, because the virus is heat labile and pathogenic to humans. No report is available on JEV infection in humans from pork. Survival of the virus in the environment is not expected because it is highly temperature sensitive, but human infection can occur during the mosquito season. Inactivated vaccines are available for humans, and are highly recommended for susceptible populations.

6 Encephalomyocarditis Virus

Encephalomyocarditis virus (EMCV) naturally infects rodents and a wide range of vertebrate species. The host range includes chimpanzees, monkeys, elephants, lions, squirrels, mongooses, raccoons and pigs. Rats and mice are believed to be the principal reservoir of the virus. Many rodents are susceptible to experimental infection, showing high levels of virus in their tissues, and infected rodents excrete virus in their feces and urine. The virus has been isolated from dried feces and from intestines of rats or mice captured on farms where swine disease had previously occurred (Gainer 1967; Acland and Littlejohns 1975). Although the virus has been isolated from mosquitoes caught in Africa, Brazil and USA, and from ticks in India, there is no evidence that natural EMCV infection in swine is vector-borne.

Swine is the domestic animal most susceptible to clinical disease by EMCV infection. EMCV infection in pigs was first reported in Panama in 1960, and subsequently in Florida between 1960 and 1966, and in Australia in 1970. The virus causes high mortality in young pigs and reproductive failures in breeding females. Sudden deaths of young pigs due to myocardial failure are common on infected farms, and myocarditis and encephalitis are evident in affected piglets. Clinical problems in swine are mostly limited to tropical areas, and endemic infection with significant economic losses has been identified in certain areas of tropical countries. The disease also has been observed in different zoo animals.

6.1 Virus Characteristics

The virus is classified as genus *Cardiovirus* of the family *Picornaviridae*. Many properties of EMCV are shared by other picornaviruses. The virus is ether-resistant and stable over a wide pH range. It is inactivated at 60°C for 30 min, but some strains have shown a marked thermal stability. EMCV replicates well in cell cultures originating from several animal species. The virus also replicates in mice and chicken embryos and is pathogenic to different laboratory animal hosts. EMCV has hemagglutinating ability with erythrocytes of guinea pig, rat, horse and sheep, and most strains require KCl–borate buffered solution for an optimal hemagglutination reaction. The EMCV virions contain a single strand of RNA of molecular weight 2.6×10^6 Da, which comprises 31% of the virion mass and is enclosed in a protein capsid shell. The viral proteins show four non-identical polypeptide bands on SDS–polyacrylamide gel electrophoresis.

6.2 Pathogenesis

The natural infection of swine most probably occurs by the oral route. Following experimental oral infection in piglets, viremia was demonstrated as early as 2 days post inoculation (dpi) and persisted for 2– days. Virus was present in the feces for as long as 9 days following oral administration. The highest virus titers were recovered from heart tissues. Liver, pancreas and kidney contained virus, usually at a greater concentration than blood. Animals that survived acute disease produced anti-EMCV antibodies. The course of infection in swine appears to be influenced by virus strain, viral dose, history and level of viral passage and susceptibility of the individual animal.

Following intramuscular infection of pregnant sows, a transplacental infection with fetal deaths was observed (Love and Grewal 1986). Infected and dead fetuses showed myocardial lesions varying from multiple small foci to large diffuse patches. Some difficulty in producing experimental reproductive disease in pregnant sows was observed with a US isolate. However, transplacental infection was successful when the virus was passaged in young pigs, rather than cell culture, before inoculation (Christianson et al. 1992). Fetal deaths following infection in sows appear to occur as early as 2 weeks post infection. It is not known whether all EMCV strains can cause both the typical myocarditis observed in young pigs and reproductive failure in breeding pigs. Pathogenic variability in swine fetuses by different EMCV isolates has been reported (Kim et al. 1989).

Young pigs dying in the acute phase may show no gross lesions, but myocardial lesions are common in infected pigs. The heart is usually enlarged, with visible yellowish or white necrotic foci (2–15 mm in diameter). The lesions are most commonly observed on the epicardium of the right ventricle. Infected fetuses become mummified in various sizes depending on the stage of infection and may be hemorrhagic, edematous or apparently normal. The myocardial lesions may be seen in some infected fetuses but it would be difficult to observe under field conditions.

Histopathologically, the most significant finding in young pigs is myocarditis with focal or diffuse accumulation of mononuclear cells, vascular congestion, edema and degeneration of the myocardial fibers with necrosis. Mineralization of necrotic heart muscle is common. Congestion with meningitis, perivascular infiltration with mononuclear cells and some neuronal degeneration may be observed in the brain. Nonsuppurative encephalitis and myocarditis were also observed in swine fetuses with natural EMCV infection.

6.3 Diagnosis

High neonatal mortality with or without a history of reproductive failure is a useful tip in the diagnosis. Dyspnea manifested as rapid abdominal breathing due to heart failure may be observed in young infected pigs. Gross lesions of white necrotic areas in the heart muscle are characteristic of EMCV infection, although such lesions also resemble those caused by vitamin E and selenium deficiency.

A definitive diagnosis should be based on virus isolation, for which heart is the best tissue. Baby hamster kidney (BHK-21), HeLa or Vero cell lines are commonly used for virus isolation. Virus isolation is usually successful from pigs during the acute phase. Microscopically, myocarditis of varying stages with infiltration of mononuclear cells along with nonsuppurative encephalitis is indicative of EMCV infection. Viral nucleic acid can be detected by nucleic acid probes (Meng et al. 1993). Detection of antibody specific to EMCV from stillborn pigs is particularly significant for fetal infection (Joo et al. 1988; Kim et al. 1989).

6.4 Control and Eradication

An important source for swine infection appears to be feed or water contaminated with virus by rats, other rodents or diseased carcasses. The mode of virus transmission is not clear, but rodent-to-pig transmission is probably common. Several outbreaks in Australia were found to be closely associated with rat and mouse plagues (Acland and Littlejohns 1975). Pig-to-pig transmission has been questioned because sentinel pigs failed to become infected after contact with experimentally infected and sick pigs (Littlejohns and Acland 1975). However, the role of the infected pigs in natural transmission, either directly or indirectly, cannot be excluded, since infected pigs have been shown to excrete the virus at least for a short period.

An inactivated vaccine for EMCV infection in swine is commercially available. The vaccine appears to be effective, since high humoral immunity is detected in vaccinated pigs. On pig farms, it is important to control rodents or minimize their contact with pigs either directly or indirectly via contamination of feed or water. The virus can be inactivated in water using common disinfectants.

6.5 Xenozoonoses

Evidence for human infection with EMCV has been demonstrated by detection of the specific antibodies in human populations (Tesh 1978). However, there is no report that EMCV causes human heart disease.

7 Porcine Circovirus

Porcine circovirus (PCV) was first isolated in 1974 as a contaminant of a porcine kidney cell line (Tischer et al. 1974) and today has emerged as one of the major pathogens of swine. It is ubiquitous in swine populations around the world and is associated with a debilitating disease referred to as post weaning multisystemic wasting syndrome (PMWS). PCV has also been incriminated in porcine dermatitis nephropathy syndrome (PDNS) and in congenital tremors in swine.

7.1 Viral Characteristics

PCV is a member of the genus *Circovirus* in the family *Circoviridae*. The virus is characterized by its nonenveloped, icosahedral particle and a unique circular single-stranded genomic DNA. Other members of this genus include beak and feather disease virus, and possibly pigeon circovirus and goose circovirus. A second genus, *Gyrovirus*, is comprised of one member, chicken anemia virus. A circovirus-like virus, designated as TT virus, has been identified in humans (Miyata et al. 1999). PCV is 17 nm in diameter as detected under the electron microscope. PCV has been divided into two types based on antigenic and genetic differences. The cell culture contaminant PCV-PK-15 has been designated as PCV type 1 (PCV1) and is avirulent. The virulent PCV associated with PMWS has been referred to as PCV2. The genome of the two PCV types is similar and consists of a 1,700 nucleotide single-stranded circular DNA. Homology among isolates within the same type is 95%–99%, while it is less than 80% among viruses of different types (Fenaux et al. 2000). The viral genome has two major open reading frames (ORFs) located in opposite orientations: ORF1 is involved in the replication of the virus genome and is relatively conserved among both types of PCV with 83% nucleotide homology between two types. The ORF2 is much more variable between the two types, with 67% nucleotide homology between two types (Morozov et al. 1998). One major structural protein encoded by ORF2 of 36 kDa in PCV-1 (Tischer et al. 1982) and 30 kDa in PCV-2 was identified (Nawagitgul et al. 2000).

The virion is highly resistant to a pH as low as 3.0 and chloroform treatment, and it is stable after exposure at 56°C and 70°C for a minimum of 15 min (Allan et al. 1994). PCV can replicate in both primary cells and continuous cell lines derived from pig tissues, as well as in Vero cells (Allan et al. 1994). It is commonly propagated in PK-15 cells. For replication, PCV requires cellular enzymes expressed during the S phase of the cell cycle. Replication of PCV is enhanced by treatment of infected cell cultures with 300 mM d-glucosamine for 40–60 min at 4–6 h post infection (Tischer et al. 1987). PCV lacks hemagglutination activity. The in vitro effectiveness of various disinfectants has been reported (Royer et al. 2001).

7.2 Pathogenesis

PMWS is characterized clinically by progressive dyspnea and emaciation in 6–18-week-old pigs. Histologic lesions consist of lymphohistiocytic to granulomatous inflammatory cell infiltrates in multiple tissues, most frequently in the lung, liver, kidney, and lymphoid organs (Fig. 7) (Harding and Clark 1997; Sorden 2000). The most characteristic lesion is deple-

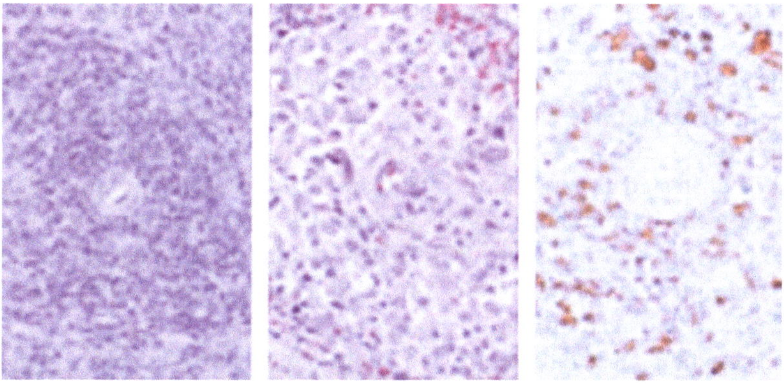

Fig. 7 Sections of spleen from a normal (*left*) and that from a PCV-infected pig with PMWS (*middle* and *right*). Sections were stained with H&E (*left* and *middle*) and or by immunohistochemistry (*right*). Note periarteriolar lymphoid sheath is present in normal porcine spleen (*left*) where as periarteriolar lymphocytes are replaced by macrophages in spleen of a pig with PMWS (*middle*). PCV2 antigen (*brown color*) is abundant in periarteriolar macrophages in pig with PMWS

tion of lymphoid tissues; in some cases, these tissues contain macrophages with intracytoplasmic clusters of basophilic inclusion bodies that ultrastructurally correspond to arrays of PCV particles (Kennedy et al. 2000). PCV2 antigen and nucleic acid are consistently demonstrable in lesions of pigs with PMWS by immunohistochemistry (Sorden et al. 1999) and in situ hybridization (Sirinarumitr et al. 2000).

Results of experimental inoculation of pigs with PCV2 have been highly variable. Gnotobiotic and less than 4-week-old colostrum-deprived pigs have in general developed more severe lesions and clinical disease than conventional pigs. For example, Bolin et al. (2001) inoculated 20–25- day-old Caesarian-delivered, colostrum-deprived (CDCD) pigs intranasally and subcutaneously with a Canadian PCV2 isolate and reproduced severe clinical disease and most of the characteristic gross and microscopic lesions associated with PMWS. This group also demonstrated PCV2 DNA in tissues from experimentally infected pigs at 125 days post inoculation, confirming persistent infection by PCV2. Inoculation of SPF or conventional pigs has induced minimal clinical signs and only mild to moderate lesions. Recently (Fenaux et al. 2002) 4-week-old SPF pigs were inoculated with cloned PCV2 plasmid DNA. Pigs developed mild respiratory disease, but wasting was not observed during the 35 day duration of the study; gross and microscopic lesions in lymphoid tissues and lungs were consistent with PMWS.

Harms et al. (2001) experimentally inoculated 3-week-old CDCD piglets with PCV2, and the antigens were detected in tissues by immunohistochemistry as early as 7 dpi. High numbers of PCV2 positive cells were found in all tested organs of all pigs from 14 to 28 dpi. The amount of PCV2 antigens in lymphoid organs and tissues was proportionate to the degree of lymphoid depletion. PCV2 DNA was detected in serum, urine, and nasal and rectal swabs from 7 to 49 dpi. Antibodies to PCV2 were first detected at 21–28 dpi.

Experimental inoculation of 1-day-old colostrum-deprived piglets (Allan et al. 2000) and weaned SPF pigs (Magar et al. 2000) demonstrated large amounts of PCV2 antigens in various tissues around 20–26 dpi. Immunofluorescent assay of frozen tissue sections demonstrated PCV2 in trachea, lung, thymus, spleen, lymph nodes, salivary gland, liver, kidney, adrenal gland, pancreas, cecum, colon and small intestine (Allan et al. 2000). PCV2 antigens were detected predominantly in the cytoplasm of cells of monocyte/macrophage lineage of most organs and with lower frequency in the nucleus of macrophages and epithelial cells (Harms et al. 2001; Magar et al. 2000). However, labeling of hepatocyte nuclei was common.

The oronasal route is believed to be the portal of entry for PCV2. In experimentally inoculated pigs (Allan et al. 1995; Harms et al. 2001; Krakowka et al. 2000; Magar et al. 2000), PCV2 antigen and/or nucleic acid are detectable in a wide variety of tissues, including lung, liver, kidney, and intestinal tract, but PCV2 is most consistently found in lymphoid tissues, including tonsil, lymph nodes, spleen, and Payer's patch (Harms et al. 2001). The predominant cell type containing PCV2 in tissues of experimentally- and naturally-infected pigs is the monocyte/macrophage. PCV2 antigen and nucleic acid have also been detected in lymphocytes and a variety of epithelial cells. Antigens of PCV2 have been detected within bronchial and bronchiolar epithelial cells as well as enterocytes lining the tip of intestinal villi by immunohistochemistry, suggesting that these cell types are sites of replication and possibly the ports of entry of the virus.

PCV2-induced PMWS is exacerbated by viral co-infections and immune stimulation. In one experiment, lymphoid tissue homogenates from pigs with PMWS that induced PMWS in gnotobiotic swine were found to contain porcine parvovirus (PPV). Subsequent studies demonstrated that co-infected pigs developed more severe clinical disease and lesions. Synergism between PCV2 and PRRSV has also been demonstrated: among 3- week-old colostrum-deprived pigs, there was moderate respiratory disease but no mortality in pigs inoculated with PRRSV, lethargy, sporadic icterus and 26% mortality in pigs inoculated with PCV2 alone, and severe lethargy and respiratory disease and 100% mortality in pigs inoculated with both PRRSV and PCV2 (Harms et al. 2001). These experimental findings are highly consistent with what is observed in field cases of PMWS; both PRRSV and PCV2 infection are demonstrated in over half of the cases of PMWS diagnosed at the Iowa State University Veterinary Diagnostic Laboratory. There is also evidence that immunization with an irrelevant antigen may potentiate the development of PWMS. Recently, Krakowka et al. (2001) inoculated gnotobiotic pigs with PCV2 and injected them with keyhole limpet hemocyanin in Freund's incomplete adjuvant. Immunized pigs developed moderate to severe PMWS whereas none of the PCV2-infected but nonimmunized pigs developed PMWS.

PCV2 has been associated with PDNS characterized by multifocal cutaneous infarction, necrotizing (leukocytoclastic) vasculitis in dermal, subcutaneous, renal, and other blood vessels, and fibrinous/necrotizing glomerulonephritis. Most affected pigs are infected with PCV2, and many have lymphoid depletion and other lesions characteristic of PMWS. While necrotizing vasculitis and glomerulonephritis are consistent with type III hypersensitivity response (mediated by deposition of immune complexes within vessel walls), this has not been proven to be the mechanism underlying PDNS (Allan and Ellis, 2000).

PCV has also been incriminated in congenital tremors, a CNS disease that is characterized by myelin deficiency and whole body tremors that appear shortly after birth. Severity of tremors varies from severe to mild and piglets die of starvation as they are unable to suckle. The disease has been reproduced by inoculation of pregnant sows with cell-free brain extracts from pigs with congenital tremors as well as cell culture propagated virus. All samples tested were PCV2 positive. Recently, in situ hybridization demonstrated PCV2 in neurons in the brains of pigs with congenital tremors (Stevenson et al. 2001).

Recently, PCV2 was shown to be vertically transmitted and involved reproductive failure. In 1999, a new sow facility in Canada was confronted with late-term abortion and farrowing of both stillborn and mummified piglets (West et al. 1999). Autopsy examination of a fetus showed that the ventricles of the heart were dilated, the liver was enlarged and firm, and hydrothorax and ascites were observed. Microscopic lesions included myocardial degeneration with mild fibrosis and diffuse infiltration of lymphocytes and macrophages. Copious amounts of PCV2 antigens were detected in both the nucleus and cytoplasm of cells throughout the myocardium. Livers of multiple fetuses contained PCV2 antigens, primarily in the sinusoid endothelial and Kupffer cells. There are other reports of PCV2-associated reproductive failure (Josephson and Charbonneau 2001). Experimental inoculation studies support the heart as a primary site of PCV2 replication in fetuses. Both PCV1 and PCV2 have been detected in boar semen, supporting the possible role of PCV2 in reproductive disorders (Larochelle et al. 2000).

7.3 Diagnosis

PCV associated PMWS should be suspected if clinical signs of wasting are observed along with histological lesions of lymphoid depletion and/or lymphohistiocytic to granulomatous inflammation in any organs. Presence of viral antigen or nucleic acids confirms the role of PCV. Viral antigens can be detected by Immunofluorescent assay in frozen sections (Allan et al. 1999, 2000; Kennedy et al. 2000) or by immunohistochemistry (Fig. 7) (Sorden et al. 1999) in formalin-fixed, paraffin-embedded tissues. An in situ hybridization technique has been developed to detect PCV2 nucleic acids in histological lesions (Sirinarumitr et al. 2000). PCV2 nucleic acids can also be detected by PCR: several PCR applications have been reported for the detection of PCV or for differentiating PCV types 1 and 2 or typing of PCV, including standard PCR (Larochelle et al. 1999), multiplex PCR for typing PCV1 and PCV2 (Larochelle et al. 1999) combination of PCR and restriction fragment length polymorphism (Hamel et al. 1998), quantitative and competitive PCR for the detection of PCV DNA in serum (Liu et al. 2000), PCR to detect PCV2 in formalin-fixed, paraffin-embedded tissues (Kim et al. 2001) and nested PCR (Larochelle et al. 2000) or combined multiplex and nested PCR for the detection of PCV2 in semen (Kim et al. 2001).

PCV is isolated by inoculating primary porcine kidney cell cultures or the porcine kidney cell line PK-15 (lines which are free of contaminating PCV). Virus replicates in nucleus and viral antigen can be observed in cytoplasm and nucleus by immunofluorescence.

The most commonly used methods to detect PCV2 antibodies are Immunofluorescent and immunoperoxidase monolayer assays (Allan et al. 1999; Dulac and Afshar 1989; Ellis et al. 1998). A recombinant ORF2-based indirect ELISA (Nawagitgul et al. 2002), and synthetic peptide-based ELISA (Walker et al. 2000), which are as sensitive and specific, have been developed.

7.4
Control and Eradication

PCV is ubiquitous in swine herds around the world. It is excreted in oronasal secretions and feces, which serve as the main source of swine infections. In utero infection of swine fetuses is also common as PCV infection has been detected in newborn pigs as well as CDCD pigs. Boars also serve as a source of PCV infection. Passively acquired antibodies are protective and PCV-free pigs have been obtained from PCV-immune sows by isolating them away from their mothers during the first 4 weeks of life and raising them in a PCV-free environment.

7.5
Xenozoonoses

Mixed results have been reported as to the evidence for PCV infections in humans. Two groups of researchers did not detect any antibodies in serum samples from the general human population (Allan et al. 2000) nor did veterinarians working with PMWS affected pigs (Ellis et al. 2000). In contrast, Tischer et al. (1995) found antibodies to PCV in 30.2% of samples from hospitalized patients with fever of unknown etiology. PCV has also been shown to infect human cell lines with limited to no replication (Allan et al. 1994). We have attempted to infect several established human cell lines with PCV2 unsuccessfully. We believe that PCV2 should be considered a potential, although a low, risk as it has been shown to produce persistent infections, to be vertically transmitted and some variability has been discovered. Furthermore, a circovirus-like virus (TT Virus) has been detected in humans, the significance of which is not known.

8 Herpesviruses

Three types of herpesviruses are prevalent in swine: Pseudorabies rabies virus (PRV), also known as Aujeskey's disease virus, porcine cytomegalovirus, and porcine lymphotropic herpesvirus. Of these PRV has been most studied but all three viruses are common in swine and cause persistent infections and represent a risk of xenozoonoses.

8.1 Pseudorabies Virus

Pseudorabies virus infections are common in swine around the world. The salient features of pseudorabies virus are its ability to cause latent infection in sensory ganglia of the nervous system and in lymphoid tissue of the tonsils. Pigs are the only natural host; however, pseudorabies virus infects cattle, sheep, goats, and cats, producing neurological clinical disease that is often fatal (Kluge et al. 1992).

8.1.1 Virus Characteristics

Pseudorabies virus is a member of the *Alphaherpesvirinae* subfamily under the family *Herpesviridae*. Virions are enveloped, 150–180 nm in diameter, and contain a 150-kb double-stranded DNA genome. The virus is well conserved with a single serotype; however, genetic differences have been observed (Paul et al. 1982). Major viral envelope proteins are gB, gC, gD, gE, gI, and gG. Virus is very labile and is sensitive to pH, temperature and common disinfectants.

8.1.2 Pathogenesis

In pigs, the outcome of PRV infection varies from subclinical infection to severe respiratory disease, neurological disease, and/or abortions depending upon the strain of PRV, the challenge dose, and the age of the pigs at the time of infection. Neonatal seronegative pigs are most susceptible and suffer from severe respiratory disease with high mortality. Pigs show clinical signs of respiratory disease and CNS signs, possibly with respiratory distress. Nursery and grow-finish pigs have fever and anorexia. Infected pigs may exhibit sneezing, coughing, and nasal discharge. In adult pigs, infections are usually subclinical with inappetance and transient fever. Abortions are common in pregnant swine. Gross lesions include none to fibrinonecrotic rhinitis, laryngitis, tracheitis, swollen and hemorrhagic lymph nodes of the upper respiratory tract, and mild keratoconjunctivitis. Microscopic lesions include pulmonary congestion with multiple foci of necrosis and hemorrhage involving septa and airways. Eosinophilic intranuclear inclusion bodies in focal necrotic areas may be detected. Maternal antibodies are protective; however, high doses of virus can overcome low maternal antibodies.

8.1.3 Diagnosis

Pseudorabies should be suspected in neonatal pigs with respiratory disease or in cases of abortions in sows. Microscopic evidence of viral encephalitis along with multifocal necrotizing pneumonia is further suggestive of PRV infection. Confirmation of the presence of PRV antigen by fluorescent antibody tests in frozen sections of tonsils, brainstem, lung or trachea can be used to confirm pseudorabies. PRV infection may also be confirmed by isolation of virus from brain, spleen or lungs. Viral isolates can be differentiated by restriction endonuclease analysis (Paul et al. 1982). Serologic evidence for PRV infection can be obtained by virus neutralization or ELISA. Differential ELISA for the differentiation of vaccinated from infected animals are commercially available.

8.1.4 Eradication and Control

PRV is shed in oronasal secretions. Virus transmission occurs via air, water, and contaminated fomites and infected pigs. The virus causes latent infections, which can be reactivated by stress. The ability of PRV to cause latent infection complicates its eradication and control. Efforts are underway in the USA and a number of other countries to eradicate pseudorabies virus. The availability of gene-deleted vaccines and companion diagnostic tests to differentiate vaccinated from infected animals have made eradication of pseudorabies a possibility. The approaches used for eradication include vaccination of pigs with gene-deleted vaccines and culling of infected animals.

8.1.5 Xenozoonoses

PRV virus has a broad host range and infects pigs, cattle, sheep, goats, cats and horses. Wild animals including raccoon, opossum, rat, and mouse also are susceptible. Nonhuman primates, such as chimpanzees and apes, are resistant to PRV infection whereas marmosets and rhesus monkeys are susceptible. Limited human infection studies have been conducted. In 1987, serologic evidence for PRV infection was observed in three humans with low level seroconversion after exposure to cats. Anusz et al. (1992) described six of seven workers in contact with cattle developing pruritus on their hands, which spread to their shoulders and backs. Herpesviruses also have been shown to recombine (Umene et al. 1999). Although unlikely, the recombination of swine herpesviruses with human herpesviruses could potentially lead to a new virus with broad host specificity potentially causing a public health crisis.

8.2 Porcine Lymphotropic Herpesvirus

Porcine lymphotropic herpesvirus (PLHV) is a recently identified gamma-herpesvirus in swine. The first evidence for the existence of a new porcine lymphotropic herpesvirus was obtained by Ehlers et al. (1999). These investigators used PCR with degenerate primers representing conserved regions of the herpesvirus DNA polymerase gene to screen peripheral blood mononuclear cells (PBMC), spleens, lungs, kidneys and livers of pigs from Germany and Spain. Specific PCR fragments were amplified from several splenic and PBMC samples. Sequence analysis of PCR fragments revealed two closely related gamma-herpesviruses (PLHV-1 and PLHV-2) with a high homology with the DNA polymerase gene of herpesviruses of the oncogenic subfamily *Gammaherpesvirinae*. In a further study conducted by the same group (Ulrich et al. 1999), a 4.6-kb fragment of the genome of both PLHV-1 and PLHV-2 viruses was sequenced. The region sequenced included the 3'-end of glycoprotein B gene, the entire DNA polymerase gene and downstream ORF. Sequence comparison showed 95% amino acid identity between PLHV-1 and

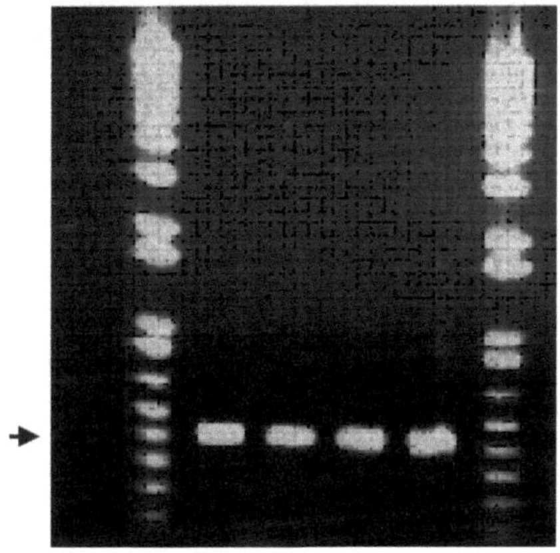

Fig. 8 Detection of PLHV by PCR in spleen of pigs. Note PLHV PCR-amplified DNA fragment of 437 bp in *lanes 2–5*. A similar band was not detected in DNA from normal spleen (*lane 1*). *Lane M* represents 1 kb molecular weight standards. All four samples were positive for PLHV by PCR

PLHV-2 DNA polymerase genes. Phylogenetic analysis showed that DNA polymerase genes of PLHV form separate clusters with other members of the *Gammaherpesvirinae* subfamily, including Epstein–Barr virus, equine herpesvirus 2, *Herpesvirus saimiri*, rhesus monkey rhadinovirus, human herpesvirus 8 associated with Kaposi's sarcoma, and murine gamma-herpesvirus 68. Another ORF located downstream of the DNA polymerase gene also was characterized. Overall, the characterized sequence showed G+C content of 37%, with suppression of CpG dinucleotide frequency. These characteristic features have been found previously in several A+T-rich lymphotropic herpesviruses of the genus Rhadinovirus (*Herpesvirus saimiri*, murine gamma-herpesvirus 68, and AlHV-1) (Albrecht et al. 1992; Ensser et al. 1997; Virgin et al. 1997).

Limited studies suggest that PLHV infections are common in swine. Ehlers et al. (1999) analyzed DNA isolated from PBMC of 39 animals and spleens of 19 animals and found 87% of PBMC and 95% of spleens were positive for PLHV. We have also evaluated 20 tissue and blood samples from eight different cases submitted to the Veterinary Diagnostic Laboratory of Iowa State University, and peripheral blood leukocytes from five animals from the Iowa State University Animal Science Swine Herd. Peripheral blood leukocytes from eight herds were positive by PCR (Fig. 7).

PLHV-1 and PLHV-2 represent two newly recognized members of the *Gammaherpesvirinae* subfamily, and represent the first gamma-herpesvirus infecting pig species. Limited PCR studies indicate a high prevalence of these viruses in both domestic and feral pigs (Fig. 8). No information is available on modes of transmission and the ability of PLHV to cause persistent and/or latent infection. However, based on the ability of herpesviruses to cause latent infections, it is highly likely that PLHV too causes persistent/latent infections. Additional studies are needed to better characterize PLHVs, to better define their epidemiology, to determine their modes of transmission and prevalence in swine herds, and to examine the feasibility of producing pigs free of PLHV. The PLHV should be considered as a xenozoonoses risk and pigs for xenotransplantation should be screened for PLHV.

8.3 Porcine Cytomegalovirus

Porcine cytomegalovirus (PCMV) infection characterized by the presence of inclusion bodies in the mucosal glands of turbinates was described by Done (1955), who later reported herpes-like particles in lesions. The name 'inclusion body rhinitis' was given because of the presence of basophilic intranuclear inclusion bodies in the nasal passages of pigs with rhinitis. PCMV is now ubiquitous in swine populations around the world. PCMV is a beta-herpesvirus belonging to the family *Herpesviridae*. Viral particles are enveloped with a diameter of 120–150 nm.

Although PCMV infection in pigs is common, clinical disease and mortality are uncommon. The severity of disease depends on the age and immune status of the pig and immunity of the dam. The two primary modes of PCMV transmission are transplacental and by droplet. Virus invades and replicates in cells of the nasal, lacrimal, and Harderian mucous glands leading to viremia. There is a predilection for cells of the reticuloendothelial system. Virus is also shed in urine.

Clinical signs in pigs under 10 days of age include: sneezing, thick white nasal exudates, inability to nurse, paresis, and death in 4–5 days. In pigs over 2 weeks of age clinical signs include: snuffles, mucopurulent nasal exudates, low morbidity, anemia, stunting and mortality. In most pigs, infection is unapparent. Gross lesions include mucopurulent nasal exudates, sinusitis, petechial hemorrhages on the kidneys, possible mild multifocal consolidation of the lung and interlobular edema. Microscopically, typical large basophilic intranuclear inclusion bodies are seen in cytomegalic cells of the tubulo-alveolar glands of the turbinates. Occasionally, similar inclusions are present in other organs, especially renal tubular epithelium, and there is desquamation of glandular epithelium, lymphoplasmacytic inflammation, loss of cilia, and lymphoid hyperplasia.

Diagnosis is based on histopathologic observation of the characteristic basophilic intranuclear inclusion bodies in the nasal mucus glands. Virus isolation is achieved by inoculation of alveolar macrophage cells from pigs with suspected material. Viral antigen can be detected by immunofluorescence using anti-PCMV serum. A porcine fallopian tube cell line has been used to adapt PCMV and used in an indirect immunofluorescence assay to detect antibodies. Recently, a PCR assay has been developed for the detection of PCMV (Fryer-Jacqueline et al. 2001). However, these techniques are not routinely available. Young pigs can be infected in the presence of maternal antibody and the infection is often subclinical. The initial site of replication is in the mucous glands of the nasal mucosa. In neonatal pigs, viremia occurs between 5 and 19 dpi, although in older pigs this period is often between 14 and 18 days. Generalized infections may occur in neonatal pigs and the virus can be found in the reticuloendothelial cells with inclusion bodies in macrophages, capillary endothelium, sinus and sinusoidal cells of lymphoid tissue (Edington 1999). In older pigs the virus is usually confined to the nasal mucosa, but has also been identified in the Harderian and lachrymal glands and renal tubules. PCMV can cross the placenta causing fetal death or generalized disease in neonatal piglets (Edington et al. 1977). The most important route of virus shedding is from the nasal secretions, but virus is also excreted in the urine and ocular (Plowright et al. 1976) and cervical fluids (Edington et al. 1977).

PCMV has been identified in pulmonary macrophages of healthy pigs, suggesting that animals may become latently infected (Edington et al. 1976a). PCMV has also been shown to be reactivated after corticosteroid treatment (Edington et al. 1976b). A PCR test based on the sequence of the DNA polymerase gene has been developed recently to detect PCMV in blood and tissue DNA samples (Hamel et al. 1999; Widen et al. 1999; Rupasinghe et al. 1999). Although a number of studies have been conducted on acute infections with PCMV, limited information is available on persistence and latent infections. Also, improved methods for the propagation and detection of this virus need to be developed.

8.3.1 Xenozoonoses

PCMV is host specific and does not replicate in cells of nonporcine origin or in rabbits, mice, hamsters, chick embryos, or cattle. The host specificity of PCMV limits its ability to be a significant xenozoonotic risk. However, human cytomegalovirus is considered an opportunistic organism and is commonly present in immunosuppressed human patients. PCMV, like other cytomegaloviruses, causes persistent infections and hence present a xenozoonoses risk. What role immunosuppression has in the susceptibility of human patients to PCMV is unknown.

9 **Porcine Parvovirus**

PPV is ubiquitous in the domesticated swine population worldwide. The salient features of PPV infections are that infections are unapparent except for reproductive failure in pregnant females. The virus crosses the placental barrier in pregnant females and infects fetuses in utero, resulting in embryonic death and resorption, fetal death and mummification, and reduction in the number of live born pigs per litter.

9.1 Virus Characteristics

PPV is a member of genus *Parvovirus* of the family *Parvoviridae* (Mengeling 1992). Other members of this family include human parvovirus, canine parvovirus, minute virus of mice, and feline panleukopenia virus. PPV is an enveloped virus of 20 nm diameter. The viral genome is single-stranded linear DNA of 5 Kb and replicates through a double-stranded replicative form. The viral capsid is composed of three structural proteins: VP1 of 82.5 kDa, VP2 of 65 kDa, and VP3 of 62 kDa. VP3 is the major viral immunogen and is responsible for viral neutralization. PPV possesses hemagglutination activity and guinea pig erythrocytes are the best source for erythrocytes for detecting this. The virus is very stable to heat, pH and treatment with common disinfectants. PPV requires mitotic cells for replication, a possible reason for its predilection for fetal tissues. PPV replicates in swine kidney cells and has been adapted in selected established cell lines. The virus produces cytopathic effects that include cell rounding, pyknosis and cell degeneration.

The PPV genome is quite stable and well conserved, based on antigenic and genetic studies, and most of the viral isolates represent a single serotype of PPV. This is in contrast to the extensive heterogeneity among feline and canine parvoviruses. However, some antigenic and genetic variation has been observed: two PPV isolates, the KBSH and Kresse strains, have minor genetic differences from the reference strain NADL. Additionally one isolate, the H-45 strain isolated from diarrheic pigs in Japan, has been shown to be distinct.

9.2
Pathogenesis

The natural route of exposure to PPV appears to be oronasal. PPV infections are usually subclinical or result in minimal clinical disease, such as mild fever and leukopenia. PPV crosses the placental barrier and infects concepti. The outcome of PPV infection depends upon the stage of the embryo/fetus at the time of PPV infection. PPV exposure during the first 2 weeks of gestation may result in embryo death and resorption and sows may return to estrus. Infection of the conceptus during the second trimester of gestation results in fetal infection and death followed by mummification (Fig. 9). As a result, a smaller litter of pigs is born. Infection of the fetus during the third semester of gestation as the fetus becomes immunocompetent does not result in fetal death, but fetuses are infected and make antibodies. Viremia, persisting usually for 7–14 days, is detected in pigs around 3 days after infection. Virus is excreted in feces and can be detected for 28 days.

9.3
Diagnosis

PPV infection in pigs is easily detected by HI, virus neutralization, or ELISA. HI is most commonly used. Virus can be isolated in primary porcine kidney cell cultures and viral antigens can be identified by an immunofluorescence test. An immunofluorescent assay has also been often used to detect viral antigens in infected tissues or to confirm PPV diagnosis in mummified fetuses. PCR, nucleic acid probes and in situ hybridization tests are available for viral nucleic acid detection.

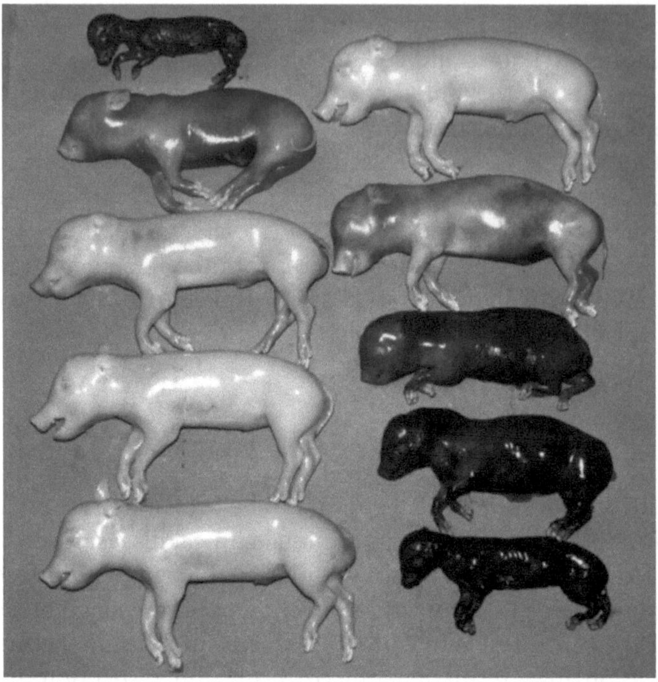

Fig. 9 Dead and mummified pigs within a litter of sows inoculated orally with PPV at 42 days of age and necropsied at 84 days of age. PPV antigen was evident in the lung sections of dead and mummified fetuses

9.4 Control and Eradication

PPV infections are widespread and almost 100% of adult pigs older than 1 year of age are infected with PPV. Pigs born to seropositive dams are protected from PPV infection and passively acquired antibodies also are protective. PPV-free pigs can be obtained from seropositive pigs by isolating them from adult pigs at around 3–4 weeks of age and raising them in clean environment free from exposure to PPV-positive pigs. Similarly, PPV-free pigs can also be obtained by Cesarean section from sows. As PPV infections are common in swine herds, extreme care should be taken to avoid PPV infection when introducing new genetic stocks.

9.5 Xenozoonoses

PPV is a common contaminant of trypsin (Croghan et al. 1973), which is derived from porcine pancreas and has been used extensively in cell culture work for production of vaccines for humans and animals. There has not been any evidence of PPV-associated disease in humans or reports of PPV-associated infections or diseases in swine handlers and veterinarians. This is in spite of the fact that porcine clotting factor has been used for many years in the treatment of hemophilia in humans. Erdman et al. (2000) found 21 of 22 lots of Hyate:C to be contaminated with PPV. None of the 98 serum samples tested from patients receiving Hyate:C treatment had antibodies to PPV. This study showed that risk of human infections with PPV is low; however, it would be wise to use PPV-free tissues for xenotransplantation as PPV produces persistent infections and crosses the transplacental barrier. The immunosuppressive properties of feline and canine parvoviruses and the adaptation of feline panleukopenia virus in dogs resulting in a major epidemic further suggest the potential of parvoviruses to cross the species barrier.

10 Coronaviruses

Four coronaviruses have been identified in pigs: transmissible gastroenteritis virus (TGEV), porcine respiratory coronavirus, porcine epidemic diarrhea virus and hemagglutinating encephalomyelitis virus. Only a brief description of these viruses, the diseases they produce, and diagnosis is provided here as they do not present a significant risk through xenotransplantation. However, there is a concern that coronaviruses present a xenozoonoses risk because of the high rate of errors during coronavirus replication through polymerase jumping, and their ability to recombine which could lead to new viruses capable of replication in both pigs and humans.

Transmissible gastroenteritis virus is the most common and best studied of the swine coronaviruses (Saif and Wesley 1999). It is a member of the family *Coronaviridae*. The virus is pleomorphic with a diameter of 160–200 nm and 12–25-nm-long surface spikes. The viral genome is about 30 kb and has three major structural proteins (S, M, and N): S is the envelope spike glycoprotein of 200 kDa, M is an integral membrane protein of 28 kDa, and N is a nucleoprotein of 48 kDa. TGEV causes gastroenteritis in neonatal pigs; it replicates primarily in the respiratory and the intestinal tract, where lesions include villous atrophy. TGEV persists for a long time in pigs and it is suspected that virus-infected pigs may serve as carriers—the virus is shed in feces for about 4 weeks; however, it has been isolated from lungs for 104 days (Underdahl et al. 1975). Virus can be isolated in a swine testis cell line or can be detected by PCR, immunofluorescence, immunohistochemistry or in situ hybridization (reviewed by Sirinarumitr et al. 1997). Viral antibodies are routinely detected by a virus neutralization test.

Porcine respiratory coronavirus (PRCV) appears to be a mutant of TGEV. It was first detected by Pensaert et al. (1986) and now is believed to be widespread around the world. Major differences between PRCV and TGEV are that a portion of S gene is missing in PRCV giving rise to smaller S protein of 180 kDa. The size of the deletion in S gene varies from 621 to 681 base pairs (Paul et al. 1994). Deletions are also present in genes 3 and 3-1. PRCV also has a different tropism from that of TGEV: TGEV replicates in the villous epithelial cells of both the small intestine and the respiratory tract whereas PRCV replicates primarily in the respiratory tract in cells such as bronchiolar epithelial cells, type II pneumocytes, alveolar and septal macrophages, and type 1 pneumocytes. PRCV and TGEV can be isolated in a swine testis cell line and the two viruses can be differentiated by reverse transcriptase–PCR (Vaughn et al. 1995; Sirinarumitr et al. 1996, 1997). Antibodies to the two viruses can be differentiated by competitive ELISA (Callebaut et al. 1989).

Porcine epidemic diarrhea virus is caused by coronavirus and is antigenically related to TGEV, however, PEDV is not present in the swine herds in the USA. The disease is characterized by watery diarrhea similar to that caused by TGEV except that PEDV replicates in both small and large intestine. PEDV is fastidious and has been adapted to grow in the Vero cell line using trypsin producing extensive syncytia. There appears to be only one serotype of the virus. Pigs are the only known hosts for PEDV.

Hemagglutinating encephalomyelitis virus (HEV) is associated with respiratory and neurologic disease in pigs. HEV is similar to other coronaviruses except that it has five major proteins including hemagglutinin. The virus replicates in pig kidney cells producing syncytia. HEV also possesses hemagglutinating activity and hemagglutinates chicken and mouse erythrocytes. The virus is quite stable as there is only one known serotype. HEV is antigenically related to Bovine coronavirus and human respiratory coronavirus OC43. HEV infections are mostly subclinical but do produce two clinical syndrome in neonatal pigs: an acute disease with encephalomyelitis or vomiting, and wasting disease. Microscopic lesions are observed in the tonsils and in the nervous and respiratory systems. Diagnosis can be made by virus isolation from tonsil, brain, and lungs. Antibodies to HEV can be detected by virus neutralization or hemagglutination inhibition tests.

Swine coronaviruses appear to be host specific. No reports are available on infections of other species with swine coronaviruses. Coronaviruses undergo mutations during replication due to polymerase jumping errors giving rise to new mutants. Porcine respiratory coronavirus is such a mutant of TGEV with different tropism. Coronaviruses have also been shown to undergo recombination. Because of their ability to recombine and mutate to give rise to new viruses with different tropisms coronaviruses should be considered a potential xenozoonoses risk.

11 Adenoviruses

Adenovirus infections are common in swine and adenoviruses appear to persist in swine tissues for long periods, but have not been shown to be associated with any significant disease. Characteristics of swine adenovirus are similar to those of other adenoviruses. Adenovirus is a member of the family *Adenoviridae*. The virus is nonenveloped, spherical and 75 nm in diameter. The viral genome is double-stranded DNA encapsulated by a protein shell comprised of 252 capsomeres. Porcine adenovirus is stable to chloroform, low pH, and temperature. Four serotypes (1–4) have been detected in pigs; serotype 4 is the most abundant. Natural infection with adenovirus is by inhalation or by the oral route. Virus transmission is via a fecal oral route and possibly by aerosol. Virus is excreted in feces and can be detected for several weeks. Experimental infection of pigs with adenovirus serotype 4 resulted in diarrhea. Lesions have also been detected in brain, lung, and kidney. Adenovirus is incriminated in respiratory disease, and is isolated from aborted fetuses. The virus replicates primarily in the tonsils and small intestine and has been shown to persist in kidneys. Meningoencephalitis was observed in pigs infected experimentally with adenovirus types 1 and 3. Heart and liver also contained chronic inflammatory changes. The primary sites of virus replication are the tonsils.

Adenovirus should be suspected if inclusion bodies are detected in the lungs, liver, or kidneys. Demonstration of viral antigen by fluorescence assay or immunoperoxidase staining in tissues confirms the role of adenovirus in the disease. Virus isolation can be accomplished in porcine kidney cell cultures. The virus does not produce any characteristic cytopathic effect, hence the viral antigen is detected by an immunofluorescence test. Adenovirus infection can be detected by virus neutralization by rising antibody titers.

No information is available on the public health risk of swine adenoviruses. However, pigs have been shown to be susceptible to human adenovirus; infection of neonatal pigs with human adenovirus resulted in bronchopneumonia (Betts et al. 1962). No data is available on whether swine adenovirus infects humans. Adenovirus does produce persistent infection so it is prudent to screen pigs and keep them free from adenovirus infection.

12 Conclusion

There have been major advances during the last decade in our understanding of pathogenesis of swine viral infections. More reliable diagnostic tests have increasingly become available for the detection of swine viruses and swine viral infections. In spite of these advances there are major gaps in research to assess the xenozoonoses risk of swine viruses. Studies are needed to determine whether swine viruses infect humans; serologic evidence of infections with swine viruses should be sought in high-risk populations such as swine producers, veterinarians, and abattoir workers. The potential of swine viruses to infect humans can be assessed by studying their ability to replicate in human cell lines as well as primary cell cultures of human origin. Nonhuman primates may also serve as good animal models to test the ability of swine viruses to infect humans. Hence, infection of nonhuman primates with swine viruses under conditions mimicking xenotransplantation will provide additional information on their potential xenozoonoses risk. Monitoring of xenotransplant human and nonhuman primate recipients for possible infections with swine viruses is essential. Such studies will require additional resources for the development of rapid and more reliable diagnostic methods.

References

Acland HM and Littlejohns IR (1975) Encephalomyocarditis virus infection of pigs. I. An outbreak in New South Wales. Aust Vet J 51:409–415

Albrecht JC, Nicholas J, Biller D, Cameron KR, Biesinger B, Newman C, Wittmann S, Craxton MA, Coleman H, et al. (1992) Primary structure of the herpesvirus saimiri genome. J Virol 66:5047–58

Allan GM and Ellis JA (2000) Porcine circoviruses: a review. J Vet Diagn Invest 12:3–14

Allan GM, Phenix KV, Todd D and McNulty MS (1994) Some biological and physicochemical properties of porcine circovirus. Zentralbl Veterinarmed [B] 41:17–26

Allan GM, McNeilly F, Cassidy JP, Reilly GA, Adair B, Ellis WA and McNulty MS (1995) Pathogenesis of porcine circovirus, experimental infections of colostrum deprived piglets and examination of pig fetal material. Vet Microbiol 44:49–64

Allan GM, Kennedy S, McNeilly F, Foster JC, Ellis JA, Krakowka SJ, Meehan B M and Adair BM (1999) Experimental reproduction of severe wasting disease by co-infection of pigs with porcine circovirus and porcine parvovirus. J Comp Pathol 121:1–11

Allan GM, McNeilly F, Ellis J, Krakowka S, Meehan B, McNair I, Walker I and Kennedy S (2000) Experimental infection of colostrum deprived piglets with porcine circovirus 2 (PCV2) and porcine reproductive and respiratory syndrome virus (PRRSV) potentiates PCV2 replication. Arch Virol 145:2421–9

Anusz Z, Szweda W, Popkko J and Trybala E (1992) Is Aujeszky's disease a zoonosis? Przegl Epidemiol 46:181–186

Bach FH, Fishman JA, Daniels N, Proimos J, Anderson B, Carpenter CB, Forrow L, Robson SC and Fineberg HV (1998) Uncertainty in xenotransplantation: individual benefit versus collective risk [see comments]. Nat Med 4:141–4

Benfield DA, Nelson E, Collins JE, Harris L, Goyal SM, Robison D, Christianson WT, Morrison RB and Gorcyca D (1992) Characterization of swine infertility and respiratory syndrome (SIRS) virus (isolate ATCC VR-2332). J Vet Diagn Invest 4:127–133

Betts AO, Jennings AR, Lamont PH and Page Z (1962) Inoculation of pigs with adenoviruses of man. Nature 193:45–46

Bolin SR, Stoffregen WC, Nayar GP and Hamel AL (2001) Postweaning multisystemic wasting syndrome induced after experimental inoculation of cesarean-derived, colostrum-deprived piglets with type 2 porcine circovirus. J Vet Diagn Invest 13:185–94

Botner A, Strandbygaard B, Sorensen KJ, Have P, Madsen KG, Madsen S and Alexandersen S (1997) Appearance of acute PRRS-like symptoms in sow herds after vaccination with a modified live PRRS vaccine. Vet Rec 141:497–499

Brown IH (2000) The epidemiology and evolution of influenza viruses in pigs. Vet Microbiol 74:29–46

Brown IH, Done SH, Spencer YI, Cooley WA, Harris PA and Alexander DJ (1993) Pathogenicity of a swine influenza H1N1 virus antigenically distinguishable from classical and European strains. Vet Rec 132:598–602

Brown IH, Chakraverty P, Harris PA and Alexander DJ (1995) Disease outbreaks in pigs in Great Britain due to an influenza A virus of H1N2 subtype. Vet Rec 136:328–329

Burke DS, Tingpalapong M, Elwell MR, Paul PS, Van Deusen RA. (1985) Japanese encephalitis virus immunoglobulin M antibodies in porcine sera. Am J Vet Res 46:2054–2057

Callebaut P, Pensaert MB and Hooyberghs J (1989) A competitive inhibition ELISA for the differentiation of serum antibodies from pigs infected with transmissible gastroenteritis virus (TGEV) or with the TGEV-related porcine respiratory coronavirus. Vet Microbiol 20:9–19

Chan KP, Rollin PE, Ksiazek TG, Leo YS, Goh KT, Paton NI, Sng EH, Ling AE (2002) A survey of Nipah virus infection among various risk groups in Singapore. Epidemiol Infect 128:93–98

Chant K, Chan R, Smith M, Dwyer DE, Kirkland P and the NSW Expert Group (1998) Probable human infection with a newly described virus in the family Paramyxoviridae. The NSW Expert Group Emerg Infect Dis 4:273–5

Chapman LE, Folks TM, Salomon DR, Patterson AP, Eggerman TE and Noguchi PD (1995) Xenotransplantation and xenogeneic infections. N Engl J Med 333:1498–501

Chew MHL, Arguin PM, Shay DK, Goh KT, Rollin PE, Shieh WJ, Zaki SR, Rota PA, Ling AE, Ksiazek TG, Chew SK and Anderson LA (2000) Risk factors for Nipah virus infection among abattoir workers in Singapore. J Infect Dis 181:1760–1763

Christianson WT, Kim HS, Yoon IJ and Joo HS (1992) Transplacental infection of midgestation sows with encephalomyocarditis virus. Am J Vet Res 53:44–47

Christopher-Hennings J, Nelson EA, Nelson JA, Hines RJ, Swenson SL, Hill HT, Zimmerman JJ, Katz JB, Yaeger MJ, Chase CCL and Benfield DA (1995) Detection of porcine reproductive and respiratory syndrome virus in boar semen by PCR. J Clin Microbiol 33:1730–1734

Chua KB, Bellini WJ, Rota PA, Harcourt BH, Tamin A, Lam SK, Ksiazek TG, Rollin PE, Zaki SR, Shieh WJ, Goldsmith CS, Gubler DJ, Roehrig JT, Eaton B, Gould AR, Olson J, Field H, Daniels P, Ling AE, Peters CJ, Anderson LJ and Mahy BWJ (2000a) Nipah virus: a recently emergent deadly paramyxovirus. Science 288:1432–1435

Chua KB, Goh KJ, Wong KT, Kamarulzaman A, Tan PSK, Ksiazek TG, Zaki SR, Paul G, Lam SK and Tan CT (2000b) Fatal encephalitis due to Nipah virus among pig-farmers in Malaysia. Lancet 354:1257–1259

Claas ECJ, Kawaoka Y, de Jong JC, Masurel N and Webster RG (1994) Infection of children with avian-human reassortant influenza virus from pigs in Europe. Virology 204:453–457

Collins JE, Benfield DA, Christianson WT, Harris L, Hennings JC, Shaw DP, Goyal SM, McCullough S, Morrison RB and Joo HS (1992) Isolation of swine infertility and respiratory syndrome virus (isolate ATCC VR-2332) in North America and experimental reproduction of the disease in gnotobiotic pigs. J Vet Diagn Invest 4:117–126

Croghan DL, Matchett A and Koski TA (1973) Isolation of porcine parvovirus from commercial trypsin. Appl Microbiol 26:431–433

Daniels P (1999) Experimental infection of pigs and cats at CSIRO-AAHL - Preliminary Observations. A working paper for WHO Meeting on Zoonotic Paramyxoviruses, Kuala Lumpur, Malaysia, 19 -21 July, 1999

Done JT (1955) An"inclusion body"rhinitis of pigs. Vet Record 70:877–878

Dulac GC and Afshar A (1989) Porcine circovirus antigens in PK-15 cell line (ATCC CCL-33) and evidence of antibodies to circovirus in Canadian pigs. Can J Vet Res 53:431–3

Easterday BC and Van Reeth K (1999) Swine influenza. In Straw BE, D'Allaire S, Mengeling WL, et al. (eds). Diseases of Swine. Iowa State University Press, Ames, IA. 8th ed. Pp. 277–290

Edington N, Plowright W and Watt RG (1976a) Generalized porcine cytomegalic inclusion disease: distribution of cytomegalic cells and virus. J Comp Pathol 86:191–202

Edington N, Watt RG and Plowright W (1976b) Cytomegalovirus excretion in gnotobiotic pigs. J Hyg (Camb) 77:283–290

Edington N, Watt RG and Plowright W (1977) Experimental transplacental transmission of porcine cytomegalovirus. J Hyg (Lond) 78:243–51

Edington N (1999) Cytomegalovirus. In Straw B, D'allaire S, Mengeling WL, et al. (Eds) Diseases of Swine, Iowa State University Press, Ames, Ia 8th Edition pp 125–131

Ehlers B, Ulrich S and Goltz M (1999) Detection of two novel porcine herpesviruses with high similarity to gammaherpesviruses. J Gen Virol 80:971–8

Ellis J, Hassard L, Clark E, Harding J, Allan G, Willson P, Strokappe J, Martin K, McNeilly F, Meehan B, Todd D and Haines D (1998) Isolation of circovirus from lesions of pigs with postweaning multisystemic wasting syndrome. Can Vet J 39:44–51

Ellis JA, Bratanich A, Clark EG, Allan G, Meehan B, Haines DM, Harding J, West KH, Krakowka S, Konoby C, Hassard L, Martin K and McNeilly F (2000) Coinfection by porcine circoviruses and porcine parvovirus in pigs with naturally acquired postweaning multisystemic wasting syndrome. J Vet Diagn Invest 12:21–7

Ensser A, Pflanz R and Fleckenstein B. (1997) Primary structure of the alcelaphine herpesvirus 1 genome. J Virol 71:6517–25

Erdman DD, Evatt BL, Anderson LJ, Torok TJ, Jamil M, Barnhart E, Tepper M, Burrill HN, Pickett AM, Mengeling WL (2000) Investigation of porcine parvovirus among persons with hemophilia receiving Hyate:C porcine factor VIII concentrate. Transfusion-Bethesda 40:708–711

Fenaux M, Halbur PG, Gill M, Toth TE and Meng XJ (2000) Genetic characterization of type 2 porcine circovirus (PCV-2) from pigs with postweaning multisystemic wasting syndrome in different geographic regions of North America and development of a differential PCR- restriction fragment length polymorphism assay to detect and differentiate between infections with PCV-1 and PCV-2. J Clin Microbiol 38:2494–503

Fenaux M, Halbur PG, Haqshenas G, Royer R, Thomas P, Nawagitgul P, Gill M, Toth TE and Meng XJ (2002) Cloned genomic DNA of type 2 porcine circovirus is infectious when injected directly into the liver and lymph nodes of pigs: Characterization of clinical disease, virus distribution, and pathologic lesions. J Virol 76:541–551

Feng WH, Laster SM, Tompkins M, Brown T, Xu JS, Altier C, Gomez W, Benfield, D and McCaw MB (2001) *In utero* infection by porcine reproductive and respiratory syndrome virus is sufficient to increase susceptibility of piglets to challenge with Streptococcus suis type II. J Virol 75:4889–4895

Fishman JA (1994) Miniature swine as organ donors for man: strategies for prevention of xenotransplant-associated infections. Xenotransplantation 1:47–57

Fryer-Jacqueline FL, Griifiths PD, Fishman JA, Emery VC and Clark DA (2001) Quantitation of porcine cytomegalovirus in pig tissues by PCR. J Clin Microbiol 39:1155–1156

Fujisaki Y, Sugimori T, Morimoto T, Miura Y, Kawakami Y and Nakano K (1975) Immunization of pigs with the attenuated S strain of Japanese encephalitis virus. National Institute Animal Health Quarterly (Tokyo) 15:55–60

Gainer JH (1967) Encephalomyocarditis virus infection in Florida, 1960–1966. J Am Vet Med Assoc 151:421–425

Goh KJ, Tan CT, Chew NK, Tan PSK, Kamarulzaman A, Sarji SA, Wong KT, Abdullah BJJ, Cua KB and Lam SK (2000) Clinical features of Nipah virus encephalitis among pig farmers in Malaysia. The New England J Med 342:1229–1235

Goldfield M, Noble G and Dowdle WR (1977) Identification and preliminary antigenic analysis of swine influenza-like viruses isolated during an influenza outbreak at Fort Dix, New Jersey. J Infect Dis 136 (Suppl):381–385

Gourreau JM, Kaiser C, Valette M, Douglas AR, Labie J and Aymard M (1994) Isolation of two H1N2 influenza viruses from swine in France. Arch Virol 135:365–382

Greig AS, Johnson CM and Bovillant AMP (1971) Encephalomyelitis of swine caused by a hemagglutinating virus. VI. Morphology of the virus. Res Vet Sci 12:305–307

Groshup MH, Brun A and Haas B (1993) Serological studies on the potential synergism of porcine respiratory and reproductive syndrome virus and influenza-, corona-, and paramyxoviruses in the induction of respiratory syndrome in swine. J Vet Med B 40:681–689

Gunzburg WH and Salmons B (2000) Xenotransplantation: is the risk of viral infection as great as we thought? Mol Med Today 6:1999–208

Halbur PG, Andrews JJ, Huffman EL, Paul PS, Meng XJ and Niyo Y (1994) Development of a streptoavidin-biotin immunoperoxidase procedure for the detection of porcine reproductive and respiratory syndrome virus antigen in porcine lung. J Vet Diagn Invest 6:254–257

Halbur PG, Paul PS, Frey ML, Landgraf J, Eernisse K, Meng X-J, Lum MA, Andrews JJ and Rathje JA (1995) Comparison of the pathogenicity of two U.S. porcine reproductive and respiratory syndrome virus isolates with that of the Lelystad virus. Vet Pathol 32:648–660

Hamel AL, Lin LL and Nayar GP (1998) Nucleotide sequence of porcine circovirus associated with postweaning multisystemic wasting syndrome in pigs. J Virol 72:5262–7

Hamel AL, Lin L, Sachvie C, Grudeski E and Nayar GPS (1999) PCR assay for detecting porcine cytomegalovirus. J Clin Microbiol 37:3767–8

Harms PA, Sorden SD, Halbur PG, Bolin SR, Lager KM, Morozov I and Paul PS (2001) Experimental reproduction of severe disease in CD/CD pigs concurrently infected with type 2 porcine circovirus and porcine reproductive and respiratory syndrome virus. Vet Pathol 38:528–39

Harcourt BH, Tamin A, Ksiazek TG, Rollin PE, Anderson LJ, Bellini WJ and Rota PA (2000) Molecular characterization of Nipah virus, a newly emergent paramyxovirus. Virology 271:334–349

Harding JC and Clark EG (1997) Recognizing and diagnosing postweaning multisystemic wasting syndrome (PMWS). Swine Health and Production 5:201–203

Harding JCS, Clark EG, Strokappe JH, Willson PI and Ellis JA (1998) Post-weaning multisystemic wasting syndrome (PMWS): epidemiology and clinical presentation. Swine Health Prod 6:249–254

Hay AJ (1998) The virus genome and its replication. In Nicholson KG, Webster RG, Hay AJ (eds), Textbook of Influenza. Blackwell Science, Oxford pp. 43–53

Haynes JS, Halbur PG, Sirinarumitr T, Paul PS, Meng XJ and Huffman EL (1997) Temporal and morphologic characterization of the distribution of porcine reproductive and respiratory syndrome virus (PRRSV) by in situ hybridization in pigs infected with isolates of PRRSV that differ in virulence. Vet Pathol 34:39–43

Heinen E, Herbst W and Schmeer N (1998) Isolation of cytopathogenic virus from a case of porcine respiratory and reproductive syndrome (PRRS) and its characterization as parainfluenza virus type 2. Arch Virol 143:2233–2239

Hill H (1990) Overview and history of mystery swine disease (swine infertility and respiratory syndrome). Proc. Mystery Swine Dis Committee Mtg, October 6, Denver, CO, pp. 29–31. Livestock Conservation Institute, Madison, WI

Hinshaw VS, Bean WJ jr, Webster RG and Easterday BC (1978) The prevalence of influenza viruses in swine and the antigenic and genetic relatedness of influenza viruses of man and swine. Virology 84:51–62

Hooper P, Zaki S, Daniels P and Middleton D (2001) Comparative pathology of the diseases caused by Hendra and Nipah viruses. Microbes and Infection 34:323–329

Hori H, Morita K and Igarashi A (1986) Oligonucleotide fingerprint analysis on Japanese encephalitis virus strains isolated in Japan and Thailand. Acta Virol 30:353–359

Hsu ST, Chang LC, Lin SY, Chuang TY, Ma CH, Inoue YK and Okuno T (1972) The effect of vaccination with a live attenuated strain of Japanese encephalitis virus on stillbirths in swine in Taiwan. Bulletin WHO 46:465–471

Janke BH (2000) Diagnosis of swine influenza. Swine Health Prod 8:79–84

Janke BH, Paul PS, Landgraf JG, Halbur PG and Huinker CD (2001) Paramyxovirus infection in pigs with interstitial pneumonia and encephalitis in the United States. J Vet Diagn Invest 13:428–433

Joo HS, Kim HS and Leman AD (1988) Detection of antibody to encephalomyocarditis virus in mummified or stillborn pigs. Arch Virol 100:131–134

Josephson G and Charbonneau G (2001) Case report of reproductive failure in a new startup operation. J Swine Health Prod 9:258–259

Karasin AI, Olsen CW and Anderson GA (2000a) Genetic characterization of an H1N2 influenza virus isolated from a pig in Indiana. J Clin Microbiol 38:2453–2456

Karasin AI, Brown IH, Carman S and Olsen CW (2000b) Isolation and characterization of H4N6 avian influenza viruses from pigs with pneumonia in Canada. J Virol 74:9322–9327

Kim HS, Christianson WT and Joo HS (1989) Pathogenic properties of encephalomyocarditis virus isolates in swine fetuses. Arch Virol 109:51–57

Kim J, Han DU, Choi C and Chae C (2001) Differentiation of porcine circovirus (PCV)-1 and PCV-2 in boar semen using a multiplex nested polymerase chain reaction. J Virol Methods 98:25–31

Kennedy S, Moffett D, McNeilly F, Meehan B, Ellis J, Krakowka S and Allan GM (2000) Reproduction of lesions of postweaning multisystemic wasting syndrome by infection of conventional pigs with porcine circovirus type 2 alone or in combination with porcine parvovirus. J Comp Pathol 122:9–24

Kluge JP, Beran GW, Hill HT, Platt KB (1992) Pseudorabies (Aujeszky's Disease) In Leman AD, Straw BE, Mengeling WL, D'Allaire S, Taylor DJ (eds). Diseases of Swine, Iowa State University Press, Ames, IA. 7th ed. pp.312–323

Krakowka S, Ellis JA, Meehan B, Kennedy S, McNeilly F and Allan G (2000) Viral wasting syndrome of swine: experimental reproduction of postweaning multisystemic wasting syndrome in gnotobiotic swine by coinfection with porcine circovirus 2 and porcine parvovirus. Vet Pathol 37:254–63

Krakowka S, Ellis JA, McNeilly F, Ringler S, Rings DM and Allan G (2001) Activation of the immune system is the pivotal event in the production of wasting disease in pigs infected with porcine circovirus-2 (PCV-2). Vet Pathol 38:31–42

Larochelle R, Antaya M, Morin M and Magar R (1999) Typing of porcine circovirus in clinical specimens by multiplex PCR. J Virol Methods 80:69–75

Larochelle R, Bielanski A, Muller P and Magar R (2000) PCR detection and evidence of shedding of porcine circovirus type 2 in boar semen. J Clin Microbiol 38:4629–4632

Lipkind M, Shohan D and Shihmanter E (1986) Isolation of paramyxovirus from pigs in Israel and its antigenic relationship with avian paramyxoviruses. J Gen Virol 67:422–439

Littlejohns IR and Acland HM (1975) Encephalomyocarditis virus infection in pigs. II. Experimental diseases. Aust Vet J 51:416–422

Liu Q, Wang L, Willson P and Babiuk L A (2000) Quantitative, competitive PCR analysis of porcine circovirus DNA in serum from pigs with postweaning multisystemic wasting syndrome. J Clin Microbiol 38:3474–3477

Love RJ and Grewal AS (1986) Reproductive failure in pigs caused by encephalomyocarditis virus. Aust Vet J 63:128–129

Magar R, Larochelle R, Thibault S and Lamontagne L (2000) Experimental transmission of porcine circovirus type 2 (PCV2) in weaned pigs: a sequential study. J Comp Pathol 123:258–269

McCormack JG (2000) Hendra, Menangle and Nipah viruses. Aust NZ J Med 30:9–10

Meng XJ, Paul PS, Vaughn EM and Zimmerman JJ (1993) Development of a Nucleic Acid Probe for the Detection of Encephalomyocarditis Virus of Swine. J Vet Diag Invest 5:254–258

Meng XJ, Paul PS, Halbur PG and Morozov I (1995) Sequence comparison of open reading frames 2 to 5 of low and high virulence United States isolates of porcine reproductive and respiratory syndrome virus. J gen Virol 76:3181–3188

Meng XJ, Paul PS, Halbur PG and Lum MA (1996) Characterization of a high-virulence US isolate of porcine reproductive and respiratory syndrome virus in a continuous cell line, ATCC CRL11171. J Vet Diagn Invest 8:374–381

Mengeling WL. Porcine parvovirus. (1992) In Leman AD, Straw BE, Mengeling WL, D'Allaire S, Taylor DJ (eds). Diseases of Swine. Iowa State University Press, Ames, IA. 7th edition pp. 299–311

Mengeling WL, Vorwald AC, Lager KM and Brockmeier SL (1996) Comparison among strains of porcine reproductive and respiratory syndrome virus for their ability to cause reproductive failure. Am J Vet Res 57:834–839

Miyata H, Tsunoda H, Kazi A, Yamada A, Khan MA, Murakami J, Kamahora T, Shiraki K and Hino S (1999) Identification of a novel GC-rich 113-nucleotide region to complete the circular, single-stranded DNA genome of TT virus, the first human circovirus. J Virol 73:3582–3586

Morimoto T (1969) Epizootic swine stillbirth caused by Japanese encephalitis virus. Proceedings of a symposium on factors producing embryonic and fetal abnormalities, death, and abortion in swine. US ARS 91–73:137–153

Morozov I, Sirinarumitr T, Sorden SD, Halbur PG, Morgan MK, Yoon KJ, Paul PS (1998) Detection of a novel strain of porcine circovirus in pigs with postweaning multisystemic wasting syndrome. J Clin Microbiol 36:2535–2541

Murray K, Selleck P, Hooper P, Hyatt A, Gould A, Gleeson L, Westbury H, Hiley L, Selvey L and Rodwell B (1995) A morbillivirus that caused fatal disease in horses and humans. Science 268:94–97

Nawagitgul P, Morozov I, Bolin SR, Harms PA, Sorden SD and Paul PS (2000) Open reading frame 2 of porcine circovirus type 2 encodes a major capsid protein. J gen Virol 9:2281–2287

Nawagitgul P, Harms PA, Morozov I, Thacker BJ, Sorden SD, Lekcharoensuk C and Paul PS (2002) Modified indirect porcine circovirus (PCV) type 2-based and recombinant capsid protein (ORF2)-based enzyme-linked immunosorbent assays for detection of antibodies to PCV. Clin Diagn Lab Immunol 9:33–40

Nelson EA, Christopher-Hennings J, Drew T, Wensvoort G, Collins JE and Benfield DA (1993) Differentiation of U.S. and European isolates of porcine reproductive and respiratory syndrome virus by monoclonal antibodies. J Clin Microbiol 31:3184–3189

Nielsen HS, Oleksiewicz MB, Forsberg R, Stadejek T, Botner A and Storgaard T (2001) Reversion of a live porcine reproductive and respiratory syndrome virus vaccine investigated by parallel mutations. J gen Virol 82:1263–1272

Ogasa A, Yokoki Y, Fujisaki Y and Habu A (1977) Reproductive disorders in boars infected experimentally with Japanese encephalitis virus. Jap J Animal Reproduction 23:171–175

Ouchi A, Nerome K, Kanegae Y, Ishida M, Nerome R, Hayashi K, Hashimoto T, Kaji M, Kaji Y and Inaba Y (1996) Large outbreak of swine influenza in southern Japan caused by reassortant (H1N2) influenza viruses: Its epizootic background and characterisation of the causative viruses. J gen Virol 77:1751–1759

Parashar UD, Sunn LM, Ong F, Mounts AW, Arif MT, Ksiazek TG, Kamaluddin MA, Mustafa AN, Kaur H, Ding LM, Othman G, Radzi HM, Kitsutani PT, Stockton PC, Arokiasam J, Gary HEJr and Anderson LJ (2000) Case-control study of risk factors for human infection with a new zoonotic paramyxovirus, Nipah virus, during a 1998–1999 outbreak of severe encephalitis in Malaysia. J Infect Dis 181:1755–1759

Patience C, Takeuchi Y and Weiss RA (1997) Infection of human cells by an endogenous retrovirus of pigs [see comments]. Nature Med 3:282–286

Patience C, Takeuchi Y and Weiss RA (1998) Zoonosis in xenotransplantation. Curr Opin Immunol 10:539–542

Patriarca RA, Kendal AR, Zakowski RC, Cox NJ, Trautman MS, Cherry JD, Auervach DM, McCusker J, Belliveau RR and Kappus KD (1984) Lack of significant person-to-person spread of swine infuenza-like virus following fatal infection in an immunocompromised child. Am J Epidemiol 119:152–158

Paul PS, Mengeling WL and Pirtle EC (1982) Differentiation of pseudorabies virus isolates by restriction endonuclease analysis. Arch Virol 73:193–198

Paul PS, Halbur PG and Vaughn E (1994) Significance of porcine respiratory coronavirus infection. Compend Cont Educ Pract Vet 16:1223–1234

Pensaert MB, Callebaut P and Vergote J (1986) Isolation of porcine respiratory non-enteric coronavirus related to transmissible gastroenteritis. Vet Quart 8:257–261

Philbey A, Kirkland DP, Ross A, Davis RJ, Gleeson AB, Love RJ, Daniels PW, Gould AR and Hyatt AD (1998) An apparently new virus (Family Paramyxoviridae) infectious for pigs, humans, and fruit bats. Emerging Infectious Diseases 2:269–271

Plagemann PG and Moenning B (1992) Lactate dehydrogenase-elevating virus, equine arteritis virus and simian hemorrhagic fever virus: A new group of positive stranded RNA viruses. Adv Virus Res 41:99–102

Plowright W, Edington N and Watt RG (1976) The behavior of porcine cytomegalovirus in commercial pig herds. J Hyg (Lond) 76:125–135

Royer RL, Nawagitgul P, Halbur PG and Paul PS (2001) Susceptibility of porcine circovirus type 2 to commercial and laboratory disinfectants. Swine Health Prod 9:281–284

Rupasinghe V, Tajima T, Maeda K, Iwatsuki HK, Sugii S and Horimoto T (1999) Analysis of porcine cytomegalovirus DNA polymerase by consensus primer PCR. J Vet Med Sci 61:1253–1255

Saif LJ and Wesley RD (1999) Transmissible gastroenteritis and porcine respiratory coronavirus. In Straw BE, D'Allaire S, Mengeling WL, et al. (Eds) Diseases of Swine, Iowa State University Press, Ames, IA 8th edition pp 295–325

Sasahara J, Hayashi S, Kumagai T, Yamamoto Y, Hirasawa K, Munekata K, Okaniwa A and Kato K (1954) On a swine virus disease newly discovered in Japan. 1. Isolation of the virus. 2. Some properties of the virus. Virus 4:131–139

Shimizu T, Kawakami Y, Fukuhaira S and Matsumoto M (1954) Experimental stillbirth in pregnant swine infected with Japanese encephalitis virus. Jap J Exp Med 24:363–375

Sirinarumitr T, Paul PS, Kluge JP and Halbur PG (1996) In situ hybridization technique for the detection of swine enteric and respiratory coronaviruses, transmissible gastroenteritis virus (TGEV) and porcine respiratory coronavirus (PRCV), in formalin-fixed paraffin-embedded tissues. J Virol Methods 56:149–160

Sirinarumitr T, Paul PS, Halbur PG and Kluge JP (1997) An overview of immunological and genetic methods for detecting swine coronaviruses, transmissible gastroenteritis virus, and porcine respiratory coronavirus in tissues. Mechanisms in the pathogenesis of enteric diseases ed. Paul, Francis and Benfield. Plenum Press, New York, pp. 37–46

Sirinarumitr T, Zhang Y, Kluge JP, Halbur PG and Paul PS (1998) A pneumo-virulent United States isolate of porcine reproductive and respiratory syndrome virus induces apoptosis in bystander cells both in vitro and in vivo. J gen Virol 79:2989–2995

Sirinarumitr T, Morozov I, Nawagitgul P, Sorden SD, Harms PA and Paul PS (2000) Utilization of a rate enhancement hybridization buffer system for rapid in situ hybridization for the detection of porcine circovirus in cell cultures and in tissues of pigs with postweaning multisystemic wasting syndrome (PMWS). J Vet Diagn Invest 12:562–565

Sorden SD, Harms PA, Nawagitgul P, Cavanaugh D and Paul PS (1999) Development of a polyclonal-antibody-based immunohistochemical method for the detection of type 2 porcine circovirus in formalin-fixed, paraffin-embedded tissue. J Vet Diagn Invest 11:528–530

Sorden SD (2000) Update on porcine circovirus and postweaning multisystemic wasting syndrome (PMWS). Swine Health Prod 8:133–136

Stephano HA (1999) Blue eye disease. In Diseases of swine, 8th edition, editors B. Straw, S. Allaire, W.Mengeling, D.Taylor. Iowa State University Press, Ames, Iowa, pp. 103–112

Stephano HA, Gay GM and Ramirez TC (1988) Encephalomyelitis, reproductive failure and corneal opacity (blue eye) in pigs, associated with a paramyxovirus infection. Vet Record 122:6–10

Stevenson GW, Kiupel M, Mittal SK, Choi J, Latimer KS and Kanitz CL (2001) Tissue distribution and genetic typing of porcine circoviruses in pigs with naturally occurring congenital tremors. J Vet Diagn Invest 13:57–62

Takashima I, Watanabe T, Ouchi N and Hashimoto N (1988) Ecological studies of Japanese encephalitis virus in Hokkaido: Inter-epidemic outbreaks of swine abortion and evidence for the virus to over winter locally. Am J Tropical Med Hygiene 38:420–427

Tchoyoson-Lim CC, Sitoh YY, Hui F, Lee KE, Ang BSP, Lim E, Lim WEH, Oh HML, Tambyah PA, Wong JSL, Tan CB and Chee TSG (2000) Nipah viral encephalitis or Japanese encephalitis? MR findings in a new zoonotic disease. Am J Neurological Res 21:455–461

Tesh RB (1978) The prevalence of encephalomyocarditis virus neutralizing antibodies among various human populations. Am J Tropical Med Hygiene 27:144–149

Tischer I, Rasch R and Tochtermann G (1974) Characterization of papovavirus- and picornavirus-like particles in permanent pig kidney cell lines. Zentralbl Bakteriol Mikrobiol Hyg [A]. 226:153–167

Tischer I, Gelderblom H, Vettermann W and Koch MA (1982) A very small porcine virus with circular single-stranded DNA. Nature 295:64–6

Tischer I, Mields W, Wolff D, Vagt M and Griem W (1986) Studies on epidemiology and pathogenicity of porcine circovirus. Arch Virol 91:271–6

Tischer I, Peters D, Rasch R and Pociuli S (1987) Replication of porcine circovirus: induction by glucosamine and cell cycle dependence. Arch Virol 96:39–57

Tischer I, Bode L, Apodaca J, Timm H, Peters D, Rasch R, Pociuli S and Gerike E (1995) Presence of antibodies reacting with porcine circovirus in sera of humans, mice, and cattle. Arch Virol 140:1427–39

Ulrich S, Goltz M and Ehlers B (1999) Characterization of the DNA polymerase loci of the novel porcine lymphotropic herpesviruses 1 and 2 in domestic and feral pigs. J Gen Virol 80:3199–3205

Umene K (1999) Mechanism and application of genetic recombination in herpesviruses. Rev Med Virol 9:171–182

Underdahl NR, Mebus CA, Stair EL and Twiehaus MJ (1975) Recovery of transmissible gastroenteritis virus from chronically infected experimental pigs. Am J Vet Res 36:1473–1476

Van Reeth K, Brown IH and Pensaert M (2000) Isolations of H1N2 influenza A virus from pigs in Belgium. Vet Rec 146:588–589

van-Vugt-Joke JFA, Storgaard T, Oleksiewicz MB and Botner A. (2001) High frequency RNA recombination in porcine reproductive and respiratory syndrome virus occurs preferentially between parental sequences with high similarity. J gen Virol 82:2615–2620

Vaughn EM, Halbur PG and Paul PS (1995) Sequence comparison of porcine respiratory coronavirus isolates reveals heterogenecity in the S, 3, 3–1 genes. J Virol 69:3176–3184

Vincent LL, Janke BH, Paul PS and Halbur PG (1997) A monoclonal-antibody-based immunohistochemical method for the detection of swine influenza virus in formalin-fixed, paraffin embedded tissues. J Vet Diagn Invest 9:191–195

Walker IW, Konoby CA, Jewhurst VA, McNair I, McNeilly F, Meehan BM, Cottrell TS, Ellis JA, Allan GM (2000) Development and application of a competitive enzyme-linked immunosorbent assay for the detection of serum antibodies to porcine circovirus type 2. J Vet Diagn Invest 12: 400–405

Virgin HW, Latreille P, Wamsley P, Hallsworth K, Weck KE, Dal-Canto AJ and Speck SH (1997) Complete sequence and genomic analysis of murine gammaherpesvirus 68. J Virol 71:5894–904

Wang LF, Yu M, Hansson E, Pritchard LI, Shiell B, Michalski WP and Eaton BT (2000) The exceptional large genome of Hendra virus: support for creation of a new genus within the family Paramyxoviridae. J Virol 74:9972–9979

Weiss RA (1998) Transgenic pigs and virus adaptation. Nature 391:327–8

Wensvoort G, Terpstra C, Pol JM, TerLaak EA, Bloemradd M, DeKluyver EP, Kragten C, Van Butten L, Den BEsten A, Wagenaar F, Broekhuijsen JM, Moonen PLJM, Zetstra T, DeBoer EA, Tibben HJ, De Jong MF, Vanit Veld P, Groenland GJR, Van Gennep JA, Voets MT, Verheijden JHM and Braamskamp J (1991) Mystery swine disease in the Netherlands: the isolation of Lelystad virus. Veterinary Quarterly 13:121–130

Wentworth DE, Thompson BL, Xu X, Regnery HL, Cooley AJ, McGregor MW, Cox NJ and Hinshaw VS (1994) An influenza A (H1N1) virus, closely related to swine influenza virus, responsible for a fatal case of human influenza. J Virol 68:2051–2058

Wentworth DE, McGregor MW, Macklin MD, Neumann V and Hinshaw VS (1997) Transmission of swine influenza virus to humans after exposure to experimentally infected pigs [see comments]. J Infect Dis 175:7–15

Wesley RD, Mengeling WL, Andreyev V and Lager LM (1996) Differentiation of vaccine (Strain RespPRRS) and field strains of porcine reproductive and respiratory syndrome virus by restriction enzyme analysis. In Proc. 27th Annual Meeting Am Assoc Swine Pract pp141–143

West KH, Bystrom JM and Wjnarowicz C (1999) Myocarditis and abortion associated with intrauterine infection of sows with porcine circovirus 2. Vet Diagn Invest 11:530–532

Widen BF, Lowings JP, Belak S and Banks M (1999) Development of a PCR system for porcine cytomegalovirus detection and determination of the putative partial sequence of its DNA polymerase gene. Epidemiol Infect 123:177–80

Wills RW, Zimmerman JJ, Yoon KJ, Swenson SL, McGinley MJ, Hill HT, Platt KB, Christopher-Hennings J and Nelson EA (1997) Porcine reproductive and respiratory syndrome virus: A persistent infection. Vet Microbiol 55:231–240

Wong SC, Ooi MH, Wong MNL, Tio PH, Solomon T and Cardosa MJ (2001) Late presentation of Nipah virus encephalitis and kinetics of the humoral immune response. J Neurol Neurosurg Psychiatry 71:552–554

Yoon IJ, Joo HS, Christianson WT, Kim HS, Collins JE, Morrison RB and Dial GD (1992) An indirect fluorescent antibody test for the detection of antibody to swine infertility and respiratory syndrome virus in swine sera. J Vet Diagn Invest 4:144–147

Yoon KJ, Wu LL, Zimmerman JJ, Hill HT and Platt KB (1996) Antibody-dependent enhancement (ADE) of porcine reproductive and respiratory syndrome virus (PRRSV) infection in pigs. Viral Immunol 9:51–63

Swine Hepatitis E Virus: Cross-Species Infection and Risk in Xenotransplantation

X. J. Meng
Center for Molecular Medicine and Infectious Diseases, Department of Biomedical Sciences and Pathobiology, Virginia Polytechnic Institute and State University, 1410 Price's Fork Road, Blacksburg, VA 24061-0342, USA
E-mail: xjmeng@vt.edu

1 Introduction 186

2 Hepatitis E Virus 186
2.1 Hepatitis E as a Disease and Its Causative Agent. 186
2.2 Biology and Classification of HEV 187
2.3 Heterogeneity and Genotypes 188
2.4 Epidemiology 190

3 Swine HEV 192
3.1 Discovery of Swine HEV 192
3.2 Genome Organization 195
3.3 Pathogenesis 196
3.4 Anti-HEV Prevalence in Swine Population 200
3.5 Experimental Infection of Nonhuman Primates with Swine HEV 201
3.6 Anti-HEV Prevalence in Pig Handlers 203
3.7 Emergence of Novel Strains of Human HEV Closely Related to Swine HEV 204

4 Animal Reservoirs for HEV: Risk for Zoonosis 205
4.1 Anti-HEV Prevalence in Animal Species 205
4.2 Genetic Identification of Animal Strains of HEV 205
4.3 Experimental Cross-Species Infection of HEV 206
4.4 Natural History of HEV: A Hypothesis 207

5 Xenozoonotic Risk of Swine HEV Infection 207
5.1 Sites of Viral Replication in Swine 207
5.2 Risk for Xenozoonosis 209
5.3 Screening for Swine HEV Infection in Xenograft Donor Pigs. 209

References. 210

Abstract Swine hepatitis E Virus (swine HEV), a ubiquitous agent recently discovered in pigs, is antigenically and genetically closely related to the human HEV. Swine HEV infection in pigs generally occurs at about 2–3 months of age, and about 80%–100% of the pigs in commercial farms in the USA were infected. Swine HEV infections have now been recognized in pigs in many other countries of the world. Interspecies transmission has been documented, as swine HEV infects non-human primates and some strains of human HEV infect pigs. Recent seroepidemiological studies showed that swine veterinarians and other pig handlers are at higher risk of HEV infection compared to normal blood donors. In addition, novel strains of human HEV recovered from hepatitis patients in the USA, Japan and Taiwan are genetically more closely related to strains of swine HEV from respective countries than to other strains of human HEV. The ubiquitous nature of the virus in pigs and the demonstrated ability of cross-species infection raise a potential concern for swine HEV infection in xenotransplantation with pig organs. This chapter discusses the recent advances in HEV research with emphases on potential zoonosis and xenozoonosis.

1 Introduction

Xenozoonosis is one of the major concerns in xenotransplantation with pig organs (Weiss 1998). The recent discovery of Swine Hepatitis E Virus (swine HEV), a virus closely-related to the human HEV, as a ubiquitous agent in pigs and the demonstration of its ability to infect across species barriers raise a potential concern for swine HEV infection in xenotransplantation with pig organs. This article discusses the recent advances in HEV research with emphases on zoonosis and xenozoonosis.

2 Hepatitis E Virus

2.1 Hepatitis E as a Disease and Its Causative Agent

Evidence for the existence of an enterically transmitted viral hepatitis distinct from the known hepatitis A came from serological studies of water-borne epidemics of hepatitis in India (Khuroo et al. 1980; Wong et al. 1980; Purcell 1996). This new form of viral hepatitis was initially referred to as enterically transmitted non-A, non-B hepatitis, and was later named hepatitis E to conform to the standard nomenclature of viral hepatitis.

Balayan et al. (1983) demonstrated the existence of a viral hepatitis E agent by transmitting hepatitis E to a human volunteer with a stool sample collected from a non-A, non-B hepatitis patient. The volunteer developed severe hepatitis, shed virus-like particles in his stool, and developed antibody response to the virus-like particles. Balayan et al. (1983) also successfully transmitted hepatitis E to nonhuman primates, and recovered virus-like particles from the infected primates. The identity of the causative agent of hepatitis E was not known until Reyes et al. (1990) isolated a cDNA from the virus responsible for hepatitis E. This new virus was named Hepatitis E Virus (HEV).

2.2 Biology and Classification of HEV

HEV is a spherical, nonenveloped virus particle approximately 32–34 nm in diameter (Purcell 1996). Electron microscopy revealed symmetrical virus particles with cup-shaped depressions on the surface, similar to caliciviruses (Ticehurst et al. 1992; Aggarwal and Krawczynski 2000; Krawczynski et al. 2000). The genome of HEV is a single-stranded positive-sense RNA molecule of approximately 7.2 kb. The viral genome consists of three open reading frames (ORFs 1, 2 and 3), and a 5′ and a 3′ noncoding region (NCR) (Tam et al. 1991; Purcell 1996; Reyes 1997; Haqshenas et al. 2001). The ORF1 encodes viral nonstructural proteins that are involved in viral replication and protein processing. Its sequence contains motifs characteristic of methyltransferases, papain-like cysteine proteases, helicases and RNA-dependent RNA polymerases (Jameel et al. 1996; Aggarwal and Krawczynski 2000). ORF2 encodes the capsid protein that contains a typical signal peptide sequence at its N terminus, and three potential glycosylation sites (Jameel et al. 1996; Zafrullah et al. 1999). It has been shown that when the ORF2 is expressed in the baculovirus system, a truncated version of ORF2 protein lacking the N-terminal 111 amino acid residues is produced (Li et al. 1997; Zhang et al. 1997). The truncated ORF2 protein was cleaved at amino acid position 111–112 (Zhang et al. 1997) but was still able to form virus-like particles (Li et al. 1997). ORF3 encodes a cytoskeleton-associated phosphoprotein (Zafrullah et al. 1997). The N terminus of ORF3 has a cysteine-rich region and can bind to HEV RNA and enters into a complex with the capsid protein (Jameel et al. 1996).

Based on its similar morphological, physiochemical and structural similarity with caliciviruses, HEV was initially classified in the family *Caliciviridae* (Purcell 1996). However, the genome of HEV, which possesses a cap structure at its 5′end (Kabrane-Lazizi et al. 1999a; Emerson et al. 2001), does not share significant sequence homology with caliciviruses. Studies have shown that the codon usage and genomic organization of HEV are more related to that of rubella virus (a togavirus) and the beet necrotic yellow vein virus (a plant furovirus) than to that of the caliciviruses (Fry et al. 1992; Koonin et al. 1992). Thus, HEV has recently been declassified from the family *Caliciviridae* and designated as an unassigned genus 'hepatitis E-like viruses' (Pringle 1998).

2.3
Heterogeneity and Genotypes

The complete nucleotide sequences of several HEV strains from Asia, Africa, Mexico and the USA have been determined. However, most HEV strains are only partially sequenced. Based upon the complete nucleotide sequences, four well-recognized major genotypes of HEV have been identified: the Burmese-like genotype consisting of Asian and African strains, the Mexican genotype consisting of a single Mexican strain, the USA genotype consisting of both U.S. human and swine HEV strains (Fig. 1; Purcell 1996; Reyes 1997; Meng et al. 1998b), and the new genotype 4 strains from Asia (Wang et al. 2000; Takahasi et al. 2002). With the aid of modern molecular biology techniques, numerous genetically distinct strains of HEV have recently been identified from patients with acute hepatitis E in both developing and industrialized countries.

In endemic regions, novel strains of HEV distinct from the known epidemic strains have been identified. Wang et al. (2000) found that a novel Chinese strain of human HEV (strain T1) is related to the Taiwanese swine and human strains of HEV (Hsieh et al. 1998, 1999). Wang et al. (1999) identified six novel isolates of HEV from Chinese patients that are seronegative for anti-HEV. These six novel Chinese isolates of HEV are genetically similar to each other but differ extensively from other known HEV strains. Huang et al. (1995) also identified two unique strains of HEV from patients in China: they shared about 89% sequence identity with each other but only 76%–78% identity with other known strains of HEV including other Chinese strains. In Nigeria, a genetically

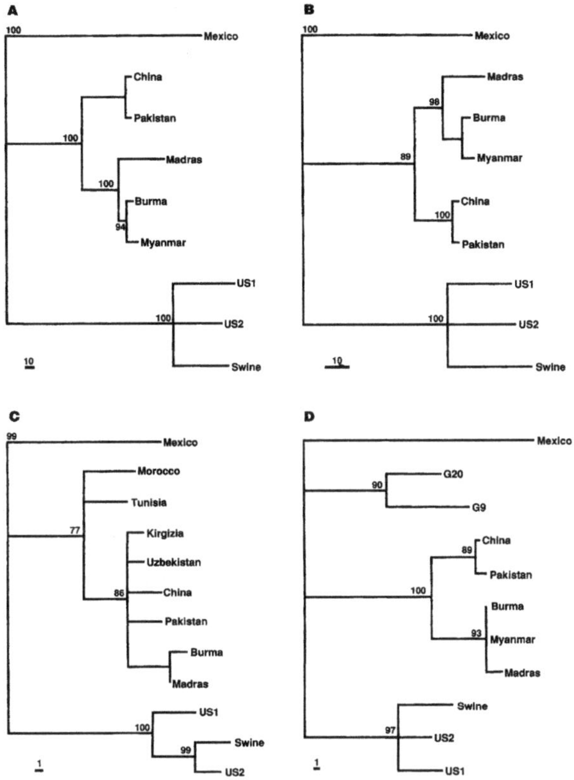

Fig. 1A–D Phylogenetic trees based on the nucleotide sequences of different regions of the HEV genome. (**A**) RNA-dependent RNA polymerase; (**B**) methyltransferase; (**C**) a stretch of 232 bp sequence in the overlap regions of ORFs 1, 2 and 3; (**D**) a 210-bp sequence in the putative RdRp region of ORF1 that corresponding to the only sequence available for strains G-9 and G-20. The *scale bars* representing the numbers of character state changes are shown, and the branch lengths are proportional to the numbers of character state changes. Bootstrap values of less than 75% are not shown. (Reproduced by permission of the American Society for Microbiology, from Meng et al. 1998b)

distinct strain of HEV was identified from native Nigerians with acute hepatitis (Buisson et al. 2000).

Until recently hepatitis E was not considered to be endemic in industrialized countries. Two cases of acute hepatitis E have recently been reported in the USA, one in Minnesota and one in Tennessee (Schlauder et al. 1998; Erker et al. 1999). The patient from Minnesota (US-1) had no history of traveling outside the USA, whereas the patient from Tennessee (US-2) had traveled to Mexico prior to the diagnosis of hepatitis E. The two virus isolates recovered from the patients are genetically distinct from other known strains of human HEV worldwide: they shared 92% nucleotide sequence identity to each other but only about 74% identity to the Burmese and Mexican strains. Similarly, several novel isolates of HEV have been identified from Taiwanese patients with no history of travel to endemic regions (Hsieh et al. 1998; Wu et al. 2000). Zanetti et al. (1999) identified a novel strain of HEV from an Italian patient with no history of traveling to endemic regions. Sequence analyses revealed that this novel Italian strain of HEV shared only about 79.5%–85.8% nucleotide sequence identity with other known strains of HEV. Schlauder et al. (1999) identified three other novel strains of HEV from patients in other nonendemic areas, two from Greece and one from Italy. The Greek and Italian strains are significantly divergent from other known strains and from each other. The source of these novel HEV strains identified from patients in industrialized countries is not clear, but given the fact that there exist several potential animal reservoirs, a zoonotic infection seems plausible.

With the identification of numerous novel strains of HEV, at least eight different genotypes of HEV have now been proposed (Schlauder et al. 1999, 2000). However, a definitive conclusion as to how many genotypes of HEV actually exist cannot be drawn because the phylogenetic analyses were based on partial sequences that are available for most strains (Schlauder et al. 1999, 2000). The nucleotide sequence difference between genotypes is about 20%–30%. However, most of the nucleotide sequence variations represent silent mutations without affecting the deduced amino acid sequences. Therefore, despite the extensive nucleotide sequence variations, all HEV strains recovered to date appear to be antigenically related (Haqshenas et al. 2002).

2.4 Epidemiology

Hepatitis E is transmitted primarily by the fecal–oral route through contaminated water or water supplies and the disease generally affects young adults (Purcell 1996; Reyes 1997; Aggarwal and Krawczynski 2000). As a fecal–orally transmitted disease, hepatitis E is an important public health concern in many developing countries where sanitation conditions are poor. Epidemics, associated with fecal contamination of water, are usually confined in Southeast and Central Asia, Northern and Western Africa as well as in Mexico. Water-borne epidemics are the most explosive form of HEV infection in these regions (Vishwanathan 1957; Khuroo 1980; Wong et al. 1980; Naik et al. 1992; Purcell 1996). The overall mortality rate caused by HEV infection is generally low with less than 1%. However, it has been reported that the mortality rate can be up to 20% in HEV-infected pregnant women (Vishwanathan 1957; Khuroo 1980; Purcell 1996; Jaiswal et al. 2001). The pathogenesis of fulminant hepatitis E in infected pregnant women is not understood. In the primate model, fulminant hepatitis in pregnant rhesus monkeys could not be experimentally reproduced: there was no increased severity of hepatitis in pregnant monkeys when compared to nonpregnant monkeys (Tsarev et al. 1995). The elevation of serum alanine aminotransferase and the presence of liver pathological lesions generally correspond to the detection of HEV serum antibodies and with decreasing levels of HEV antigen in hepatocytes, suggesting that the pathogenesis of hepatitis E may be immunologically mediated and that hepatitis results from a host immune response to infected cells rather than damage to the hepatocytes by the virus itself (Purcell 1996; Aggarwal and Krawczynski 2000). Epidemics of hepatitis E are actually uncommon and most acute hepatitis E cases have occurred as endemic or sporadic forms. In industrialized countries, most cases occurred primarily in travelers recently returned from endemic regions (Purcell 1996; Reyes 1997; Kabrane-Lazizi et al. 2001). However, sporadic cases of acute hepatitis E with no known epidemiological risk factors have recently been reported from patients in several industrialized countries (Purcell 1996; Reyes 1997; Schlauder et al. 1998, 1999, 2000; Erker et al. 1999; Meng 2000a, 2000b; Aggarwal and Krawczynski 2000; Takahashi et al. 2001).

The availability of serological assays for detecting HEV antibodies has greatly aided the understanding of HEV epidemiology, although the relative sensitivity and specificity of these assays are not known. It has been shown that anti-HEV prevalence in endemic countries is much lower than expected, generally ranging from 3% to 27% (Purcell 1996), although much higher seroprevalence rates have been reported in some endemic regions such as Egypt with more than 60% seroprevalence (Fix et al. 2000). The anti-HEV prevalence is found to be age specific (Arankalle et al. 1995; Meng et al. 2002), and the highest attack rate is among young adults 15–40 years of age in endemic regions (Aggarwal and Krawczynski 2000). A surprisingly high anti-HEV prevalence in industrialized countries, where hepatitis E was generally considered nonendemic, has been reported. Thomas et al. (1997) reported that IgG anti-HEV was detected in about 21% of the blood donors from Baltimore, MD. In Northern California, about 1.2%–1.4% of blood donors were found to be positive for IgG anti-HEV, and 31%–38% of the seropositive individuals had no history of international travel (Mast et al. 1997). In Japan, the prevalence of the IgG anti-HEV in healthy individuals ranged from 1.9% to 14.1%, depending on the geographical location (Li et al. 2000). Similar results have also been reported in other industrialized countries (Hsieh et al. 1998; Fagan and Harrison 2000; Meng 2000a, b). The existence of a population of individuals in industrialized countries who are positive for anti-HEV has led to a hypothesis that an animal reservoir for HEV exists, and that hepatitis E is a zoonosis.

3 Swine HEV

3.1 Discovery of Swine HEV

The first evidence of HEV infection in swine came from a study by Balayan et al. (1990) who have reportedly infected domestic swine with a Central Asian strain of human HEV. Subsequently, Clayson et al. (1995) reported the detection of IgG anti-HEV in 18 of 55 swine and HEV RNA from sera and feces in three of 47 swine in Nepal. However, the identity of the virus infecting swine was not determined in those studies.

Fig. 2A–C A prospective study of natural swine HEV infection in pigs in a commercial swine farm: seroconversion of piglets to HEV. Anti-HEV responses of three representative piglets are presented. **A** Piglet born to a seropositive sow with a high titer of IgG anti-HEV. **B** Piglet born to a seropositive sow with a lower titer of IgG anti-HEV. **C** Piglet born to a seronegative sow. The ELISA optical density value of IgG anti-HEV in breeder sows is indicated (*S*). (Reproduced by permission of the National Academy of Science, from Meng et al. 1997)

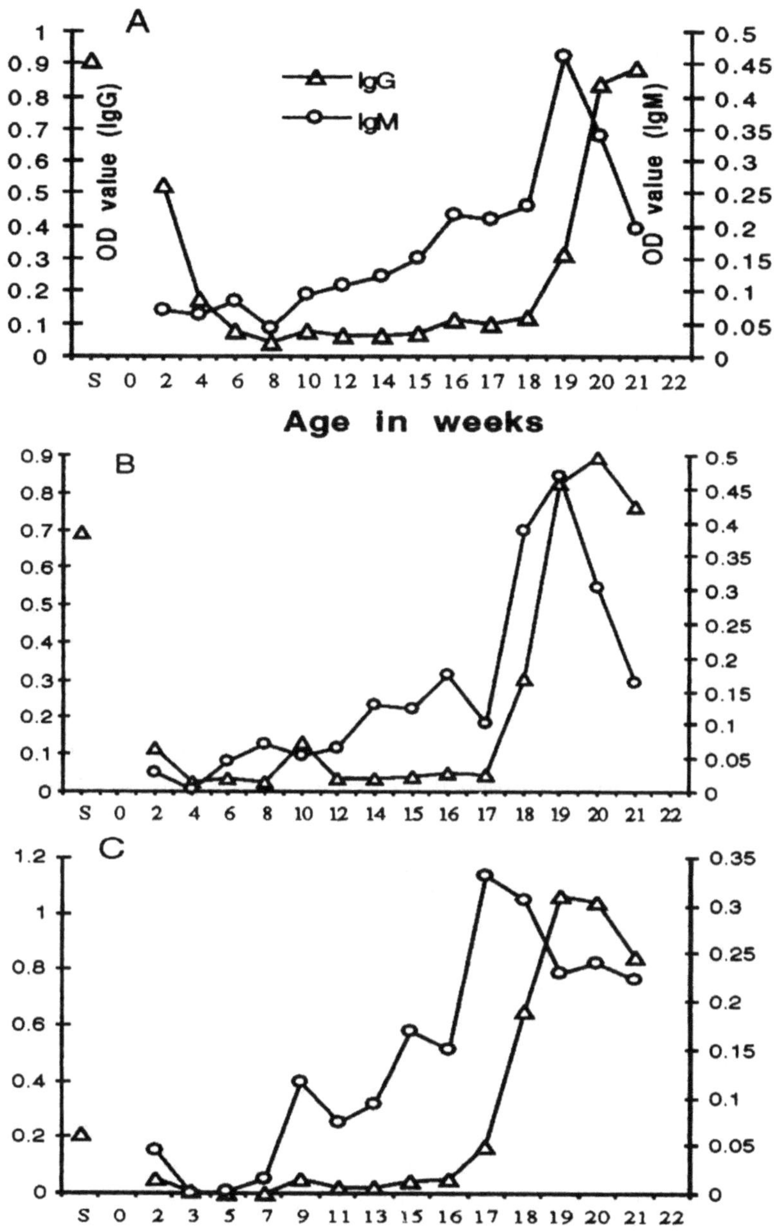
A
IgG
IgM
OD value (IgG)
OD value (IgM)
Age in weeks
B
C

Meng et al. (1997) isolated and characterized the first animal strain of HEV, swine HEV, from a pig in the USA. To identify swine HEV, Meng et al. (1997) conducted a prospective study in a commercial swine farm in Illinois. Twenty piglets born to both anti-HEV seronegative and seropositive sows were selected, tagged and mixed with other piglets in the same herd. The piglets were closely monitored for more than 5 months for evidence of HEV infection, including seroconversion by an ELISA, and viremia and fecal virus shedding by a reverse transcription (RT)-polymerase chain reaction (PCR) using degenerate HEV primers. The first piglet seroconverted at the age of 14 weeks, followed within a few weeks by seroconversion of piglets in other pens housed in the same building (Fig. 2). The pattern of anti-HEV appearance, starting with piglets grouped near the first seropositive piglet, then followed by more distal ones, was consistent with seroconversion induced by an infectious agent. By 21 weeks of age, 16 of the 20 study piglets had seroconverted. A virus genetically related to human HEV, designated swine HEV, was identified from the acute phase sera of the naturally infected piglets (Meng et al. 1997). Koch's postulates were fulfilled as swine HEV infection was experimentally reproduced in specific pathogen-free (SPF) pigs, and swine HEV was recovered from experimentally infected SPF pigs (Meng et al. 1998a, b; Halbur et al. 2001). Since the identification of swine HEV from a pig in the USA (Meng et al. 1997), numerous strains of swine HEV have been genetically identified from pigs in other countries including Taiwan (Hsieh et al. 1999; Wu et al. 2000, 2002), New Zealand (Garkavenko et al. 2001), Canada (Yoo et al. 2001), Japan (Okamoto et al. 2001) and the Netherlands (Van der Poel et al. 2001). In the USA, Huang et al. (2002a) tested fecal and serum samples of pigs of 2–4 months of age from 37 different USA swine farms for swine HEV RNA. Thirty-four of the 96 pigs (35%) and 20 of the 37 swine herds (54%) tested were positive for swine HEV RNA. Sequence analyses revealed that the 27 USA swine HEV isolates identified in the study (Huang et al. 2002) had 88%–100% nucleotide sequence identity to each other and 89%–98% identities with the prototype USA swine HEV. The USA swine HEV isolates are only distantly related to the Taiwanese strains of swine HEV with about 74%–78% nucleotide sequence identities, to most known human strains of HEV worldwide (<79% sequence identities), and to avian HEV with 54%–56% sequence identities.

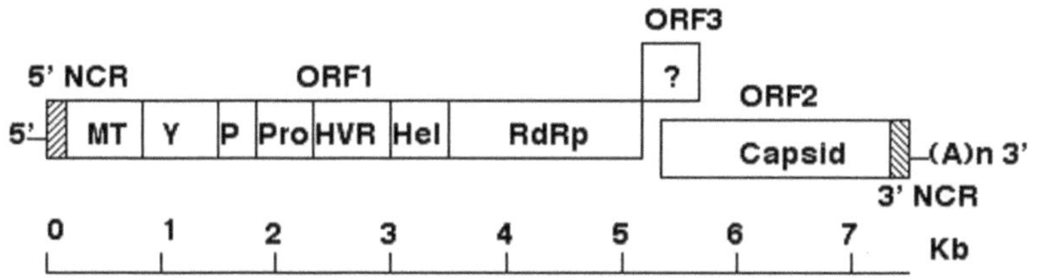

Fig. 3 Genomic organization of swine HEV. The positive sense RNA molecule encodes three open reading frames (*ORF*): ORF1 encodes nonstructural proteins, ORF2 putative capsid protein and ORF3 a small protein of unknown function. *NCR*, noncoding region; *MT*, methyltransferase; *Y*, "Y" domain; *P*, a papain-like cysteine protease; *Pro*, a proline-rich domain that may provide flexibility; *HVR*, a hypervariable region; *Hel*, helicase; *RdRp*, RNA-dependent RNA polymerase

3.2
Genome Organization

The complete genomic sequence of swine HEV has been determined (Meng et al. 1997, 1998b; Haqshenas and Meng 2001; Okamoto et al. 2001). The genome is a polyadenylated, single-stranded positive-sense RNA molecule of approximately 7.2 kb (Meng et al. 1998b). Sequence analyses revealed that the genome of swine HEV contains three ORFs, a 5′ NCR and a 3′ NCR (Fig. 3). ORF1 is predicted to encode the nonstructural proteins. Based on the sequence comparison with human HEV, several putative functional domains and motifs have been assigned to the ORF1 of swine HEV (Meng et al. 1998b). The methyl transferase domain located at the 5′end, followed by a Y domain (a sequence of unknown function), a papain-like cysteine protease (P), a proline-rich domain that may provide flexibility, a hypervariable region (HVR), a helicase, and an RNA-dependent RNA polymerase. ORF2 encodes the putative capsid protein that contains a typical signal peptide sequence at its N terminus and three potential glycosylation sites. ORF3, a small ORF of less than 400 nucleotides, overlaps both ORF1 and ORF2 (Meng et al. 1997, 1998b). The function of ORF3 of swine HEV is unknown. The ORF3 of human HEV is a cytoskeleton-associated phosphoprotein that may be involved in virus replication (Zafrullah et al. 1997).

3.3 Pathogenesis

Little is known about the pathogenesis of swine HEV infection. Swine HEV is presumably transmitted through the fecal–oral route. Feces from infected pigs appear to be the principal source of the virus. Meng et al. (1998b) demonstrated that a sentinel uninoculated pig, housed in the same room with a swine HEV-inoculated pig, became infected about 2 weeks after the experimentally inoculated pig became infected. It is believed that pigs acquire infection through direct contact with infected pigs or through ingestion of feces-contaminated feed or water. However, experimental reproduction of swine HEV infection in pigs via the oral route of inoculation has not yet been successful. Kasorndorkbua et al. (2002) demonstrated that even a $10^{4.5}$ 50% pig infectious dose of swine HEV was insufficient to infect pigs via the oral route. However, SPF pigs can be readily infected by swine HEV via the intravenous route of inoculation (Meng et al. 1998a, 1998b; Halbur et al. 2001; Kasorndorkbua et al. 2002). The high anti-HEV prevalence in pigs suggested that swine HEV is readily transmissible in the swine population, and thus other route(s) of swine HEV transmission cannot be ruled out.

In pigs naturally infected by swine HEV, clinical illness was not observed and the infection was subclinical. In a prospective study of swine HEV infection in a commercial farm, four piglets at an early stage of natural infection were necropsied (Meng et al. 1997). Gross lesions were not apparent in 19 different tissues or organs examined during necropsy. Microscopically, all four piglets necropsied had evidence of hepatitis characterized by mild to moderate multifocal and periportal lymphoplasmacytic hepatitis with mild focal hepatocellular necrosis. In addition, all piglets had lymphoplasmacytic enteritis, and three piglets also had mild multifocal lymphoplasmacytic interstitial nephritis (Meng et al. 1997).

In SPF pigs experimentally infected with swine HEV, evidence of clinical disease or elevation of liver enzymes or bilirubin was not observed (Meng et al. 1998a; Halbur et al. 2001). Mild-to-moderate multifocal lymphoplasmacytic hepatitis and focal hepatocellular necrosis were observed in infected pigs (Fig. 4). HEV RNA was detected in feces, liver tissue and bile of infected pigs from 3 to 27 days postinoculation (dpi) (Table 1).

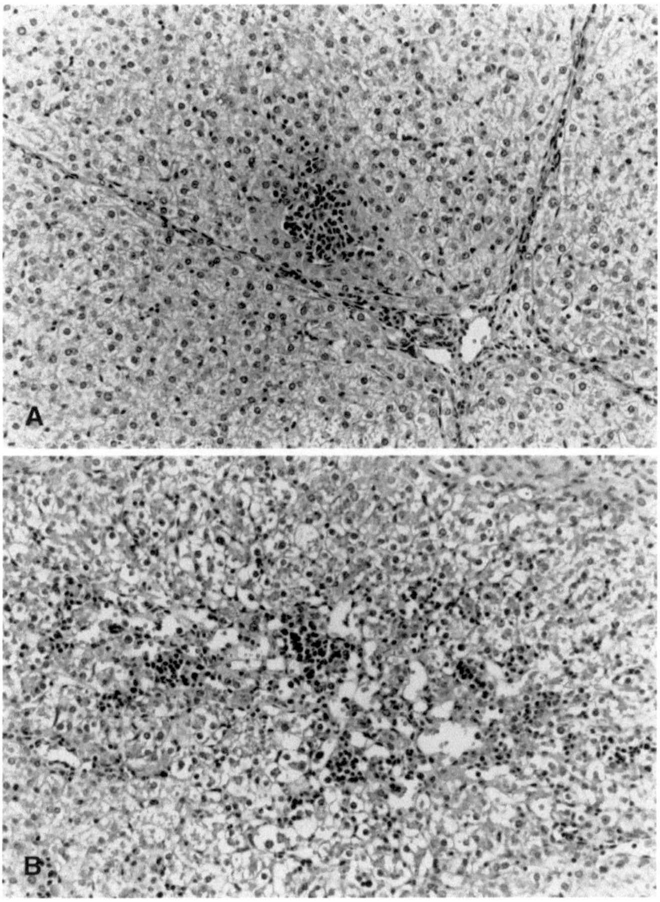

Fig. 4. A Liver of a pig experimentally infected with swine HEV. There is mild focal infiltration of lymphocytes, plasma cells, and macrophages and mild diffuse inflammation in hepatic sinusoids at 14 dpi. Hepatocytes are mildly swollen and vacuolated. **B** Liver of a pig experimentally infected with the US-2 strain of human HEV. There is severe lymphoplasmacytic and histiocytic hepatitis and severe vacuolar degeneration and swelling of hepatocytes at 14 dpi. (Reproduced by permission of the American Society for Microbiology, from Halbur et al. 2001) H&E

Table 1 Detection of hepatitis E virus (HEV) RNA in feces, serum, liver, and bile of SPF pigs experimentally infected with swine HEV and the US-2 strain of human HEV[a]

		Days postinoculation								
Inoculum	Sample	0	3	7	14	20	27	35	42	55
None	Feces	0/17[b]	NT[c]	NT	NT	NT	NT	NT	NT	0/2
	serum	0/17	NT	NT	NT	NT	NT	NT	NT	0/2
	Liver	NT	0/3	0/3	0/3	0/3	0/3	NT	NT	0/2
	Bile	NT	0/3	0/3	0/3	0/3	0/3	NT	NT	0/2
Swine HEV[d]	Feces	0/18	NT	15/15	12/12	4/9	1/6	0/3	0/3	0/3
	Serum	0/18	NT	9/15	8/12	1/9	0/6	NT	NT	0/3
	Liver	NT	2/3	3/3	1/3	1/3	0/3	NT	NT	0/3
	Bile	NT	3/3	3/3	3/3	2/3	1/3	NT	NT	0/3
Human HEV[e]	Feces	0/19	NT	16/16	13/13	9/10	3/7	2/4	0/4	0/4
	Serum	0/19	NT	15/16	13/13	5/10	0/7	NT	NT	0/4
	Liver	NT	3/3	3/3	3/3	2/3	2/3	NT	NT	0/4
	Bile	NT	3/3	3/3	3/3	3/3	3/3	NT	NT	0/4

[a] Modified by permission of the American Society for Microbiology, from Halbur et al. 2001.
[b] Numbers positive/numbers tested.
[c] Samples not collected or tested at this dpi.
[d] USA strain of swine HEV (Meng et al. 1997).
[e] US-2 strain of human HEV (Schlauder et al. 1998).

Table 2 Seroprevalence of IgG anti-HEV from pigs in different geographic regions

Geographic origin	Herd	Pig age	No. positive/ no. tested (%)	Reference
USA	A	6–12 weeks	0/16 (0)	Meng et al. 1997
		20 weeks	8/8 (100)	
		26 weeks	5/8 (63)	
		Adult	14/25 (56)	
	B	3–8 weeks	0/24 (0)	
		13 weeks	10/12 (83)	
		6 months	8/8 (100)	
		Adult	16/17 (94)	
	C	2 months	1/8 (13)	
		3 months	8/8 (100)	
		4 months	4/8 (50)	
		5 months to adult	16/16 (100)	
	9 herds	6 months to 3 years	90/90 (100)	
	2 herds	Adult	20/25 (80)	
Spain	6 herds	3 weeks to 2 months	2/10 (20)	Pina et al. 2000
		5–6 months	7/24 (29)	
		6 months to 4 years	6/26 (23)	
Australia	2 herds	Mixed	12/40 (30)	Chandler et al. 1999
	2 herds	16 weeks	45 (92–95)	
	Wild pigs	Unknown	15/59 (17)	
Taiwan	10 herds	mixed	102/275 (37)	Hsieh et al. 1999
Canada (Quebec)	37 herds	Nursery	82/310 (26)	Meng et al. 1999
	16 herds	Adult	34/90 (38)	
Canada (Ontario)	10 herds	Nursery	1/230 (<1)	Meng et al. 1999
	4 herds	Adult	12/82 (15)	
Canada (5 provinces)	81 herds	6 months	594/998 (60)	Yoo et al. 2001
Korea	Multiple	1–2 months	6/40 (15)	Meng et al. 1999
		3–6 months	39/80 (49)	
		Sows	12/20 (60)	

Table 2 (continued)

Geographic origin	Herd	Pig age	No. positive/ no. tested (%)	Reference
Nepal		Mixed	18/55 (33)	Clayson et al. 1995
China	A	1–2 months	9/21 (43)	Meng et al. 1999
	B	3–5 months	8/30 (27)	
	C	6 months to adult	5/21 (24)	
Thailand	A	1–2 months	0/20 (0)	Meng et al. 1999
		3–4 months	13/20 (65)	
	B	6 months	7/10 (70)	
		Sows	2/10 (20)	
	C	Adult	1/5 (20)	
	D	Sows	0/10 (0)	
Vietnam	Unknown	Unknown	36%	Tien et al. 1997
India (1988)	Unknown	Unknown	102/137 (74)	Arankalle et a. 2001
India (1993)	Unknown	Unknown	53/97 (55)	Arankalle et al. 2001

3.4 Anti-HEV Prevalence in Swine Population

Seroepidemiological studies demonstrated that swine HEV is ubiquitous in pigs in the USA, and that about 80%–100% of the pigs in commercial farms in the USA were infected (Meng et al. 1997). The infection generally occurs at about 2–3 months of age. Similar findings were also reported in other countries, both endemic and nonendemic. A recent serosurvey of pigs in two industrialized countries (Canada and Taiwan) and two developing countries (China and Thailand) showed that about 20%–90% of the pigs older than 3 months of age were positive for IgG anti-HEV (Meng et al. 1999). In the Kathmandu Valley of Nepal where hepatitis E is endemic, about 33% of the swine tested were positive for anti-HEV (Clayson et al. 1995). In Australia, anti-HEV was detected in 92%–95% of 4-month-old commercial pigs and 17% of wild-caught pigs (Chandler et al. 1999). Pina et al. (2000) found that about 25% of the Spanish pigs were positive for anti-HEV. In New Zealand, about 91% of the swine herds tested were positive for anti-HEV (Garkavenko et al. 2001). Arankalle et al. (2001) recently found that about 55%–74% of the pigs in India are also positive for IgG anti-HEV. These data indicated that swine HEV infection in pigs is common worldwide (Table 2). Even some high biosecurity SPF swine farms in the USA also tested positive for anti-HEV (X.J. Meng, P.G. Halbur, S.U. Emerson and R.H. Purcell, unpublished results). The ubiquitous nature of swine HEV infection in pigs suggests a need to adequately screen for swine HEV in xenograft donor pigs.

3.5 Experimental Infection of Nonhuman Primates with Swine HEV

Rhesus monkeys and a chimpanzee have been experimentally infected with swine HEV (Meng et al. 1998b). The two rhesus monkeys inoculated intravenously with a $10^{4.5}$ 50% pig infectious dose of swine HEV seroconverted to HEV 4 weeks postinoculation and were still seropositive at the end of the 16-week experiment. Viremia and fecal excretion of swine HEV were detected in inoculated rhesus monkeys. The peak PCR titer of swine HEV in the feces of inoculated rhesus monkeys was 10^6 genomic equivalents per gram of feces (Meng et al. 1998b). There was a slight elevation of serum liver enzymes (alanine aminotransferase and isocitrate dehydrogenase) in the two inoculated primates. Focal necroinflammatory changes, consistent with mild acute viral hepatitis, were observed in liver biopsy specimens near the time of serum liver enzyme elevations (Fig. 5). The chimpanzee inoculated with swine HEV also became infected. Swine HEV RNA was detected in feces of the inoculated chimpanzee. Seroconversion to HEV occurred at 6 weeks postinoculation, although viremia was not detected by RT–PCR. The serum levels of liver enzymes in the infected chimpanzee were not significantly elevated. Both rhesus monkeys and the chimpanzee infected with swine HEV remained clinically normal, and there were no clinical signs of hepatitis. The swine HEV recovered from an experimentally infected rhesus monkey was successfully transmitted to additional nonhuman primates (X.J. Meng, S.U. Emerson and R.H. Purcell, unpublished results). Infection of nonhuman primates, the surrogates of man, with swine HEV demonstrated the ability of swine HEV to infect across species barriers and the possibility of human infection with swine HEV.

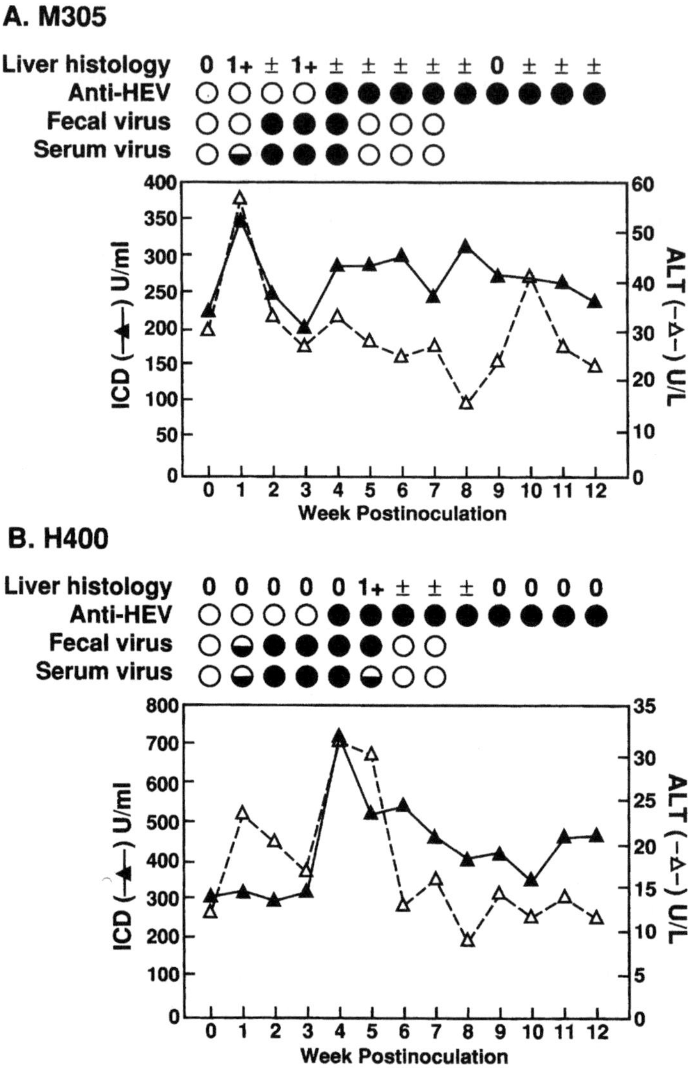

Fig. 5A, B Experimental infection of rhesus monkeys with swine HEV. Levels of serum liver enzymes (ALT and ICD) are plotted. Presence (*filled circle*) or absence (*open circle*) of anti-HEV and swine HEV RNA in serum and feces is indicated. *Half-filled circles* indicated detection of swine HEV RNA only by a nested PCR. The degree of liver lesions observed in liver biopsies is indicated (scale of 0–4+). (Modified by permission of American Society for Microbiology, from Meng et al. 1998b)

3.6
Anti-HEV Prevalence in Pig Handlers

A very limited number of pig handlers from two HEV endemic countries was tested for anti-HEV prevalence (Meng et al. 1999). It was found that 11 of 11 pig handlers tested from China were positive for IgG anti-HEV, although 17 of 35 (55%) of the normal blood donors from the same geographic region were also positive. In Thailand, five of seven pig handlers tested were seropositive. A definitive conclusion as to whether swine handlers have a higher risk of HEV infection cannot be drawn because of the limited number of pig handlers tested and because of the high seroprevalence background in endemic countries. Recently, several seroepidemiological studies of pig handlers were conducted in industrialized countries, where hepatitis E was not considered to be endemic. In Taiwan, Hsieh et al. (1999) found that about 27% of the Taiwanese pig handlers were positive for anti-HEV compared to only about 8% of the control subjects. More recently, a total of 468 swine veterinarians and 400 normal USA blood donors were tested for IgG anti-HEV using recombinant capsid antigens from the prototype strain of swine HEV and a Pakistani strain of human HEV (Sar-55) (Meng et al. 2002). Among the 295 swine veterinarians tested from the eight USA states from which normal blood donor samples were available, about 23% (swine HEV antigen) or 26% (Sar-55 antigen) of swine veterinarians were positive for IgG anti-HEV compared to 17% (swine HEV antigen) or 18% (Sar-55 antigen) of normal blood donors. Swine veterinarians in the eight USA states were 1.51 times more likely when tested with swine HEV antigen [95% confidence interval (CI), 1.03–2.20] and 1.46 times more likely when tested with Sar-55 human HEV antigen (95% CI, 0.99–2.17) to be anti-HEV positive than normal USA blood donors. There was a difference in anti-HEV prevalence in both swine veterinarians and normal blood donors among the eight selected states, with subjects from Minnesota (a major swine state) six times more likely to be anti-HEV positive than those from Alabama (a traditionally nonswine state). Drobeniuc et al. (2001) recently tested 264 swine farmers and 255 control subjects with no occupational exposure to swine in Moldova, a country without a reported case of hepatitis E, for IgG anti-HEV prevalence. They found that anti-HEV prevalence was higher in swine farmers (51%) than that in control subjects (25%) (95% CI, 1.62–2.64). HEV infection was associated with an occupational history of cleaning barns or assisting sows at birth, years of exposure to swine, and a history of drinking raw milk. Taken together, these data strongly suggested that swine veterinarians and other pig handlers are at risk of potential zoonotic infection.

3.7 Emergence of Novel Strains of Human HEV Closely Related to Swine HEV

Numerous novel strains of HEV closely related to swine HEV have recently been identified from patients with acute hepatitis E. In the USA, two cases of acute hepatitis E have been reported (Schlauder et al. 1998; Erker et al. 1999). The two USA isolates of HEV (US-1 and US-2) are genetically distinct from other known strains of HEV worldwide (about 80% amino acid sequence identity in ORF1) but are most closely related to the USA strain of swine HEV recovered from a pig in Illinois (about 98% sequence identity in ORF1). It is not known, however, if the two patients had any occupational exposures to pigs. Kabrane-Lazizi et al. (2001) recently reported another USA strain of HEV that is genetically most similar to the USA swine HEV from a patient who had recently returned from vacation in Thailand. Several novel isolates of HEV have been identified from patients in Taiwan with no history of travel to endemic regions (Hsieh et al. 1998, 1999; Wu et al. 2000). These Taiwanese isolates are genetically distinct from other known strains of HEV (about 70%–75% nucleotide sequence identity) but are most closely related to Taiwanese strains of swine HEV recovered from Taiwanese pigs (about 97% sequence identity). Pina et al. (2000) found that the Spanish E11 strain of HEV of possibly swine origin is closely related to two Spanish strains of human HEV but is less related to other known strains of HEV. An indigenous Japanese strain of human HEV (JRA1) was identified from a Japanese hepatitis patient who had no history of traveling abroad (Takahashi et al. 2001). The Japanese JRA1 strain of human HEV was most closely related to the Japanese strains of swine HEV identified from pigs (89% nucleotide sequence identity) but had only 73%–76% sequence identity to Asian and Mexican strains of human HEV. The close genetic relatedness between swine HEV and human HEV in the same geographic region suggested that these novel strains of human HEV may be of swine origin, and that swine HEV may infect humans.

4 Animal Reservoirs for HEV: Risk for Zoonosis

4.1 Anti-HEV Prevalence in Animal Species

In addition to pigs, serological evidence of HEV infection of other animal species has also been documented. Kabrane-Lazizi et al. (1999b) found that about 77% of the rats from Maryland, 90% from Hawaii and 44% from Louisiana were positive for IgG anti-HEV. The prevalence of anti-HEV in rats was age-specific and increased in parallel with the estimated age of the rats. Favorov et al. (2000) also reported the detection of anti-HEV among rodents in the USA. The highest rate of anti-HEV prevalence in rats was found in the genus *Rattus*. The high anti-HEV prevalence in rats suggested that rats might transmit the virus to swine or vice versa (Meng et al. 2000a, 2000b) since rodents are often found in proximity to swine farms. In Vietnam where HEV is endemic, anti-HEV was detected in 44% of chickens, 36% of pigs, 27% of dogs and 9% of rats (Tien et al. 1997). Favorov et al. (1998) showed that about 29%–62% of cows from Somali, Tajikistan and Turkmenistan, about 42%–67% of the sheep and goats from Turkmenistan and about 12% of cows from Ukraine were positive for anti-HEV. In India, anti-HEV antibodies were detected in 4%–7% of cattle, 55%–74% of pigs and 2%–22% of rodents (Arankalle et al. 2001). Tsarev et al. (1995) also reported the detection of naturally acquired anti-HEV in rhesus macaques. Taken together, these serological data suggested that these animal species have been exposed to HEV (or a related agent). Karetnyi et al. (1999) reported that the anti-HEV prevalence in field workers from the Iowa Department of Natural Resources is significantly higher than that in blood donors, suggesting that human populations with occupational exposure to wild animals may have increased risks of HEV infection.

4.2 Genetic Identification of Animal Strains of HEV

In addition to swine HEV from pigs, strains of HEV from other animal species have also been genetically identified. A variant strain of HEV was reportedly identified from tissue and fecal samples of wild-trapped rodents from Kathmandu Valley, Nepal (Tsarev et al. 1998). Sequence analyses revealed that the HEV sequence recovered from rodents was most closely related to the HEV isolates from patients in Nepal. Payne et al. (1999) reported the identification of a virus associated with big liver and spleen disease (BLS) of chickens in Australia. The BLS virus shared about 62% nucleotide sequence identity with human HEV. Recently, Haqshenas et al. (2001) identified an avian strain of HEV, designated avian HEV, from chickens with hepatitis-splenomegaly syndrome in the USA. The avian HEV shared about 50%–60% nucleotide sequence identity with human and swine strains of HEV, and about 80% identity with the chicken BLS virus (Huang et al. 2002b). The avian HEV has been shown to share antigenic epitopes in the capsid protein with human and swine HEV (Haqshenas et al. 2002). Genetic identification of HEV strains from swine, chickens and rodents further strengthens the argument that animal reservoirs for HEV exist, and that hepatitis E is a zoonosis.

4.3 Experimental Cross-Species Infection of HEV

It has been demonstrated that swine HEV can cross species barriers and infect nonhuman primates, therefore possibly humans. Conversely, a human strain of HEV (strain US-2) has also been shown to infect SPF pigs (Meng et al. 1998b; Halbur et al. 2001). The inoculated pigs rapidly became viremic and seroconverted to HEV, suggesting that the US-2 strain of human HEV is already competent to replicate in swine and may be of swine origin. Evidence of clinical disease or elevation of liver enzymes or bilirubin was not found in infected pigs. Enlarged hepatic and mesenteric lymph nodes were observed in infected pigs. Multifocal lymphoplasmacytic hepatitis and focal hepatocellular necrosis were also observed in infected SPF pigs. Hepatic inflammation and hepatocellular necrosis peaked in severity at 20 dpi, and were still moderately severe at 55 dpi in infected pigs. A Central Asian strain of human HEV has been reported to infect Russian domestic swine (Balayan et al. 1990), and the infected swine developed jaundice. However, others were unable to infect SPF swine with similar strains of human HEV. Meng et al. (1998a) failed to infect crossbred SPF swine with two well-characterized epidemic strains of human HEV (a Mexican strain and a Pakistani strain). Similarly, Platt et al. (1998) were unable to infect SPF swine with the Mexican strain of human HEV, and Arankalle et al. (2001) failed to infect pigs with an Indian strain of human HEV (AKL-90). It is possible that these epidemic strains may have a more limited host range than do swine HEV or other HEV strains of animal origin. Cross-species infection of HEV has also been reported in other animal species. Lambs were reportedly infected with human HEV isolates (Usmanov et al. 1994). Similarly, Wistar rats were reportedly infected with a human stool suspension containing infectious HEV (Maneerat et al. 1996).

4.4 Natural History of HEV: A Hypothesis

The natural history of HEV is not known. The ability of swine HEV to infect across species, the genetic identification of novel HEV strains from chickens and rats, and the existence of numerous other animal species that are positive for anti-HEV further complicated the understanding of the natural history of HEV. It is known that human-to-human transmission of HEV is uncommon. Therefore, a speculative scenario for HEV transmission is that HEV is constantly circulating among different animal species including swine (Fig. 6). HEV infects humans through direct contact with infected domestic or farm animals or with feces-contaminated water or water supplies. If this happens in a developing country, it may result in an endemic or epidemic due to the poor sanitation conditions. However, if this happens in an industrialized country, it will occur only as a sporadic case of acute hepatitis E because of the good sanitation conditions. It will be important to determine whether there are basic differences in host range or pathogenicity between epidemic/endemic strains in humans and enzoonotic strains that are primarily circulating in animal species. Understanding the natural history of HEV is important for the prevention and control of hepatitis E and for the generation of xenograft donor pigs free of HEV.

5 Xenozoonotic Risk of Swine HEV Infection

5.1 Sites of Viral Replication in Swine

The initial site of swine HEV replication in pigs is still unknown. In primates and pigs experimentally infected with swine HEV, virus replica-

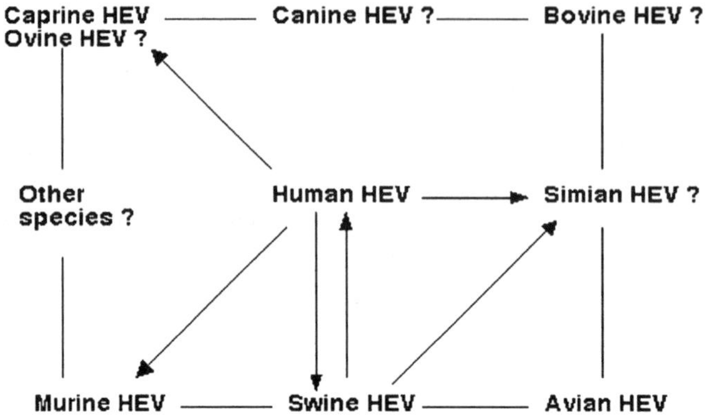

Fig. 6 Natural history of HEV: a hypothesis. *Arrows* indicate documented inter-species transmissions. Strains of HEV have been genetically identified from human, rodents, chickens and pigs. HEV antibodies have been detected in monkeys, sheep, goats, cattle and dogs but the identities of the seropositivity in these species have not yet been determined

tion in the liver has been documented (Meng et al. 1998b; Halbur et al. 2001). However, the mechanism by which the virus reaches the liver is not yet understood. It is believed that the virus is released to the gall bladder from hepatocytes by unknown mechanisms and then is excreted in feces. It is suggested that the virus probably replicates in the intestinal tract prior to infecting the liver (Fagan and Harrison 2000). Using a swine model, Williams et al. (2001) recently studied the potential extra-hepatic sites of HEV replication in pigs experimentally infected with swine HEV and the US-2 strain of human HEV. As a positive-strand RNA virus, HEV produces an intermediate negative-strand viral RNA during virus replication. By using a negative strand-specific RT–PCR, replicative negative-strand HEV RNA was detected in the liver as well as in several extrahepatic tissues and organs including small intestine, colon, spleen, kidney, tonsil, and hepatic and mesenteric lymph nodes. Although the significance of the extrahepatic sites of virus replication is not known, the data do raise additional concerns for xenotransplantation with pig organs other than the liver. Aside from the xenozoonosis concern, pigs recovered from swine HEV infection may have a damaged liver or other organs which would limit its usefulness for xenotransplantation. Microscopic lesions of hepatitis were observed in pigs and primates experimentally infected by swine HEV (Meng et al. 1998b; Halbur et al. 2001). Lymphoplasmacytic interstitial nephritis and enteritis were also observed in pigs naturally infected by swine HEV (Meng et al. 1997).

5.2
Risk for Xenozoonosis

Swine HEV appears to be ubiquitous in pigs worldwide and has the ability to infect humans. Thus, xenozoonosis due to the transmission of swine HEV from pig xenografts to human transplant recipients and the potential subsequent transmission of the virus to others are possible. Although swine HEV appears to cause only subclinical infection in pigs and primates under experimental conditions (Meng et al. 1998b; Halbur et al. 2001; Kasorndorkbua et al. 2002), it may become pathogenic in immunosuppressed xenograft recipients. However, unlike some other porcine viruses such as the porcine endogenous retrovirus, xenograft donor pigs free of swine HEV can be generated through strict breeding procedures. A recent study showed that piglets negative for swine HEV can be successfully generated through segregated early weaning from pregnant SPF sows experimentally infected with swine HEV (B. Thacker, personal communication). Therefore, the potential xenozoonotic infection by swine HEV in xenotransplantation is preventable through adequate screening and strict breeding procedures for donor pigs.

5.3
Screening for Swine HEV Infection in Xenograft Donor Pigs

The discovery of swine HEV has added yet another virus to the growing list of zoonotic viruses that should be screened before tissues and organs from swine can be used for xenotransplantation. Sensitive and easy-to-perform assays must be developed to screen for swine HEV infection in donor pigs. Currently, the diagnosis of swine HEV infection is primarily based on PCR and serological assays. However, the sensitivity and specificity of these assays are not known. The recombinant human HEV capsid antigen cross-reacted well with antibodies to swine HEV in ELISA assays, and has been used to detect anti-HEV in swine (Meng et al. 1997, 1999, 2002; Hsieh et al. 1998, 1999; Chandler et al. 1999; Wu et al. 2000; Yoo et al. 2001). Recently, the capsid protein of the USA strain of swine HEV has also been expressed and used in an ELISA to detect anti-HEV

(Meng et al. 2002). The ELISA results based on the recombinant swine HEV antigen correlated well with those obtained with a recombinant antigen from the Sar-55 strain of human HEV (Engle et al. 2002; Meng et al. 2002).

Serological assays alone are inadequate in screening swine HEV infection in donor pigs since anti-HEV antibodies generally occur in pigs at least 2 weeks after infection. Viremia and fecal virus shedding occur in infected pigs much earlier than the appearance of anti-HEV antibodies and thus, seronegative pigs could actually be infected with swine HEV (Meng et al. 1997, 1998a). A sensitive and specific RT–PCR assay should be used in combination with serological assays to screen donor pigs. RT–PCR has been successfully used to detect different strains of swine HEV from infected pigs (Meng et al. 1997; Hsieh et al. 1999; Wu et al. 2000; Okamoto et al. 2001; Van der Poel et al. 2001; Yoo et al. 2001). However, the specificity of the current RT–PCR assays in detecting swine HEV in pigs from different geographic regions is not known. Human strains of HEV isolated from different geographic locations varied extensively in their genomic sequences. Recent studies indicated that swine HEV strains identified from pigs in different geographic regions also vary considerably in their genomic sequences (Hsieh et al. 1999; Pina et al. 2000; Wu et al. 2000; Huang et al. 2002a). Therefore, genetic identification and characterization of additional field strains of swine HEV from different geographic regions will be critical for developing a universal RT–PCR assay that can detect all strains of swine HEV that may exist in xenograft donor pigs.

Acknowledgements. The author thanks R.H. Purcell and S.U. Emerson of the National Institutes of Health, Bethesda, MD and P.G. Halbur of Iowa State University, Ames, IA, for their support and collaborations. The author also thanks T.E. Toth for critical review of the manuscript. The author's research on HEV is supported by grants from the National Institutes of Health (AI01653, AI46505, AI050611), from the National Pork Board, from the U.S. Department of Agriculture (NRI 2002-35204-12531) and from Fort Dodge Animal Health Inc.

References

Aggarwal R, Krawczynski K (2000) Hepatitis E: An overview and recent advances in clinical and laboratory research. J Gastroenterol Hepatol 15:9–20

Arankalle VA, Tsarev SA, Chadha MS, Alling DW, Emerson SU, Banerjee K, Purcell RH (1995) Age-specific prevalence of antibodies to hepatitis A and E viruses in Pune, India, 1982 and 1992. J Infect Dis 171:447–450

Arankalle VA, Chadha MS, Tsarev SA, Emerson SU, Risbud AR, Banerjee K, Purcell RH (1994) Seroepidemiology of water-born hepatitis in India and evidence for a third enterically-transmitted hepatitis agent. Proc Natl Acad Sci USA 91:3428–3432

Arankalle VA, Joshi MV, Kulkarni AM, Gandhe S, Chobe L, Rautmare S, Mishra A, Padbidri V (2001) Prevalence of anti-hepatitis E virus antibodies in different Indian animal species. J Viral Hepat 8:223–227

Balayan MS, Andjaparidze AG, Savinskaya SS, Ketiladze ES, Braginsky DM, Savinov AP, Poleschuk VF (1983) Evidence for a virus in non-A, non-B hepatitis transmitted via the fecal-oral route. Intervirology 20:23–31

Balayan MS, Usmanov RK, Zamyatina DI, Karas FR (1990) Brief report: experimental hepatitis E infection in domestic pigs. J Med Virol 32:58–59

Buisson Y, Grandadam, Nicand ME, Cheval P, Van Cuyck-Gandre H, Innis B, Rehel P, Coursaget P, Teyssou R, Tsarev S (2000) Identification of a novel hepatitis E virus in Nigeria. J Gen Virol 81:903–909

Chandler JD, Riddell MA, Li F, Love RJ, Anderson DA (1999) Serological evidence for swine hepatitis E virus infection in Australian pig herds. Vet Microbiol 68:95–105

Clayson ET, Innis BL, Myint KS, Narupiti S, Vaughn DW, Giri S, Ranabhat P, Shrestha MP (1995) Detection of hepatitis E virus infections among domestic swine in the Kathmandu Valley of Nepal. Am J Trop Med Hyg 53:228-232

Drobeniuc J, Favorov MO, Shapiro CN, Bell BP, Mast EE, Dadu A, Culver D, Iarovoi P, Robertson BH, Margolis HS (2001) Hepatitis E virus antibody prevalence among persons who work with swine. J Infect Dis 184:1594–1597

Emerson SU, Zhang M, Meng XJ, Nguyen H, Huang Y, Purcell RH (2001) Recombinant hepatitis E virus genomes infectious for primates: Importance of capping and discovery of a cis-reactive element. Proc Natl Acad Sci USA 98:15270–15275

Engle RE, Yu C, Emerson SU, Meng XJ, Purcell RH (2002) Hepatitis E virus (HEV) capsid antigens derived from viruses of human and swine origin are equally efficient for detecting anti-HEV by enzyme immunoassay. J Clin Microbiol 40: 4576–4580

Erker JC, Desai SM, Schlauder GG, Dawson GJ, Mushahwar IK (1999) A hepatitis E virus variant from the United States: molecular characterization and transmission in cynomolgus macaques. J Gen Virol 80:681–690

Fagan EA, Harrison TJ (2000) Viral Hepatitis. Springer-Verlag New York Inc. P.62–88

Favorov MO, Kosoy MY, Tsarev SA, Childs JE, Margolis HS (2000) Prevalence of antibody to hepatitis E virus among rodents in the United States. J Infect Dis 181:449–455

Favorov MO, Nazarova O, Margolis HS (1998) Is hepatitis E an emerging zoonotic disease? Am J Trop Med Hyg 59:242

Fix AD, Abdel-Hamid M, Purcell RH, Shehata MH, Abdel-Aziz F, Mikhail N, El Sebai H, Nafeh M, Habib M, Arthur RR, Emerson SU, Strickland GT (2000) Prevalence of antibodies to hepatitis E in two rural Egyptian communities. Am J Trop Med Hyg 62:519-523

Fry KE, Tam AW, Smith MM, Kim JP, Luk KC, Young LM, Piatak M, Feldman RA, Yun KY, Purdy MA, et al. (1992) Hepatitis E virus (HEV): strain variation in the nonstructural gene region encoding consensus motifs for an RNA-dependent RNA polymerase and an ATP/GTP binding site. Virus Genes 6:173–185

Garkavenko O, Obriadina A, Meng J, Anderson DA, Benard HJ, Schroeder BA, Khudyakov YE, Fields HA, Croxson MC (2001) Detection and characterization of swine hepatitis E virus in New Zealand. J Med Virol 65:525-529

Halbur PG, Kasorndorkbua C, Gilbert C, Guenette D, Potters MB, Purcell RH, Emerson SU, Toth TE, Meng XJ (2001) Comparative pathogenesis of infection of pigs with hepatitis E viruses recovered from a pig and a human. J Clin Microbiol 39 918–923

Haqshenas G, Shivaprasad HL, Woolcock P, Read DH, Meng XJ (2001) Genetic identification and characterization of a novel virus related to the human hepatitis E virus from chickens with Hepatitis-Splenomegaly Syndrome in the United States. J Gen Virol 82:2449–2462

Haqshenas G, Meng XJ (2001) Determination of the nucleotide sequences at the extreme 5' and 3' ends of swine hepatitis E virus genome. Arch Virol 146:2461–2467

Haqshenas G, Huang FF, Fenaux M, Guenette DK, Pierson FW, Larsen CT, Shivaprasad HL, Toth TE, Meng XJ (2002) The putative capsid protein of the newly identified avian hepatitis E virus shares antigenic epitopes with that of swine and human hepatitis E viruses and the chicken big liver and spleen disease virus. J Gen Virol 83: 2201–2209

Hsieh SY, Yang PY, Ho YP, Chu CM, Liaw YF (1998) Identification of a novel strain of hepatitis E virus responsible for sporadic acute hepatitis in Taiwan. J Med Virol 55:300–304

Hsieh SY, Meng XJ, Wu YH, Liu ST, Tam AW, Lin DY, Liaw YF (1999) Identity of a novel swine hepatitis E virus in Taiwan forming a monophyletic group with Taiwan isolates of human hepatitis E virus. J Clin Microbiol 37:3828–3834

Huang CC, Nguyen D, Fernandez J, Yun KY, Fry KE, Bradley DW, Tam AW, Reyes GR (1992) Molecular cloning and sequencing of the Mexico isolate of hepatitis E virus (HEV). Virology 191:550–558

Huang FF, Haqshenas G, Guenette DK, Halbur PG, Schommer S, Pierson FW, Toth TE, Meng XJ (2002a) Detection by RT-PCR and genetic characterization of field isolates of swine hepatitis E virus from pigs in different geographic regions of the U.S. J Clin Microbiol 40: 1326–1332

Huang FF, Haqshenas G, Shivaprasad HL, Guenette DK, Woolcock PR, Larsen CT, Pierson FW, Elvinger F, Toth TE, Meng XJ (2002b) Heterogeneity and seroprevalence of a newly identified avian hepatitis E virus from chickens in the United States. J Clin Microbiol 40: 4197–4202

Huang R, Nakazono N, Ishii K, Kawamata O, Kawaguchi R, Tsukada Y (1995) Existing variations on the gene structure of hepatitis E virus strains from some regions of China. J Med Virol 47:303–308

Jaiswal SP, Jain AK, Naik G, Soni N, Chitnis DS (2001) Viral hepatitis during pregnancy. Intl J Gynaecol Obstet 72:103–108

Jameel S, Zafrullah M, Ozdener MH, Panda SK (1996) Expression in animal cells and characterization of the hepatitis E virus structural proteins. J Virol 70:207–216.

Kabrane-Lazizi Y, Meng XJ, Purcell RH, Emerson SU (1999a) Evidence that the genomic RNA of hepatitis E virus is capped. J Virol 73:8848–8850

Kabrane-Lazizi Y, Fine JB, Elm J, Glass GE, Higa H, Diwan A, Gibbs CJ Jr., Meng XJ, Emerson SU, Purcell RH (1999b) Evidence for wide-spread infection of wild rats with hepatitis E virus in the United States. Am J Trop Med Hyg 61:331–335

Kabrane-Lazizi Y, Zhang M, Purcell RH, Miller KD, Davey RT, Emerson SU (2001) Acute hepatitis caused by a novel strain of hepatitis E virus most closely related to United States strains. J Gen Virol 82:1687–1693

Karetnyi YV, Gilchrist MJ, Naides SJ (1999) Hepatitis E virus infection prevalence among selected populations in Iowa. J Clin Virol 14:51–55

Kasorndorkbua C, Halbur PG, Guenette DK, Toth TE, Meng XJ (2002) Use of a swine bioassay and a RT-PCR assay to assess the risk of transmission of swine hepatitis E virus in pigs. J Virol Methods 101:71–78

Khuroo MS (1980) Study of an epidemic of non-A, non-B hepatitis: possibility of another human hepatitis virus distinct from post-transfusion non-A, non-B type. Am J Med 68:818–824

Koonin EV, Gorbalenya AE, Purdy MA, Rozanov MN, Reyes GR, Bradley DW (1992) Computer-assisted assignment of functional domains in the nonstructural polyprotein of hepatitis E virus: delineation of an additional group of positive-strand RNA plant and animal viruses. Proc Natl Acad Sci USA 89:8259–8263

Krawczynski K, Aggarwal R, Kamili S (2000) Hepatitis E. Infect Dis Clin North Am 14:669–687

Li TC, Yamakava Y, Suzuki K, Tatsumi M, Azeez Razak MA, Uchida T, Takeda N, Miyamura T (1997). Expression and self-assembly of empty virus-like particles of hepatitis E virus. J Virol 71:7207–7213

Li TC, Zhang J, Shinzawa H, Ishibashi M, Sata M, Mast EE, Kim K, Miyamura T, Takeda N (2000) Empty virus-like particle-based enzyme-linked immunosorbent assay for antibodies to hepatitis e virus. J Med Virol 62:327–333

Maneerat Y, Clayson ET, Myint KSA, Young GD, Innis BL (1996) Experimental infection of the laboratory rat with the hepatitis E virus. J Med Virol 48:121–128

Mast EE, Kuramoto IK, Favorov MO, Schoening VR, Burkholder BT, Shapiro CN, Holland PV (1997) Prevalence of and risk factors for antibody to hepatitis E virus seroreactivity among blood donors in Northern California. J Infect Dis 176:34–40

Meng XJ, Purcell RH, Halbur PG, Lehman JR, Webb DM, Tsareva TS, Haynes JS, Thacker BJ, Emerson SU (1997) A novel virus in swine is closely related to the human hepatitis E virus. Proc Natl Acad Sci USA 94:9860–9865

Meng XJ, Halbur PG, Haynes JS, Tsareva TS, Bruna JD, Royer RL, Purcell RH, Emerson SU (1998a) Experimental infection of pigs with the newly identified swine hepatitis E virus (swine HEV), but not with human strains of HEV. Arch Virol 143:1405–1415

Meng XJ, Halbur PG, Shapiro MS, Govindarajan S, Bruna JD, Mushahwar IK, Purcell RH, Emerson SU (1998b) Genetic and experimental evidence for cross-species infection by the swine hepatitis E virus. J Virol 72:9714–9721

Meng XJ, Dea S, Engle RE, Friendship R, Lyoo YS, Sirinarumitr T, Urairong TK, Wang D, Wong D, Yoo D, Zhang Y, Purcell RH, Emerson SU (1999) Prevalence of antibodies to the hepatitis E virus in pigs from countries where hepatitis E is common or is rare in the human population. J Med Virol 58:297–302

Meng XJ (2000a) Zoonotic and xenozoonotic risks of hepatitis E virus. Infect Dis Rev 2:35–41

Meng XJ (2000b) Novel strains of hepatitis E virus identified from humans and other animal species: Is hepatitis E a zoonosis? J Hepatol 33:842–845

Meng XJ, Wiseman B, Elvinger F, Guenette DK, Toth TE, Engel R, Emerson SU, Purcell RH (2002) Prevalence of antibodies to the hepatitis E virus in veterinarians working with swine and normal blood donors in the United States and other countries. J Clin Microbiol 40:117–122

Naik SR, Aggarwal R, Salunke PN, Mehrotra NN (1992) A large waterborne viral hepatitis E epidemic in Kanpur, India. Bull WHO 70:597–604.

Okamoto H, Takahashi M, Nishizawa T, Fukai K, Muramatsu U, Yoshikawa A (2001). Analysis of the complete genome of indigenous swine hepatitis E virus isolated in Japan. Biochem Biophys Res Commun 289:929–936

Payne CJ, Ellis TM, Plant SL, Gregory AR, Wilcox GE (1999) Sequence data suggests big liver and spleen disease virus (BLSV) is genetically related to hepatitis E virus. Vet Microbiol 68:119–125

Pina S, Buti M, Cotrina M, Piella J, Girones R (2000) HEV identified in serum from humans with acute hepatitis and in sewage of animal origin in Spain. J Hepatol 33:826–833

Platt KB, Yoon KJ, Zimmerman JJ (1998) Susceptibility of swine to hepatitis E virus and its significance to human health. Swine Research Report, Iowa State University, Ames, IA, 125–126

Pringle C (1998) Minutes of the 27th International Committee on Taxonomy of Viruses Meeting. Arch Virol 143:1449–1459

Purcell RH (1996) Hepatitis E virus. In: Fields BN, Knipe DM, Howley PM et al. (eds) Fields Virology. 3rd ed. Vol 2. Lippincott-Raven Publishers, Philadelphia p.2831–2843

Reyes GR, Purdy MA, Kim JP, Luk KC, Young LM, Fry KE, Bradley DW (1990) Isolation of a cDNA from the virus responsible for enterically transmitted non-A, non-B hepatitis. Science 247:1335–1339

Reyes GR (1997) Overview of the epidemiology and biology of the hepatitis E virus. In: Willson RA (eds) Viral Hepatitis. Marcel Dekker, Inc., NY, pp.239–258

Schlauder GG, Dawson GJ, Erker JC, Kwo PY, Knigge MF, Smalley DL, Rosenblatt JE, Desai SM, Mushahwar IK (1998) The sequence and phylogenetic analysis of a novel hepatitis E virus isolated from a patient with acute hepatitis reported in the United States. J Gen Virol 79:447–456

Schlauder GG, Desai SM, Zanetti AR, Tassopoulos NC, Mushahwar IK (1999) Novel hepatitis E virus (HEV) isolates from Europe: evidence for additional genotypes of HEV. J Med Virol 57:243–251

Schlauder GG, Frider B, Sookoian S, Castano GC, Mushahwar IK (2000) Identification of 2 novel isolates of hepatitis E virus in Argentina. J Infect Dis 182:294–297

Takahashi K, Iwata K, Watanabe N, Hatahara T, Ohta Y, Baba K, Mishiro S (2001) Full-genome nucleotide sequence of a hepatitis E virus strain that may be indigenous to Japan. Virology 287:9–12

Takahashi K, Kang JH, Ohnishi S, Hino K, Mishiro S (2002) Genetic heterogeneity of hepatitis E virus recovered from Japanese patients with acute sporadic hepatitis. J Infect Dis 185: 1342–1345

Tam AW, Smith MM, Guerra ME, Huang CC, Bradley DW, Fry KE, Reyes GR (1991) Hepatitis E virus (HEV): molecular cloning and sequencing of the full-length viral genome. Virology 185:120–131

Thomas DL, Yarbough PO, Vlahov D, Tsarev SA, Nelson KE, Saah AJ, Purcell RH (1997) Seroreactivity to hepatitis E virus in areas where the disease is not endemic. J Clin Microbiol 35:1244–1247

Ticehurst J, Popkin TJ, Bryan JP, Innis BL, Duncan JF, Ahmed A, Iqbal M, Malik I, Kapikian AZ, Legters LJ, et al. (1992) Association of hepatitis E virus with an outbreak of hepatitis in Pakistan: serologic responses and pattern of virus excretion. J Med Virol. 36:84–92

Tien NT, Clayson HT, Khiem HB, Sac PK, Corwin AL, Myint KS, Vaughn DW (1997) Detection of immunoglobulin G to the hepatitis E virus among several animal species in Vietnam. Am J Trop Med Hyg 57:211 (abstract)

Tsarev SA, Tsareva TS, Emerson SU, Rippy MK, Zack P, Shapiro M, Purcell RH (1995) Experimental hepatitis E in pregnant rhesus monkeys: failure to transmit hepatitis E virus (HEV) to offspring and evidence of naturally acquired antibodies to HEV. J Infect Dis 172:31–37

Tsarev SA, Shrestha MP, He J, Scott RM, Vaughn DW, Clayson ET, Gigliotti S, Longer CF, Innis BL (1998) Naturally acquired hepatitis E virus (HEV) infection in Nepalese rodents. Am J Trop Med Hyg 59:242 (abstract)

Usmanov RK, Balayan MS, Dvoinikova OV, Alymbaeva DB, Zamiatina NA, Kazachkov LuA, Belov VI (1994) An experimental infection in lambs by the hepatitis E virus. Voprosy Virusologii 39:165–168

Van der Poel W, Verschoor F, van der Heide R, Herrera, MI, Vivo A, Kooreman M, de Roda Husman A (2001) Hepatitis E virus sequences in swine related to sequences in humans, the Netherlands. Emerg Infect Dis 7:970–976

Vishwanathan R (1957) Infectious hepatitis in Delhi (1955–1956): A critical study: epidemiology. Indian J Med Res 45 (suppl 1):1–29

Wang Y, Ling R, Erker JC, Zhang H, Li H, Desai S, Mushahwar IK, Harrison TJ (1999) A divergent genotype of hepatitis E virus in Chinese patients with acute hepatitis. J Gen Virol 80:169–177

Wang Y, Zhang H, Ling R, Li H, Harrison TJ (2000) The complete sequence of hepatitis E virus genotype 4 reveals an alternative strategy for translation of open reading frames 2 and 3. J Gen Virol 81:1675–1686

Williams TPE, Kasorndorkbua C, Halbur PG, Haqshenas G, Guenette DK, Toth TE, Meng XJ (2001) Evidence of extrahepatic sites of replication of the hepatitis E virus in a swine model. J Clin Microbiol 39:3040–3046

Weiss RA (1998) Transgenic pigs and virus adaptation. Nature 391:327–328

Wong DC, Purcell RH, Sreenivasan MA, Prasad SR, Pavri KM (1980) Epidemic and endemic hepatitis in India: evidence for a non-A, non-B hepatitis virus etiology. Lancet 2:876–879

Wu JC, Sheen IJ, Chiang TY, Sheng WY, Wang YJ, Chan CY, Lee SD (1998) The impact of traveling to endemic areas on the spread of hepatitis E virus infection: epidemiological and molecular analyses. J Med Virol 27:1415–1420

Wu JC, Chen CM, Chiang TY, Sheen IJ, Chen JY, Tsai WH, Huang YH, Lee SD (2000) Clinical and epidemiological implications of swine hepatitis E virus infection. J Med Virol 60:166–171

Wu JC, Chen CM, Chiang TY, Tsai WH, Jeng WJ, Sheen IJ, Lin CC, Meng XJ (2002) Spreead of hepatitis E virus among different-aged pigs: two year survery in Taiwan. J Med Virol 66: 488–492

Yoo D, Willson P, Pei Y, Haynes MA, Deckert A, Dewey CE, Friendship RM, Yoon Y, Gottschalk M, Yason C, Giulivi A (2001) Prevalence of hepatitis E virus antibodies in Canadian swine herds and identification of a novel variant of swine hepatitis E virus. Clin Diagn Lab Immunol 8:1213–1219

Zafrullah M, Ozdener MH, Panda SK, Jameel S (1997) The ORF3 protein of hepatitis E virus is a phosphoprotein that associated with the cytoskeleton. J Virol 71:9045–9053

Zafrullah M., Ozdener MH, Kumar R, Panda SK, Jameel S (1999) Mutational analysis of glycosylation, membrane translocation, and cell surface expression of the hepatitis E virus ORF2 protein. J Virol 73:4074–4082

Zanetti AR, Schlauder GG, Romano L, Tanzi E, Fabris P, Dawson GJ, Mushahwar IK (1999) Identification of a novel variant of hepatitis E virus in Italy. J Med Virol 57:356–360

Zhang Y, McAtee P, Yarbough PO, Tam AW, Fuerst T (1997) Expression, characterization, and immunoreactivities of a soluble hepatitis E virus putative capsid protein species expressed in insect cells. Clin Diagn Lab Immunol 4:423–428

Molecular Cloning and Functional Characterization of Infectious PERV and Development of Diagnostic Tests

M. Niebert · R. R. Tönjes
Paul-Ehrlich-Institut, Paul-Ehrlich-Straße 51–59, 63225 Langen, Germany
E-mail: toera@pei.de

1 Introduction 218

2 Detection of PERV 220

3 Transcriptional Regulation and Genetic Distribution of PERV 227

4 Risk Assessment 229

5 Summary 232

References. 232

Abstract Pigs are the donor animals of choice for xenotransplantation (XTx) and xenogeneic cell therapy measurements. Most known porcine pathogens can be controlled by conventional means like vaccination, medication or specific pathogen-free breeding conditions. As pigs have co-evolved very closely with humans for a few millennia it is not very likely that even asymptomatic pathogens have escaped attention. Porcine endogenous retroviruses (PERV) are different from conventional pathogens as they are chromosomally fixed in every cell of the animal, hence PERV cannot be easily controlled. While PERV show no phenotype in the porcine host, recent data demonstrate that some polytropic proviruses can be activated by external stimuli and that those can productively infect human cells in vitro. In evaluation of the retrovirological safety of XTx, we determined the number of replication-competent PERV to be limited and to exhibit a heterogeneous distribution, therefore suggesting that they could be removed by conventional breeding. The transcriptional regulation of some PERV due to repetitive elements in their long terminal repeats enables their adaptation to new host cells. The diagnostic tools available, based on immunological and polymerase chain reaction techniques, were shown to be sensitive in both the animal and in vitro, but must still show their potential in human XTx recipients, where they are confronted with very low antigen expression and the phenomenon of microchimerism.

1 Introduction

Porcine endogenous retroviruses (PERV) belong to the gamma-retroviruses and are mainly constituted of three classes (A, B and C; Patience et al. 2001) which encode the open reading frames (ORFs) for group-specific antigen (*gag*), polymerase/protease polyprotein (*pol*) and envelope protein (*env*; see Fig. 3A). The latter gene demonstrates the largest differences between individual proviruses and determines the host range as well as the taxonomic differentiation of PERV classes. Genes coding for accessory proteins are not common among gamma-retroviruses (Coffin 1996). The *gag* gene is colinear with the *pro/pol* ORF and the stop codon separating both genes is suppressed by $tRNA_{Gln}$. The *env* gene partially overlaps with *pro/pol* and forms a new ORF.

The differences in length of the PERV genes described to date have no impact on the highly conserved structural motifs of gamma-retroviruses. Particularly, the *env* genes bear motifs such as the variable regions A and B (VRA, VRB) and the proline rich region (PRO) of the gp70 protein that determine the host range via receptor interaction (Battini et al. 1995, 1999; LeTissier et al. 1997). The structural genes are flanked on both sides by long terminal repeats (LTRs), which act as viral promoters and, together with the integrase, facilitate the integration into the host genome. PERV classes A and B are polytropic and have the capacity to infect nonporcine cells including primate and human cells, while class C is ecotropic and is restricted to porcine targets (LeTissier et al. 1997; Patience et al. 1997; Takeuchi et al. 1998). Therefore, terms of xenotransplantation (XTx), only polytropic PERV-A and PERV-B pose a serious risk. In addition to the three classes mentioned that include several replication-competent proviruses (Akiyoshi et al. 1998; Wilson et al. 1998; Czauderna et al. 2000; Tönjes et al. 2000; Herring et al. 2001b; Krach et al. 2001; Niebert et al. 2002), other PERV sequences have been found and are designated D to G, however, only the *env* sequences of these are known so far (LeTissier et al. 1997; Patience et al. 1997).

The PERV virion resembles that of typical gamma-retroviruses which are divided into groups based on their morphology apparent in negatively-stained electron microscopy (EM) pictures: enveloped, extracellular particles with a condensed, centric core and barely visible envelope spikes (see Fig. 2A).

Data on the evolution of PERV are limited. Both the timepoint of proviral integration into the pig germline as well as the frequency of integration events is unknown. However, functional copies of several different proviruses are inherited in different breeds of pigs and those obviously do not cause any harm to their natural hosts as no symptoms of illness can be observed. This status is true for most endogenous retroviruses (ERV; Coffin 1984). Furthermore, ERV may even confer some kind of advantage to their hosts such as being protective against infections by other retroviruses (Limjoco et al. 1993). There are two different types of PERV LTRs: simple one and one with a complex repeat pattern in the U3 region. It cannot be judged yet which type of LTR existed initially or whether both types evolved in parallel. Since the LTRs harboring the repeat structure demonstrate a significantly stronger promoter activity, the repeatless LTRs might display an adaptation to the host to reduce the effect of viral replication.

Porcine cells, tissue or organs are considered the first choice for XTx applications, including perfusions of extracorporeal complete livers or bioartificial assist devices, skin grafts or even whole organ transplants (Fishman 1994; Bach et al. 1995; Hunkeler et al. 1999), since primates are no longer evaluated as donor species (Reiss 2000).

In addition to immunological barriers and putative physiological incompatibilities, the possible xenozoonotic transmission of unknown porcine infectious agents remains one of the most prominent problems in XTx (Michaels and Simmons 1994; Fishman 1997). Unlike other infectious agents, PERV cannot be eliminated from pig herds dedicated for XTx by conventional means, e.g., by breeding under specific pathogen-free (SPF) conditions or vaccination, as PERV are transmitted vertically from generation to generation.

Many experiments show that PERV are able to productively infect human cells in vitro (Akiyoshi et al. 1998; Wilson et al. 1998; Czauderna et al. 2000; Tönjes et al. 2000; Van der Laan et al. 2000; Krach et al. 2001; Niebert et al. 2002), although no case of zoonotic transmission in vivo has been reported up to now. Whereas a retrospective study of human xenotransplant recipients reported no evidence of viral transfer (Paradis et al. 1999), transplantation of porcine islet cells into diabetic NOD/SCID mice resulted in widespread PERV infection of treated animals (Van der Laan et al. 2000). These data indicate that in XTx, micro-organisms including PERV will be confronted with an even more immunosuppressed environment compared to regular allotransplantation. In general, viral infections are less controlled by the immune system in the course of transplantations.

The biology, regular life cycle and putative pathways of PERV are summarized in Fig. 1.

2
Detection of PERV

In pigs and in productively infected cell lines it is easy to detect both PERV DNA sequences and PERV proteins (Fig. 2B), although none of the detection methods used can readily discriminate replication-competent from defective PERV. The generation of retroviral particles can be observed in vitro by EM and immunodetection methods (Fig. 2). Estimations on full-length proviral PERV range from 30 to 50 copies per haploid genome (LeTissier et al. 1997; Akiyoshi et al. 1998).

To date, several studies have attempted to determine the number of full-length PERV using increasingly sophisticated techniques. The initial studies relied purely on PCR techniques, but these were not able either

Fig. 1 Life-cycle of PERV and putative heterologous pathways. (*A*) Ancestors of PERV as exogenous free virus particles must have infected pigs a long time ago. (B_1) Since then, PERV could be freely transmitted horizontally between individuals; however, it remains to be shown whether reinfections still happen today. PERV can be transmitted to human cells in vitro, but (B_2) it is unclear if xenotropic infections occur in vivo. (*C*) After integration into the germ line, PERV is transmitted vertically to every offspring and (*E*) is present in every cell. For XTx, porcine organs (D_1) together with the proviruses would be transferred to humans and (D_2) by using genetically engineered pigs to reduce the host-versus-graft reaction these immunosuppressive features could be exploited by the virus. Even though the porcine genome comprises 30–50 copies of proviral PERV on different chromosomes (*F*), only a fraction of provirus (*G*) is functional (*H*), and thus infectious, replication competent and polytropic. If porcine cells, tissues or organs are transplanted to humans, the time of exposure might be greatly enhanced. (*I*) In addition, it is possible that PERV recombine with other human pathogens, either exogenous or endogenous, to form new viruses. At present it is hard to predict whether xenotransplanted materials harboring either genetically modified PERV or recombinant PERV have the capacity to infect humans (*J*) and if so will these infections will result in severe illness

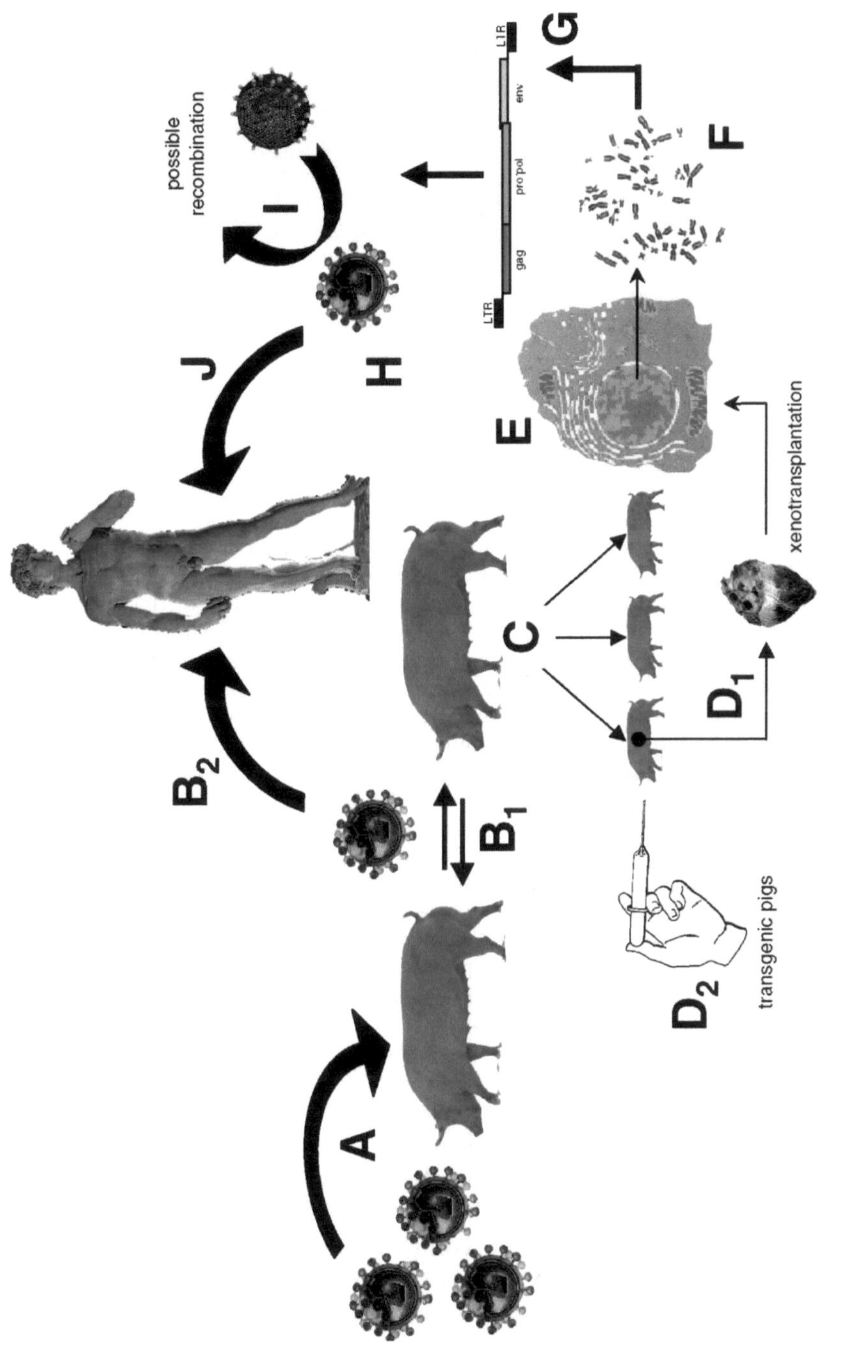
A
B1
B2
C
D1
D2
transgenic pigs
xenotransplantation
E
F
G
LTR
gag
pro pol
env
LTR
H
I
J
possible recombination

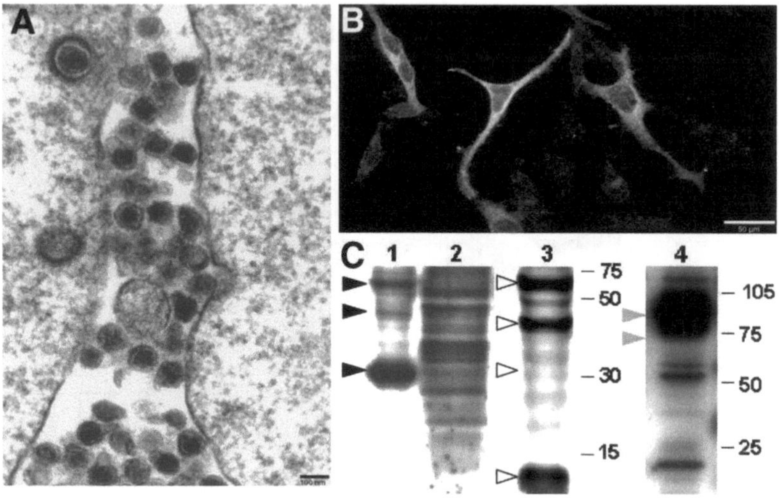

Fig. 2A–C Visualization and detection of PERV. **A** Electron microscopy of ultra-thin sections of human 293 cells transfected with molecular clone 293-PERV-A(42) producing PERV virions. **B** Indirect immunofluorescence analysis of HeLa cells transfected with molecular clone Bac-PERV-A(130A12) and stained with antiserum α-Gag p10 (Krach et al. 2000) 24 days post-transfection. **C** Immunoblotting analysis of PERV particles in tissue culture supernatants detected with various antisera. Lane *1*, sample derived from 293 cells transfected with molecular clone 293-PERV-A(42). Lane *2*, nontransfected 293 cells; antiserum α-Gag p30b (N. Fischer et al. 2003). *Black arrowheads* mark the Gag precursor (60 kDa), an intermediate (p40; weak) consisting of the capsid protein (p30) and the nucleocapsid (p10; not detected due to antibody used). Lane *3*, sample derived from 293 cells transfected with molecular clone 293-PERV-A(42); antiserum α-Gag p10. *White arrowheads* indicate Gag precursor, an intermediate consisting of capsid protein and nucleocapsid (p30 plus p10), the capsid protein, and the nucleocapsid with apparent molecular masses of 60, 40, 30, and 10 kDa, respectively. Lane *4*, sample derived from 293 cells transfected with molecular clone 293-PERV-B(33)/ATG; antiserum directed against Env α-gp70(B) (N. Fischer et al. 2003). *Gray arrowheads* indicate the Env precursor (80 kDa) and the mature Env gp70 (70 kDa)

to detect mutations within otherwise full-length proviruses, or to determine whether different amplification products belonged to the same provirus (Bosch et al. 2000; Deng et al. 2000). Subsequent studies aimed to screen for all viral genes and to detect ORFs; however, those attempts failed to prove the replication competence of the proviruses found by these methods (Herring et al. 2001b). To isolate and to characterize replication-competent PERV, we have initially used a genomic library of human embryonic kidney cell line 293 that was infected with PERV released from pig kidney cell line PK15 (Patience et al. 1997; Czauderna et al. 2000). Subsequently, PK15 cells were analyzed directly by genomic cloning techniques for the existence of productive proviral PERV (Krach et al. 2001). Eventually, the genome of primary fibroblast cells derived from a large white pig bearing a defined haplotype (H01) was constructed in bacterial artificial chromosomes (BAC) and investigated (Rogel-Gaillard et al. 1999; Niebert et al. 2002).

Each BAC clone was individually tested for the presence of all three ORFs and if positive, subjected to a functional assay in cell culture, where viral protein expression was measured over several weeks by immunofluorescence staining using Gag p10 (Krach et al. 2000) and reverse transcriptase (RT) assays. The functional clones determined in the course of this analysis are summarized in Table 1 and their genetic properties are discussed below (Niebert et al. 2002).

All studies conducted so far report different numbers for the two polytropic PERV classes A and B. For example, a recent study reports six class B proviral PERV but no full-length class A PERV (Herring et al. 2001b), whereas our strategies have mainly revealed class A proviruses in both PK15 and large white libraries. This fact may represent a strong founder effect of the herd initially used to produce the library. As a consequence, the methods to screen for replication-competent PERV described here and in other publications must be applied to that herd finally selected for XTx.

One general problem found by all studies is the choice of genome source: many approaches use large white pigs, either unmodified (as the most native situation) or genetically modified in the case of transgenic animals (as these are most likely to be used for XTx). However, additional sources, which may be more suitable for XTx exist, e.g., minipigs.

To screen specifically for the isolated replication-competent PERV in different pig genomes, we have determined the flanking genomic sequences of the full-length proviruses (Table 1) by inverse PCR (Czauderna et al. 2000). While PCR amplification of PERV genes yields multiple signals, at least parts of the flanking sequences are unique to each different provirus. This approach allows screening of individual pigs as well as different pig breeds for the presence of specific proviruses. As a consequence, the selection of pigs that show a lower prevalence of functional PERV appears possible. Those animals might be used directly for XTx and to assess the breeding rates of PERV-free pigs.

Table 1 Summary of functional analyses using various molecular PERV clones. Analyses were conducted based on the replication-competent native PERV proviruses isolated from a genomic library of large white pig and from a genomic library of the PK15 cell line. The almost replication-competent clone Bac-PERV-B(192B9) is included

Molecular clone	PERV class	Chromosomal position[b]	IFA for Gag p10[c]	RT assay[d]	Present in large white pig[e]	Present in minipig[e]	Present in d/d minipig[e]	Present in westran pig[e]	Present in wild boar[e]
Bac-PERV-A(130A12)[a]	A	1q2.4	+	+	13 of 35	2 of 2	0 of 15	2 of 10	4 of 14
Bac-PERV-A(151B10)	A	1q2.3	+	+	14 of 35	1 of 2	0 of 15	1 of 10	3 of 14
Bac-PERV-A(463H12)	A	3p1.5	+	+	7 of 35	0 of 2	0 of 15	0 of 10	3 of 14
Bac-PERV-B(192B9)	B	7p1.1	transient	–	29 of 35	1 of 2	0 of 15	2 of 10	2 of 14
PK15-PERV-A(58)	A	n.a.	+	+	24 of 35	2 of 2	0 of 15	3 of 10	3 of 14
PK15-PERV-B(213)	B	12q1.5	+	+	18 of 35	2 of 2	0 of 15	2 of 10	5 of 14

[a] The prefixes of molecular clones (column 1) indicate the genomic source of the provirus. Bac-, Genomic library of large white pig propagated in bacterial artificial chromosomes; PK15-, genomic library of PK15 cell line propagated in bacteriophage lambda.

[b] Chromosomal position indicates the localization of the PERV isolated from BAC clones performed by fluorescent in situ hybridization analyses (Rogel-Gaillard et al. 1999).

[c] IFA denotes the reactivity of infected cells using specific antiserum directed against PERV protein Gag p10 in indirect immunofluorescence analyses.

[d] RT assays indicate the reactivity of cell culture supernatants in this test over a time course of approximately 48 days.

[e] In columns 6 to 10 the presence of specific PERV is tested in five different, geographically separate subspecies of *Sus scrofa*. The d/d minipigs (column 8) are genetically related to Yucatan minipigs (column 7), but exhibit a defined swine leukocyte antigen haplotype and have been described as nontransmitters of PERV. Westran pigs (column 9) are bred in Australia. Presence in genomes was tested using flanking genomic sequences and PERV sequences in specific PCR analyses.

n.a., Not applicable; +, positive result; -, negative result; transient, expression can be observed only during the first 72 h post-transfection.

To detect infectious PERV in the course of XTx is a completely different matter. Detection of minimal amounts of viral genetic information, both free RNA and integrated proviral DNA, is an established method in HIV diagnostics and was also shown for PERV (Clemenceau et al. 2001; Herring et al. 2001a; Takefman et al. 2001). The status post XTx is the presence of microchimerism, i.e., solitary cells derived from the transplant will stray throughout the body and might escape immune responses for years, which will always yield a positive signal when looking for PERV sequences. Therefore, to discriminate between a PERV infection and the existence of PERV sequences that are present in every porcine cell, the flanking sequences of the proviruses and as a control the flanking sequences of any porcine gene could be used for detection, whereby a positive signal would indicate the porcine genome as being the source of the signal. A similar method has been described where a PCR specific for PERV and another porcine gene has been performed simultaneously (Herring et al. 2001a). Subsequently, the relative intensities of the PCR signals have been compared to yield information about the source of the PERV sequences.

For diagnostic purposes, however, the most desirable method would be the simultaneous immunological detection of two or more different PERV proteins by fast and sensitive assays such as Western blotting or enzyme linked immunosorbent assay (ELISA), that would indicate a productive infection of the XTx recipient.

So far, specific antisera directed against different epitopes of both PERV Gag and Env proteins have been developed (Matthews et al. 1999; Paradis et al. 1999, Galbraith et al. 2000; Krach et al. 2000, Stephan et al. 2001; Tacke et al. 2001; Fischer et al. 2003; Fig. 2C). These antisera have been used both in experimental assays for porcine tissue and for infected cell lines demonstrating high levels of viral expression as well as in limited clinical diagnostics. However, it is not clear whether the sensitivity of detection is sufficient for low level replication of PERV in patients, or if there might be any cross-reactions with foreign proteins (Tacke et al. 2001).

As the envelope protein of PERV-A and PERV-B shows some homologies, only a recently developed antiserum is able to specifically react with class B but not with class A Env proteins and therefore can discriminate between the two humantropic PERV (N. Fischer et al. 2003).

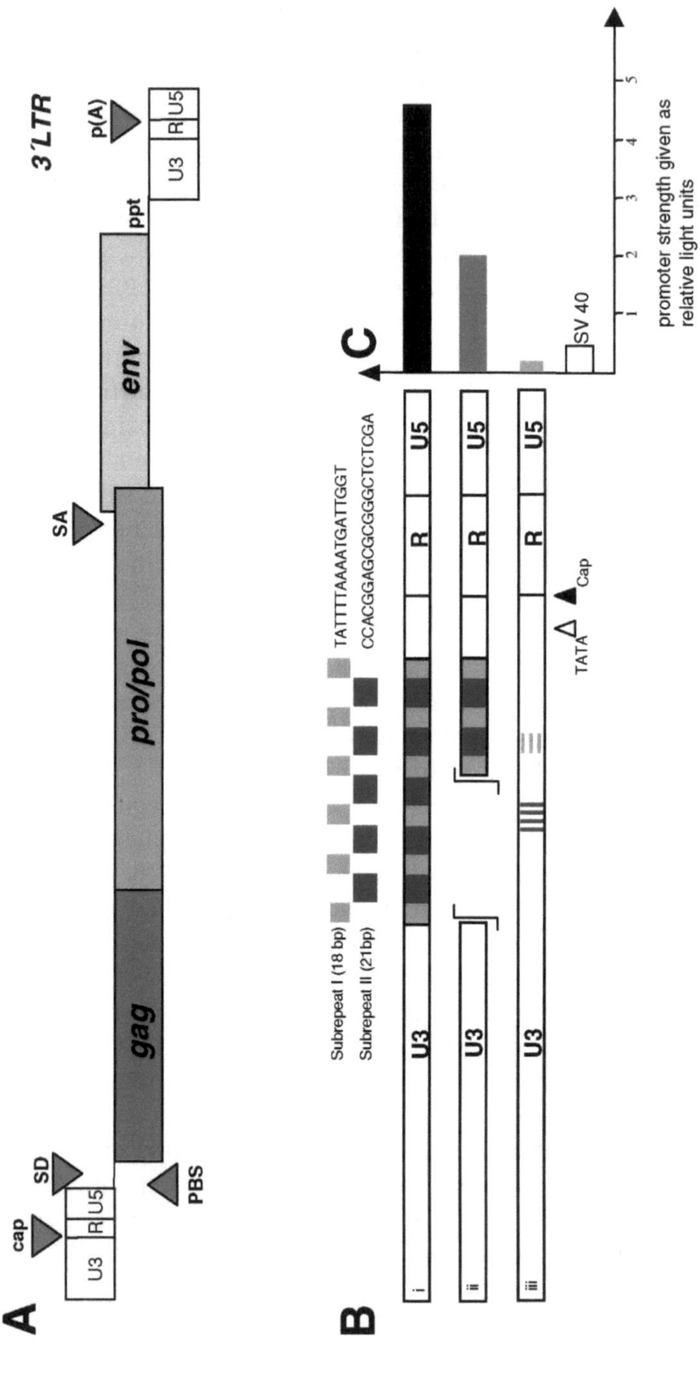
A
5´LTR
cap
U3
R
U5
SD
PBS
gag
pro/pol
SA
env
ppt
3´LTR
p(A)
U3
R
U5
B
Subrepeat I (18 bp)
TATTTTAAAATGATTGGT
Subrepeat II (21bp)
CCACGGAGCGCGGCTCTCGA
i
ii
iii
U3
R
U5
TATA
Cap
C
SV 40
1
2
3
4
5
promoter strength given as relative light units

3 Transcriptional Regulation and Genetic Distribution of PERV

The genetic organization of PERV is similar to most other gamma-retroviruses as described in this volume. Therefore, this section will concentrate mostly on some special features of the PERV LTRs as well as on the prevalence of PERV.

Sequence analyses revealed two different structures of PERV LTRs in the context of retroviral genes (Fig. 3A). One type of LTR shows a distinct repeat pattern of 39 base pair (bp) repeats in U3 and the other type is devoid of these repeats. The repeat structure in PERV LTRs has a significant impact on the activity of the viral promoter. In general, it can be stated that the more repeats are present in an LTR the higher is the promoter strength as measured in reporter gene assays (Fig. 3B, C; Scheef et al. 2001). A statistical analysis of the repeat box revealed a multitude of possible transcription factor binding sites, most prominently NF-Y. As the composition of the repeat structure does not always mediate higher replication rates in functional assays, we assume that other factors such as interaction of Env with the receptor and virus core assembly combined with a variety of transcription factors are involved.

As the repeat box shows all functions of a classical enhancer element (Scheef et al. 2001) it is not surprising that viruses completely lacking

Fig. 3A–C Genetic structure of PERV. **A** PERV, as a gamma-retrovirus, contains three genes encoding ORFs for Gag, Pro/Pol and Env. The proviral genes are shown as *boxes* and are flanked by LTRs. The transcriptional start site (*cap*), primer binding site (*PBS*), splice donor (*SD*), splice acceptor (*SA*) and the poly(A) addition site (p(A)) are indicated (*arrowheads*). *ppt*, Poly-purine tract. **B** Structures of different LTRs as they are found in the porcine genome. Within the U3 region of the LTR there is a sequence stretch composed of alternating 18-bp and 21-bp subrepeats forming a 39-bp repeat box. The number of repeats present in PERV LTRs largely influences the strength of the viral promoter. LTRs isolated from different molecular clones (*i* and *ii*) surpass the activity of SV40 promoter used as a constitutive control (Scheef et al. 2001). A particular type of LTR (*iii*) only displays rudimentary repeat structures which are distributed in U3 without any pattern (*hatched boxes*). This LTR shows comparably low promoter activities. **C** Relative promoter activities deduced from reporter gene assays (Dual Luciferase Kit, Promega) using human cell line 293 transfected with plasmid constructs containing the appropriate LTR. In general, the more repeats are present in the PERV LTR the stronger is the promoter activity. Results given represent idealized data (Scheef et al. 2001)

the repeats demonstrate a suboptimal replication performance in both reporter and functional assays (Fig. 3C). Interestingly, the LTR structure of a given virus is not static as the number of repeats changes dynamically during infection (Scheef et al. 2001). Although there are proviruses with different LTR structures present in the porcine genome (Niebert et al. 2002) we assume that this reflects a process of adaptation of the virus toward the host cell. During serial passaging, starting with a molecular clone with a defined LTR structure, the accumulation of numerous different repeat structures leading to a dominant number of 39-bp repeat boxes in U3 depending on the infected host cell was observed (Scheef et al. 2001).

The mechanism of repeat multimerization is unknown. In contrast to the hypothesis which suggests the slippage of RT (Martiney et al. 1999), we suppose that the mechanism for PERV is similar to that described for *Mus dunni* (Wolgamot and Miller 1999). In brief, a homologous misannealing during reverse transcription requires the availability of other short repeat sequences flanking the repeat region, a pattern which exists as described for PERV where an additional 18-bp subrepeat is located downstream of the 39-bp repeat box (Fig. 3B, i and ii).

The distribution and prevalence of intact PERV within the porcine population is also of particular interest. By screening a BAC library (see above) we have discovered four unique full-length proviruses which are chromosomally assigned (Table 1; Niebert et al. 2002). Three of them show productive infection upon introduction into cells in culture, while one was disabled by two in-frame stop mutations in *pol* in an otherwise intact proviral context (Fig. 3A). Further analysis of these clones by performing PCR with primers derived from the flanking genomic sequences showed that all proviruses were polymorphic in different individuals, and demonstrated slight alterations within their coding sequences. As a consequence, the individual proviruses are present in some pigs and absent in others and one provirus present in a defined chromosomal position may have slight mutations in individual pigs and in different subspecies. Most notably, the polymorphisms in the fourth BAC clone that is located in the swine leukocyte antigen region on pig chromosome 7 reveal an intact *pol* ORF in some large white pigs (Niebert et al. 2002).

We have characterized also two clones derived from a library of porcine cell line PK15 that show large homologies to the BAC clones mentioned above, but revealed different genomic flanking sequences. Yet, these two clones were not chromosomally assigned, therefore, it is not clear if these clones are different from the BAC clones or whether the genomic flanking sequences are different due to massive rearrangements during passaging of the cells over decades, as PK15 cells are malignant and transformed (Echard 1974). For these six PERV clones, their distribution among individual pigs as well as different breeds, i.e., large white pigs, minipigs, Westran pigs and wild boars, were analyzed (Table 1).

Although the LTRs are subjected to significant sequence shuffling during several rounds of infection, only minor point mutations are observed in the retroviral genes *gag*, *pol* and *env* (N. Fischer, M. Niebert and R.R. Tönjes, unpublished results).

The cellular receptor(s) used by PERV is currently unknown. Interference studies using appropriate *env* sequences revealed that the different PERV classes use different receptors, thereby explaining the different cell and species tropisms observed in pseudotype assays (Takeuchi et al. 1998). At present, there are no data describing what kind of proteins are involved and whether PERV are able to utilize some kind of co-receptor. However, by deduction from other highly homologous gamma-retroviruses, membrane-spanning transporter molecules are the most likely candidates for the PERV receptor.

The pseudotype assays also demonstrate that PERV could easily interact with other retroviruses, at least gamma types, as murine leukemia virus (MuLV) sequences were used for pseudotyping (Takeuchi et al. 1998).

4
Risk Assessment

PERV does not give any indications of pathogenesis in either its natural host or in infected cells of either animal or human lineage. However, PERV can infect heterologous cells in heavily immunosuppressed mice (Van der Laan et al. 2000). Thus, it is difficult to assess the possible in XTx. In general, as a retrovirus, PERV might be able to transform infected cells, which was extensively shown for MuLV (Leibovitch et al. 1987; Gimbel et al. 1996; Li et al. 1998). In addition, immunosuppressive properties of the virus are discussed (Tacke et al 2001). However, another important, but least assessable, risk is posed by the possible recombination of PERV with endogenous or exogenous human pathogens, giving rise to absolutely new and unexpected viruses (Micheals and Simmons 1994; Stoye and Coffin 1995; Fishman 1997). Putative recombination with human endogenous retroviruses (HERV) does not pose a serious risk due to the absence of infectious sequences such as HERV-K (Tönjes et al. 1996, 1999; Mayer et al. 1998; ; Turner et al. 2001) or the presence of heavily deleted gamma-type sequences such as HERV-R (Venables et al. 1995).

Experiments have shown that PERV can pseudotype MuLV particles (Takeuchi et al. 1998). Hence, other gamma-retroviruses would be the first ones to investigate but they do not pose extraordinary risks to humans by themselves (Cornetta et al. 1990).

In the course of XTx it will be important to monitor the transplant recipients and their close contacts for infection with PERV using the methods described above. Although xenotransplants today are rejected within hours or days, they might become viable for routine clinical application in the future. Therefore, with increasing lifespans the XTx recipient must be monitored. This scenario poses logistic as well as ethical problems which are discussed in detail elsewhere (Fox and McHale 1998; Woods 1998; Reiss 2000; Bach et al. 2001)

It is known that the promoter strength of the PERV LTR is regulated by a set of transcription factors; the factors present in human cells are better suited for the virus as promoter assays have demonstrated stronger activities of LTRs in human than in porcine cells (Scheef et al. 2001). In XTx, there are two additional sets of effector molecules, immunosuppressive drugs and human hormones or cytokines.

We have investigated the effects of several immunosuppressive drugs commonly used in clinical transplantation on the promoter strength of PERV LTR (Scheef et al. 2002). None of the drugs tested (e.g., cyclosporin A) caused a significant increase in promoter activity. Hence, we conclude that these drugs do not enhance the xenozoonotic risk of PERV.

To assess the risks of infection and recombination it is essential to know the exact number and location of all replication-competent PERV; this was one of our major goals and was also that of others (see above; Czauderna et al. 2000; Herring et al. 2001b; Niebert et al. 2002).

The knowledge and subsequent removal of replication-competent PERV would eliminate the risks of malignant transformation and immunosuppression, but not the risk of recombination, as any other infectious agent could pick up pieces of PERV genomic sequences from replication-incompetent but expressed proviruses that harbor otherwise intact ORFs.

To generate PERV-free pigs it is feasible to either use conventional breeding or genetic engineering procedures. In particular, the latter is used to generate pigs having properties that are better tolerated immunologically by the human recipient. However, the use of genetically engineered animals to reduce organ rejection, e.g., hDAF transgenic pigs or alpha-1,3-galactosyl transferase knock-out pigs (Sandrin and McKenzie 1994; Miyagawa et al. 1999; Capello et al. 2000; Bennet et al. 2001; Carrington et al. 2000; Lai et al. 2002), could make the situation even worse by allowing the virus to exploit the engineered immunosuppressive features (Hiasa et al. 1999; Takefman et al. 2002).

Inbred minipigs (Fishman 1994) actually harbor full-length retroviruses; however, some of the strains investigated obviously produce virions of the ecotropic class PERV-C only and no infectious PERV-A or PERV-B (Oldmixon et al. 2002). This effect is probably controlled by a yet unknown genetic mechanism but even the generally more harmless class PERV-C might transfer genes or parts of sequences to other viruses and therefore pose some risks in the course of XTx.

Assuming the worst case scenario in which PERV spreads to humans in spite of all the precautions taken, therapeutic means of combating the virus would be required. As PERV show highly conserved functional motifs in retroviral enzymes, protease and polymerase, it is likely that the virus is susceptible to conventional anti-retroviral reagents commonly used to treat other viruses, especially HIV. Initial data have been provided recently and refer to agents such as zidovudine (Powell et al. 2000; Qari et al. 2001). Therefore, it appears feasible to act against heterologous PERV expression in the unlikely case of xenozoonotic transmission.

A special case, regarding both biosafety and short-term feasibility of XTx measures, are extracorporeal assist devices, most often used to support or to mimic liver functions. By use of filter membranes with defined pore sizes the transmission of viral particles can be inhibited (Hunkeler et al. 1999) and the recombination of viral genomes is impeded if larger nucleic acids can be retained. In addition, the spatial separation of tissues, cells and body liquids dramatically improves the immunologic properties of such devices (Pitkin and Mullon 1999), therefore, there are some commercial interests in pursuing these approaches.

In conclusion, it may be stated that the virological barriers to XTx are not as serious as initially thought. The number of replication-competent proviruses is limited and the generation of PERV-free pigs seems possible. In addition, recombination events appear unlikely and the most closely related viruses do not pose serious risks by themselves. Initial experiments indicate that antiretroviral agents are effective against PERV and because XTx recipients must be closely monitored for transplant rejection on a routine basis, it does not appear to be restrictive to also monitor for viral infection.

5
Summary

There is a limited number of replication-competent PERV comprising three to six proviral loci present in porcine genome sources investigated so far. By means of strong founder effects concerning the pig herd analyzed, the number and localization of PERV may vary considerably.

PERV are able to productively infect some human cell lines. The host-range of PERV is determined by interaction of the envelope protein with cellular receptor(s) and to a lesser extent by the transcriptional environment of the LTRs. The virus actively adapts to its host cell by varying the number of 39-bp repeats in the U3 region of its LTR. The mechanism of repeat multimerization is unknown.

Immunosuppressive drugs do not appear to mediate any significant effect on PERV promoter activity, however, the number of compounds tested is limited and effects of human hormones and cytokines have not been investigated. On the other hand, PERV replication can be inhibited by antiretroviral agents commonly used in HIV therapy such as zidovudine.

While there remain unaddressed concerns regarding solid organ XTx, notably the possibility of long-term viral adaptation in immunosuppressive backgrounds and viral recombination, the use of porcine tissues in extracorporeal assist devices, extracorporeal organ perfusions as well as the transplantation of encapsulated islet cells should be safe, particularly when proper precautions are taken.

References

Akiyoshi DE, Denaro M, Zhu H, Greenstein JL, Banerjee PT and Fishman JA (1998) Identification of a full-length cDNA for an endogenous retrovirus of miniature swine. J Virol 72:4503–4507

Bach FH, Ivinson AJ and Weeramantry HE (2001) Ethical and legal issues in technology: xenotransplantation. Am J Law Med 27:283–300

Bach FH, Robson SC, Winkler H, Ferran C, Stuhlmeier KM, Wrighton CJ and Hancock WW (1995). Barriers to xenotransplantation. Nat. Med. 1:869–873

Battini JL, Danos O and Heard JM (1995). Receptor-binding domain of murine leukemia virus envelope glycoproteins. J. Virol. 69:713–719

Battini JL, Rasko JEJ and Miller D (1999) A human cell-surface receptor for xenotropic and polytropic murine leukimia viruses: possible role in G-protein-coupled signal transduction. Proc. Natl. Acad. Sci. 96:1385–1390

Bennet W, Bjorkland A, Sundberg B, Brandhorst D, Brendel MD, Richards A, White DJ, Nilsson B, Groth CG and Korsgren O (2001) Expression of complement regulatory proteins on islets of Langerhans: a comparison between human islets and islets isolated from normal and hDAF transgenic pigs. Xenotransplantation 2:100–105

Bosch S, Arnould C and Jestin A (2000) Study of full-length porcine endogenous retrovirus genomes with envelope gene polymorphism in a specific-pathogen-free Large White swine herd. J Virol 74:8575–8581

Cappello F, Stassi G, Lazzereschi D, Renzi L, Di Stefano C, Marfe G, Giancotti P, Wang HJ, Stoppacciaro A, Forni M, Bacci ML, Turchi V, Sinibaldi P, Rossi M, Bruzzone P, Pretagostini R, Della Casa G, Cortesini R, Frati L and Lavitrano M (2000) hDAF expression in hearts of transgenic pigs obtained by sperm-mediated gene transfer. Transplant Proc 32:892–894

Carrington CA and dos Santos Cruz G (2000) Effect of cell surface concentration of human DAF on transgenic pig aortic endothelial cells on the degree of protection afforded against human complement deposition. Expert Opin Pharmacother 3:757–769

Clemenceau B, Jegou D, Martignat L and Sai P (2001) Long-term follow-up failed to detect in vitro transmission of full-length porcine endogenous retroviruses from specific pathogen-free pig islets to human cells. Diabetologia 44:2044–2055

Coffin JM (1984) Endogenous viruses. 2nd ed. In "RNA tumor viruses" (R. Weiss, N. Teich, H. Varmus, and J. Coffin, Eds.), pp. 1109–1203. Cold Spring Harbor Laboratory Press, New York.

Coffin JM (1996) Retroviridae: The viruses and their replication. In: Fields virology, 3rd ed; Edit.: Fields BN, Knipe DM, Howley PM et al. 1767–1847

Cornetta K, Moen RC, Culver K, Morgan RA, McLachlin JR, Sturm S, Selegue J, London W, Blaese RM and Anderson WF (1990) Amphotropic murine leukemia retrovirus is not an acute pathogen for primates. Hum Gene Ther 1:15–30

Czauderna F, Fischer N, Boller K, Kurth R and Tönjes RR (2000) Establishment and characterization of molecular clones of porcine endogenous retroviruses replicating on human cells. J. Virol. 74:4028–4038

Deng YM, Lee HJ, Moran C, Jin JH, Tuch BE and Rawlinson WD (2000) Mapping dispersed repetitive loci using semi-specific PCR cloning and somatic cell hybrid mapping. Nucleic Acid Res 28: E103

Echard G (1974) Chromosomal banding patterns and karyotype evolution in three pig kidney cell strains (PK15, F and RP). Chromosoma 45:133–49

Fischer N, Krach U, Niebert M and Tönjes RR (2003) Detection of porcine endogenous retrovirus (PERV) using highly specific antisera against Gag and Env. Virology (in press)

Fishman JA (1994). Miniature swine as organ donors for man: stratagies for prevention of xenotransplant-associated infections. Xenotransplantation 1:47–57
Fishman JA (1997) Xenosis and xenotransplantation: addressing the infectious risks posed by an emerging technology. Kidney Int. 51:41–45
Fox M and McHale J (1998) Xenotransplantation: the ethical and legal ramifications. Med Law Rev 6:42–61
Galbraith DN, Kelly HT, Dyke A, Reid G, Haworth C, Beekman J, Shepherd A and Smith KT (2000) Design and validation of immunological tests for the detection of Porcine endogenous retrovirus in biological materials. J Virol Methods 90:115–124
Gimbel W, Schmidt J, Brack-Werner R, Luz A, Strauss PG, Erfle V and Werner T (1996) Molecular and pathogenic characterization of the RFB osteoma virus: lack of oncogene and induction of osteoma, osteopetrosis, and lymphoma. Virology 224:533–538
Herring C, Cunningham DA, Whittam AJ, Fernandez-Suarez XM and Langford GA (2001a) Monitoring xenotransplant recipients for infection by PERV. Clin. Biochem. 34:23–27
Herring C, Quinn G, Bower R, Parsons N, Logan NA, Brawley A, Elsome K, Whittam A, Fernandez-Suarez XM, Cunningham D, Onions D, Langford G and Scobie L (2001b) Mapping full-length porcine endogenous retroviruses in a large white pig. J Virol 75:12252–12265
Hiasa A, Watanabe M, Okada H, Ikenaka K, Fujita T, Yoshimatsu T, Kanematsu T and Shiku H (1999) Retroviruses prepared from human DAF expressing murine packaging cells acquire resistance against human serum. Int J Oncol 14:1091–1096
Hunkeler D, Sun AM, Korbutt S, Rajotte RV, Gill RG, Calafiore R and Morel P (1999). Bioartificial organs and acceptable risk. Nature Biotechn. 17:1045
Krach U, Fischer N, Czauderna F and Tönjes RR (2001). Comparison of replication-competent molecular clones of porcine endogenous retrovirus class A and class B derived from pig and human cells. J Virol 75:5465–5472
Krach U, Fischer N, Czauderna F, Kurth R and Tönjes RR (2000) Generation and testing of a highly specific anti-serum directed against porcine endogenous retrovirus nucleocapsid. Xenotransplantation 7:1–10
Lai L, Kolber-Simonds D, KW Park, HT Cheong, JL Greenstein, GS Im, Samuel M, A Bonk, Rieke A, Day BN, Murphy CN, Carter DB, Hawley RJ and Prather RS (2002) Production of {alpha}-1,3-Galactosyltransferase Knockout Pigs by Nuclear Transfer Cloning. Science 295:1089–1092
Leibovitch MP, Leibovitch SA, Hillion J, Guillier M and Harel J (1987) Expression of C-type virus in non differentiating rat myoblasts correlates with neoplastic progression. Biochem Biophys Res Commun 142:1111–1119
LeTissier P, Stoye JP, Takeuchi Y, Patience C and Weiss RA (1997). Two sets of human-tropic pig retroviruses. Nature 389:681–682
Li M, Xu F, Muller J, Hearing VJ and Gorelik E (1998) Ecotropic C-type retrovirus of B16 melanoma and malignant transformation of normal melanocytes. Int J Cancer 76:430–436
Limjoco TI, Dickie P, Ikeda H and Silver J (1993) Transgenic Fv4 mice resistant to Friend virus. J Virol 67:4163–4168

Martin U, Kiessig V, Blusch JH, Haverich A, von der Helm K, Herden T and Steinhoff G (1998) Expression of pig endogenous retrovirus by primary porcine endothelial cells and infection of human cells. Lancet 352:692–694

Martiney MJ, Rulli K, Beaty R, Levy LS and Lenz J (1999) Selection of reversion and suppressors of a mutation in the CBF binding site of a lymphomagenic retrovirus. J Virol 73:7599–7606

Matthews AL, Brown J, Switzer W, Folks TM, Heneine W and Sandstrom PA (1999) Development and validation of a Western immunoblot assay for detection of antibodies to porcine endogenous retrovirus.Transplantation 67:939–943

Mayer J, Sauter M, Rácz A, Scherer D, Mueller-Lantzsch N and Meese E (1999) An almost-intact human endogenous retrovirus K on humanchromosome 7 Nature Genetics 21:257–258

Michaels MG and Simmons RL (1994) Xenotransplant-associated zoonoses. Transplantation 57:1–7

Miyagawa S, Tanemura M, Koyota S, Koma M, Ikeda Y, Shirakura R and Taniguchi N (1999) Masking and reduction of the Galactose-alpha1,3-Galactose (alpha-Gal) epitope, the major xenoantigen in swine, by the glycosyltransferase gene transfection. Biochem Biophys Res Commun 264:611–614

Niebert M, Rogel-Gaillard C, Chardon P and Tönjes RR (2002). Characterization of chromosomally assigned replication-competent gamma porcine endogenous retroviruses derived from a large white pig and expression in human cells. J Virol 76: 2714–2720

Oldmixon BA, Wood JC, Ericsson TA, Wilson CA, White-Scharf ME, Andersson G, Greenstein JL, Schuurman HJ and Patience C (2002) PERV Transmission Characteristics of an Inbred Herd of Miniature Swine. J Virol 76: 3045–3048

Paradis K, Langford G, Long Z, Heneine W, Sandstrom P, Switzer WM, Chapman LE, Lockey C, Onions D, The XEN 111 Study Group and Otto E (1999). Search for cross-species transmission of porcine endogenous retrovirus in patients treated with liver pig tissue. Science 285:1236–1241.

Patience C, Switzer WM, Takeuchi Y, Griffiths DJ, Goward ME, Heneine W, Stoye JP and Weiss RA (2001). Multiple groups of novel retroviral genomes in pigs and related species. J Virol 75:2771–2775

Patience C, Takeuchi Y and Weiss RA (1997) Infection of human cells by an endogenous retrovirus of pigs. Nature Medicine 3:282–286

Pitkin Z and Mullon C (1999) Evidence of absence of porcine endogenous retrovirus (PERV) infection in patients treated with a bioartificial liver support system. Artif Organs 23:829–833

Powell SK, Gates ME, Langford G, Gu ML, Lockey C, Long Z and Otto E (2000) Antiretroviral agents inhibit infection of human cells by porcine endogenous retroviruses. Antimicrob. Agents Chemother. 44:3432–3433

Qari SH, Magre S, Garcia-Lerma JG, Hussain AI, Takeuchi Y, Patience C, Weiss RA and Heneine W (2001) Susceptibility of the porcine endogenous retrovirus to reverse transcriptase and protease inhibitors. J Virol 75:1048–1053

Reiss MJ (2000) The ethics of xenotransplantation. J Appl Philos 17:253–262

Rogel-Gaillard C, Bourgeaux N, Billault A, Vaiman M and Chardon P (1999) Construction of a swine BAC library: application to the characterization and mapping of the porcine type C endoviral elements. Cytogenet. Cell Genet. 85:205–211

Sandrin MS and McKenzie IF (1994) Gal alpha (1,3)Gal, the major xenoantigen(s) recognised in pigs by human natural antibodies. Immunol Rev 141:169–190

Sandrini MS, Fodor WL, Mouhtouris E, Osman N, Cohney S, Rollins SA, Guilmette ER, Setter E, Squinto SP and McKenzie IF (1995) Enzymatic remodelling of the carbohydrate surface of a xenogeneic cell substantially reduce human antibody binding and complement mediated cytolysis. Nature Medicine 1:1261–1267.

Scheef G, Fischer N, Krach U and Tönjes RR (2001) The number of a U3 repeat box acting as an enhancer in long terminal repeats of polytropic replication-competent porcine endogenous retroviruses dynamically fluctuates during serial virus passages in human cells. J Virol 75:6933–6940

Scheef G, Fischer N, Flory E, Schmitt I and Tönjes RR (2002) Transcriptional regulation of porcine endogenous retroviruses released from porcine and infected human cells by heterotrimeric protein complex NF-Y and impact of immunosuppressive drugs. J Virol 76:12553–12563

Stephan O, Schwendemann J, Specke V, Tacke SJ, Boller K and Denner J (2001) Porcine endogenous retroviruses (PERVs): generation of specific antibodies, development of an immunoperoxidase assay (IPA) and inhibition by AZT. Xenotransplantation 8:310–316

Stoye JP and Coffin JM (1995) The danger of xenotransplantation. Nature Medicine 1:1100

Tacke SJ, Bodusch K, Berg A and Denner J (2001) Sensitive and specific immunological detection methods for porcine endogenous retroviruses applicable to experimental and clinical xenotransplantation. Xenotransplantation 8:125–135

Takefman DM, Spear GT, Saifuddin M and Wilson CA (2002) Human CD59 incorporation into porcine endogenous retrovirus particles: Implications for the use of transgenic pigs for xenotransplantation. J Virol. 76:1999–2002.

Takefman DM, Wong S, Maudru T, Peden K and Wilson CA (2001) Detection and characterization of porcine endogenous retrovirus in porcine plasma and porcine factor VIII. J Virol 75:4551–4557

Takeuchi Y, Patience C, Magre S, Weiss RA, Banerjee PT, LeTissier P and Stoye JP (1998) Host range and interference studies of three classes of pig endogenous retrovirus. J. Virol. 72:9986–9991

Tönjes RR, Czauderna F and Kurth R (1999) Genome wide screening, cloning, chromosomal assignment and expression of full-length human endogenous retrovirus type K (HERV-K). J Virol 73:9187–9195

Tönjes RR, Czauderna F, Fischer N, Krach U, Boller K, Chardon P, Rogel-Gaillard C, Niebert M, Scheef G, Werner A and Kurth R (2000) Molecularly cloned porcine endogenous retroviruses replicate on human cells. Transplant Proc. 32:1158–1161

Tönjes RR, Löwer R, Boller K, Denner J, Hasenmaier B, Kirsch H, König H, Korbmacher C, Limbach C, Lugert R, Phelps RC, Scherer J, Thelen K, Löwer J and Kurth R (1996) HERV-K: the biologically most active human endogenous retrovirus family. J Acquir Immune Defic Syndr Hum Retrovirol 13:261–267

Turner G, Barbulescu M, Su M, Jensen-Seaman MI, Kidd KK and Lenz J (2001) Insertional polymorphisms of full-length endogenous retroviruses in humans. Curr Biol 11:1531–1535

Van der Laan LJW, Lockey C, Griffeth BC, Fraisier FS, Wilson CA, Onions DE, Hering BJ, Long Z, Otto E, Torbett BE and Salomon DR (2000) Infection by porcine endogenous retrovirus after islet xenotransplantation in SCID mice. Nature 407:90–94

Venables PJW, Brookes SM, Griffiths D, Weiss RA and Boyd MT (1995) Abundance of an endogenous retroviral envelope protein in placental trophoblasts suggests a biological function. Virology 211:589–592

Weiss RA (1998) Transgenic pigs and virus adaptation. Nature 391:327–328

Weiss RA (2000) Ancient and modern retroviruses. Acta Microbiol Immunol Hung 47:403–410

Wilson CA, Wong S, Muller J, Davidson CE, Rose TM and Burd P (1998) Type C retrovirus released from porcine primary peripheral blood mononuclear cells infects human cells. J Virol 72:3082–3087

Wilson CA, Wong S, Van Brocklin M and Federspiel M (2000) Extended analysis of the in vitro tropism of porcine endogenous retrovirus. J Virol 74:49–56

Wolgamot G and Miller AD (1999) Replication of Mus dunni endogenous retrovirus depends on promoter activation followed by enhancer multimerization. J. Virol. 73:9803–9809

Woods T (1998) Have a heart: xenotransplantation, nonhuman death and human distress. Soc Anim 6:47–65

Xenotransplantation—Federal Regulatory Considerations

E. T. Bloom
Laboratory of Immunology and Virology (HFM-518),
Division of Cellular and Gene Therapies,
Center for Biologics Evaluation and Research,
Food and Drug Administration, 1401 Rockville Pike, Rockville, MD 20852, USA
E-mail: Bloom@cber.fda.gov

1 Introduction 240

2 FDA Regulatory Review 241
2.1 Regulations 242
2.2 Guidance Documents 244
2.3 Advisory Committees and Public Meetings 246

3 Collaboration with Other Federal Components 247
3.1 Public Health Service Guideline on Infectious Disease Issues in Xenotransplantation. 247
3.2 Secretary's Advisory Committee on Xenotransplantation and Other Public Meetings 248
3.3 National Xenotransplantation Database 248

4 International Collaboration 249

5 Conclusions 250

References 250

Abstract Xenotransplantation may offer benefits to individual patients, but may also pose significant risks, to the recipient and to the public at large. The United States Food and Drug Administration endeavors to meet the challenge of regulating xenotransplantation to allow its development while safeguarding the public health. The approach includes using the existing FDA regulatory framework, publishing xenotransplantation-specific guidance documents, obtaining public input, and collaborating with other public health agencies and international bodies in order to develop and maintain a safe and rational program for the regulation of xenotransplantation.

1
Introduction

The worldwide shortage of human organs and tissues for allotransplantation (United Network of Organ Sharing 1997) combined with recent advances in transplantation immunobiology, surgery and medicine, have renewed interest in the clinical use of xenotransplantation, the use of living nonhuman animal materials for the treatment of human diseases. In addition to whole organ transplants, cellular implants (Fink et al. 2000) and ex vivo use of living material from animal sources (Dapolito and Auchincloss Jr 2000; Pitkin and Mullon 1999; Wang et al.1998; Chen et al.1997) have been suggested for treatment of disease in human patients. To encompass the full spectrum of xenotransplantation products, the U.S. Public Health Service (PHS) and the U.S. Food and Drug Administration (FDA) have defined xenotransplantation as any procedure that involves the transplantation, implantation, or infusion into a human recipient of either (a) live cells, tissues, or organs from a nonhuman animal source or (a) human body fluids, cells, tissues or organs that have had ex vivo contact with live nonhuman animal cells, tissues, or organs. Xenotransplantation product is defined as the live cells, tissues or organs used in xenotransplantation.

According to these definitions, xenotransplantation includes, for example, the transplantation of a nonhuman animal liver into a human patient with liver failure, the implantation of nonhuman neuronal cells into the brain of a patient with Parkinson's disease, and the infusion of nonhuman bone marrow cells into a patient with an immunodeficiency. However, it also includes the extracorporeal circulation of a patient's blood over nonhuman animal cells, tissues or organs directly or contained in a device, and human skin cells that have been expanded ex vivo on a layer of nonhuman animal cells and then used in humans for skin reconstruction. These latter procedures are included in the definition of xenotransplantation because infectious disease risks that may be associated with any contact with live nonhuman animal material may be similar to those associated with the use of direct implantation.

Although the potential for xenotransplantation to treat human disease may be substantial, the use of xenotransplantation products in humans poses risks not only to the patient but also to the public. Risks to the patient include rejection of the xenotransplantation product by the recipient's immune system with loss of graft function (Logan 2000; Lambrigts et al. 1998), and the possibility that physiologic incompatibility may preclude appropriate performance of the xenotransplantation product in the recipient (Breimer 1999; Goddard and Foweraker 2000). Of broader public health concern is the possibility that a novel xenogeneic infectious agent that may be capable of causing serious disease could be transmitted to the recipient, and then to the recipient's close contacts and other members of the public (Onions and Witt 2000; Chapman 1999). Balancing the potential risks of xenotransplantation with the possibility of clinical benefit has presented challenges for the development of a rational and scientific xenotransplantation regulatory policy.

2 FDA Regulatory Review

In the United States of America, FDA is responsible for evaluating the risks and the scientific and potential clinical merit of xenotransplantation clinical trials and determining whether proposed trials may proceed. FDA regulates xenotransplantation products under the Public Health Service Act (1944) and the Federal Food, Drug and Cosmetic Act (1938).

FDA review of xenotransplantation clinical protocols is performed by teams of physicians and scientists who combine expertise in clinical medicine and trial design, virology, immunology, veterinary medicine, pharmacology, and infectious disease. Review comprises critical evaluation of preclinical and clinical protocols and data and manufacturing information, and is an ongoing process throughout clinical and product development.

FDA personnel also conduct laboratory investigations that are essential to FDA regulatory activities. For example, following the demonstration that an established pig cell line expressed porcine endogenous retrovirus (PERV) capable of infecting human cells in vitro (Patience et al. 1997), FDA scientists made the key discovery that freshly isolated porcine lymphocytes could be activated to produce PERV infectious for human cells in vitro (Wilson et al. 1998). In October 1997, FDA placed all ongoing clinical trials involving porcine xenotransplantation products on clinical hold until the sponsors of the trials developed methods for the detection of infectious PERV in their porcine xenotransplantation products and demonstrated that they could monitor patients for evidence of PERV infection. After satisfactorily addressing FDA's concerns, several clinical investigations were allowed to resume.

FDA monitors and thoroughly considers scientific progress in xenotransplantation for its impact on regulatory policy. For example, FDA scientists and its advisors considered the report by Paradis et al. (1999) that PERV infection could not be demonstrated definitively in samples from any of the approximately 160 human patients who had been treated with xenotransplantation products. The agency and its advisors concluded that this significant body of work offered only very limited assurance of the safety of porcine xenotransplantation products (see transcript of 1/13/00 meeting of the FDA Xenotransplantation Subcommittee of the Biological Response Modifiers Advisory Committee at http://www.fda.gov/ohrms/dockets/ac/cber00.htm; Table 1). Therefore, FDA did not change its policy with regard to the need for monitoring for PERV infection with the use of porcine xenotransplantation products. Similarly, FDA considered the report by Van der Laan et al. (2000), which included an FDA scientist as a collaborator. The investigators reported PERV infection of human cells after exposure to primary pig islets in vitro, as well as limited infection of some murine tissues after transplantation of pig islets in vivo. While this report suggests that an immunosuppressed mouse model may provide useful data in the future regarding in vivo infectivity of PERV, the data did not indicate widespread viremia or pathogenic consequences of infection in this model. FDA continues to be vigilant to developments in this line of investigation.

2.1 Regulations

In the USA all clinical use of xenotransplantation products is regulated by FDA. As with all regulated products, FDA applies existing regulations found in Title 21 of the Code of Federal Regulations (21 CFR) to xenotransplantation. Most investigational xenotransplantation products are regulated as biological drugs and therefore the drug regulations, found in the 300 series of 21 CFR, apply. Additional information regarding requirements for licensed biological products can be found in the 600 series of 21 CFR. In certain cases, xenotransplantation products are considered to be biological devices, in which case the device regulations found in 21 CFR, the 800 series, apply.

Table 1 Internet sites for recent xenotransplantation guidance documents and meeting transcripts[a]

Subject (date)	Site
FDA Regulations	
The Code of Federal Regulations	http://www.access.gpo.gov/nara/cfr/cfr-table-search.html
Proposed Rule: Availability for Public Disclosure and Submission to FDA for Public Disclosure of Certain Data and Information Related to Human Gene Therapy or Xenotransplantation	http://www.fda.gov/cber/rules/frgene011801.htm or http://www.fda.gov/cber/rules/frgene011801.pdf
FDA Guidance Documents (general site: http://www.fda.gov/cber/guidelines.htm)	
Public Health Issues Posed by the Use of Nonhuman Primate Xenografts in Humans (4/6/99)	http://www.fda.gov/cber/gdlns/xenoprim.txt or http://www.fda.gov/cber/gdlns/xenoprim.pdf
Precautionary Measures to Reduce the Possible Risk of Transmission of Zoonoses by Blood and Blood Products from Xenotransplantation Product Recipients and Their Contacts (12/23/99)	http://www.fda.gov/cber/gdlns/zooxeno.txt or http://www.fda.gov/cber/gdlns/zooxeno.pdf
Source Animal, Product, Preclinical, and Clinical Issues Concerning the Use of Xenotransplantation Products in Humans (2/7/01)	http://www.fda.gov/cber/gdlns/clinxeno0201.htm or http://www.fda.gov/cber/gdlns/clinxeno0201.pdf
FDA Advisory Committee Meetings (general site: http://www.fda.gov/ohrms/dockets/ac)	
BRMAC Xenotransplantation Subcommittee (12/17/97)	http://www.fda.gov/ohrms/dockets/ac/cber97 t.htm
BRMAC Xenotransplantation Subcommittee (6/3–4/99)	http://www.fda.gov/ohrms/dockets/ac/99mtbc.htm
BRMAC Xenotransplantation Subcommittee (1/13/00)	http://www.fda.gov/ohrms/dockets/ac/00mtbc.htm
BPAC Committee (3/16–17/00)	http://www.fda.gov/ohrms/dockets/ac/00mtbc.htm
Collaboration with DHHS Components	
PHS Guideline on Infectious Disease Issues in Xenotransplantation (1/19/01)	http://www.fda.gov/cber/gdlns/xenophs0101.pdf
Secretary's Advisory Committee on Xenotransplantation	http://www4.od.nih.gov/oba/Sacx.htm
PHS Workshops	
Cross-species infectivity and pathogenesis (7/21–22/97)	http://www.niaid.nih.gov/dait/cross-species/default.htm
Developing Public Health Service Policy in Xenotransplantation (1/21–22/98)	http://www.fda.gov/ohrms/dockets/dockets/96m0311/96m0311.htm

[a] All guidance documents and most transcripts can also be accessed through the FDA Xenotransplantation Action Plan Internet site, http://www.fda.gov/cber/xap/xap.htm.

On 18 January 2001, FDA published a proposed rule in the Federal Register (66 FR 4688) 'Availability for Public Disclosure and Submission to FDA for Public Disclosure of Certain Data and Information Related to Human Gene Therapy or Xenotransplantation' for public comment. The rule proposes to amend the investigational new drug application regulations (IND regulations, 21 CFR section 312) to allow disclosure of certain information submitted in xenotransplantation and gene therapy INDs. The proposed rule applies to xenotransplantation and gene therapy because these are areas of clinical research with the potential for unique public health risks or modification of the human genome. Both have histories of public access to the information and public discussion through various public forums including advisory committee meetings, publications and the Internet. Public availability of appropriate information would facilitate further education and discussion of important public health issues as well as allow FDA to participate in such public discussions, which is very difficult under the agency's current public disclosure regulations. Finally, public availability would promote public awareness of current information throughout the conduct of each xenotransplantation clinical trial.

2.2 Guidance Documents

Since FDA published 'Points to Consider for Human Cell and Gene Therapy Products,' in 1991, a number of documents that pertain to xenotransplantation have followed. This 1991 document has recently (30 March 1998) been revised and republished as the 'Guidance for Industry: Guidance for Human Somatic Cell Therapy and Gene Therapy,' (available at http://www.fda.gov/cber/guidelines.htm). FDA explicitly stated its intention to regulate the use in humans of living cells of xenogeneic origin in the 14 October 1993 publication, 'Application of Current Statutory Authorities to Human Somatic Cell Therapy Products and Gene Therapy Products,' (Food and Drug Administration 1993).

More recently, FDA has published three guidance documents specifically aimed at providing advice to sponsors involved in or planning xenotransplantation clinical trials. The first of these 'Public Health Issues Posed by the Use of Nonhuman Primate Xenografts in Humans' was published on 6 April 1999 and can be accessed at http://www.fda.gov/cber/guidelines.htm. It was developed in response to concerns articulated by scientists and other members of the public regarding the use of nonhuman primate xenotransplantation products and was published after consultation with other components of DHHS. In this document, FDA stated that (a) an appropriate federal xenotransplantation advisory committee should address novel protocols and issues raised by the use of nonhuman primate xenotransplantation products, (b) clinical protocols proposing the use of nonhuman primate xenografts should not be submitted to FDA until sufficient scientific information exists addressing the risks posed by nonhuman primate xenotransplantation products, and (c) the agency believes that there is not sufficient information at present to assess the risks posed by nonhuman primate xenotransplantation and that it will be necessary for there to be public discussion before these issues can be adequately addressed. This guidance document was published for immediate implementation with public comment solicited.

The second guidance document 'Precautionary Measures to Reduce the Possible Risk of Transmission of Zoonoses by Blood and Blood Products from Xenotransplantation Product Recipients and Their Contacts,' was published as a draft for public comment on 23 December 1999 (http://www.fda.gov/cber/guidelines.htm). It proposed that xenotransplantation recipients and certain of their contacts should be deferred from donating whole blood and blood components, including source plasma, and source leukocytes. it also recommended questions that could be asked of prospective blood donors in order to identify such individuals. FDA advisors discussed this document at two public meetings, the 13 January 2000 meeting of the Xenotransplantation Subcommittee of the Biological Response Modifiers Advisory Committee (BRMAC) and the 16–17 March 2000 meeting of the Blood Products Advisory Committee (BPAC). Transcripts of these meetings can be found at http://www.fda.gov/ohrms/dockets/ac/00mtbc.htm. FDA has received numerous written public comments regarding this document, and it is being revised by the agency taking into consideration the full range of public commentary.

The third guidance document 'Source Animal, Product, Preclinical, and Clinical Issues Concerning the Use of Xenotransplantation Products in Humans,' was published as a draft for public comment on 7 February 2001. Beyond the recommendations set forth in the PHS Guideline (see discussion below), which are intended to minimize the potential public health risks of xenotransplantation, the FDA guidance document offers more specific advice for IND sponsors. For example, it includes additional advice concerning source animal characterization, patient monitoring and informed consent, and testing for PERV. It also provides guidance in areas of xenotransplantation clinical and product development not addressed by the PHS Guideline, including development of preclinical studies, product characterization and quality control, and manufacturing facility issues. Both documents can be accessed at http://www.fda.gov/cber/guidelines.htm.

2.3 Advisory Committees and Public Meetings

The public health concerns and risks that may be posed by xenotransplantation make it important that appropriate expert scientific advice is sought, knowledge is brought to bear, and public input is solicited and considered. BRMAC is an FDA advisory committee, and in 1997 its Xenotransplantation Subcommittee was constituted. Both the parent committee and the subcommittee have met several times since 1994 specifically to discuss various aspects of xenotransplantation. For example, BRMAC met in 1995 to discuss the administration of baboon bone marrow for the treatment of AIDS. The committee recommended that treatment of only one patient be attempted and also gave specific advice regarding the qualification of the source animal. The Subcommittee met on 3–4 June 1999 to consider new data and public health issues concerning cross-species transplantation (transcript available on the at http://www.fda.gov/ohrms/dockets/ac/99mtbc.htm). It met again on 13 January 2000 to discuss the proposed FDA guidance on blood donor deferral for xenotransplantation recipients and their contacts and to discuss a specific xenotransplantation product that is produced by co-culture of human cells with an irradiated but metabolizing murine cell line (transcript available at http://www.fda.gov/ohrms/dockets/ac/00mtbc.htm). FDA proposed guidance on blood donor deferral was presented and discussed again in March 2000 at the FDA Blood Products Advisory Committee (transcript available at http://www.fda.gov/ohrms/dockets/ac/00mtbc.htm).

3
Collaboration with Other Federal Components

3.1
Public Health Service Guideline on Infectious Disease Issues in Xenotransplantation

The Draft PHS Guideline on Infectious Disease Issues in Xenotransplantation was developed through the combined efforts of multiple components of the Department of Health and Human Services (DHHS) including FDA, Centers for Disease Control and Prevention (CDC), National Institutes of Health (NIH), Health Resources and Services Administration (HRSA) and the DHHS Office of the Assistant Secretary for Planning and Evaluation (OASPE). Advice and input from the U.S. Departments of Agriculture and Defense was also sought and received during various stages of development of the guideline. The draft guideline, which was published 26 September 1996, identified general principles for the prevention and control of infectious diseases that may be associated with xenotransplantation and that may pose a public health hazard (U.S. Public Health Service 1996). For example, the document addressed source animal selection, patient informed consent and education, and post-transplant isolation and monitoring of patients. This guideline has been revised in response to written commentary, input from public meetings including scientific advice, advances in the relevant science, and evolving international policy. It received final government clearance on 19 January 2001, and is available at http://www.fda.gov/cber/guidelines.htm. The revised guideline clarifies and elaborates on a variety of issues. Examples of where clarifications have been made include areas dealing with the designation of responsibility for the design and conduct of clinical protocols, clinical protocol review and oversight, patient informed consent and education and education of contacts, deferral of donation for allograft and blood donation, xenotransplantation product sources and testing, source animal screening and qualification, and maintenance of biological specimen archives and health records. It also suggests the formation of the Secretary's Advisory Committee on Xenotransplantation and the development of a National Xenotransplantation Database.

3.2 Secretary's Advisory Committee on Xenotransplantation and Other Public Meetings

The Secretary's Advisory Committee on Xenotransplantation (SACX), proposed in the 'PHS Guideline on Infectious Disease Issues in Xenotransplantation,' met for the first time in February 2001. It has been developed by the cooperating DHHS components including CDC, FDA, HRSA, NIH and OASPE, and it is housed at the Office of Biotechnology Affairs (OBA) of NIH. Information regarding the SACX can be accessed at http://www4.od.nih.gov/oba. The purpose of the SACX is to advise the Secretary on issues posed by xenotransplantation, including scientific, social, ethical, and economic issues, and it will provide an additional public forum for discussions of this broad spectrum of issues. The committee is composed of 18 individuals with a broad range of expertise including, for example, clinical medicine, surgery, immunology, virology, veterinary medicine, animal welfare, ethics, economics, patient advocacy, and law, appropriate to address these diverse areas.

The U.S. PHS, including FDA, has also co-sponsored or participated in numerous other national conferences that included public discussion of key issues in xenotransplantation. For example, the Institute of Medicine met in June 1995 to discuss issues of science, ethics and public policy in xenotransplantation (Institute of Medicine 1996). The PHS has also held two major public workshops on xenotransplantation. The first, 'Cross-Species Infectivity and Pathogenesis' was held in July 1997 (available at http://www.niaid.nih.gov/dait/cross-species/default.htm). The second, held in January 1998, was titled 'Developing Public Health Service Policy in Xenotransplantation,' (transcript at http://www.fda.gov/ohrms/dockets/dockets/96m0311/96m0311.htm).

3.3 National Xenotransplantation Database

The Draft PHS Guideline on Infectious Disease Issues in Xenotransplantation identified the need for a centralized database or registry for the collection and maintenance of pertinent information on xenotransplantation clinical trials. The revised Guideline describes a pilot National Xenotransplantation Database (NXD), with the anticipation that the pilot will eventually be expanded to collect data from all clinical trials in xenotransplantation and include information on all facilities providing animals or xenogeneic organs, tissues, or cells for use in manufacturing clinical xenotransplantation products. The NXD is planned as a means for rapid recognition, accurate assessment, and appropriate timely response in the event of the identification of an infectious agent or clinical event associated with a xenotransplantation product that may have public health consequences.

The main functions of the NXD will be to (a) identify rates of occurrence and clustering of health events that may represent outcomes from xenogeneic infections (b) allow accurate linkage of these clinical events to exposure, e.g., animal source (c) provide a framework for the assessment of patient outcomes and to identify areas for laboratory and clinical research and (d) provide a database for the assessment of long-term safety.

The US PHS has undertaken a pilot study of the database in order to determine the needs for routine data collection and reporting. The mature NXD will be compatible with the FDA Investigational New Drug application process. Information derived from the database may be made available to medical and scientific communities and to the public as permitted by Federal statutes and regulations such as the Privacy Act, the Freedom of Information Act, the Food Drug and Cosmetic Act and other FDA regulations pertaining to the nondisclosure of proprietary information.

4 International Collaboration

Finally, to establish and promote international cooperation in xenotransplantation, particularly in regard to infectious disease issues, the USA has participated in international policy development. As recent examples, representatives of FDA and CDC attended a meeting in October 2000, cosponsored by the Organization of Economic Cooperation and Development (OECD), World Health Organization (WHO), and Health Canada to initiate international consideration of surveillance in the area of xenotransplantation. FDA has also participated at meetings of the Council of Europe Working Party on Xenotransplantation in a process intended to develop a European guideline on xenotransplantation. Tibell has recently reviewed how different countries in Europe are individually approaching the regulation of xenotransplantation (Tibell 2001).

5 Conclusions

Xenotransplantation may offer benefits to individual patients, but may also pose significant risks to the recipient and to the public at large. Therefore the challenge in regulating xenotransplantation is to allow the development of a potentially beneficial new technology, while safeguarding the public health. U.S. public policy has been to exercise a cautious approach, including FDA regulation of xenotransplantation, the publication of guidance documents, and seeking scientific and public input within the USA in an atmosphere of international collaboration and cooperation.

References

Breimer ME (1999) Physiologic incompatibilities in discordant xenotransplantation. Transplant Proc 31:905–908

Chapman LE (1999) Xenogeneic infections and public health. Clin Exp Pharmacol Physiol 26:1005–1008

Chen S, Kahaku E, Watanabe F, Hewitt W, Eguchi S, Middleton Y, Arkadotoulos N, Rozga J, Solomon B, Demetriou A (1997) Treatment of severe liver failure with a bioartificial liver. Ann N Y Acad Sci 831:350–360

Dapolito G, Auchincloss H, Jr. (2000) Report of the Food and Drug Administration Subcommittee on Xenotransplantation: meeting of 13 January 2000, Center for Biologics Evaluation and Research. Xenotransplantation 7:75–79

Fink JS, Schumacher JM, Ellias SL, Palmer P, Saint-Hilaire M, Shannon K, Penn R, Starr P, VanHorne C, Kott HS, Dempsey PK, Fischman AJ, Raineri R, Manhart C, Dinsmore J, Isacson O (2000) Porcine xenografts in Parkinson's disease and Huntington's disease patients: preliminary results. Cell Transplant 9:273–278

Food and Drug Administration H (1993) Application of current statutory authorities to human somatic cell therapy products and gene therapy products. Federal Register 58:53248–53251

Goddard MJ, Foweraker JE (2000) Xenotransplantation - 2000. J Clin Pathol 53:44–48

Institute of Medicine (1996) Xenotransplantation: Science, Ethics, and Public Policy. National Academy Press, Washington, D.C.

Lambrigts D, Sachs DH, Cooper DKC (1998) Discordant organ xenotransplantation in primates. World experience and current status. Transplantation 66:547–561

Logan JS (2000) Prospects for xenotransplantation. Curr Opin Immunol 12:563–568

Onions D, Witt CJ (2000) Xenotransplantation: an overview of microbiolgoical risks and potentials for risk management. Rev Sci Tech OIE 19:289–301

Paradis K, Langford G, Long Z, Heneine W, Sandstrom P, Switzer WM, Chapman LE, Lockey C, Onions D, The XEN 111 Study Group, Otto E (1999) Search for cross-species transmission of porcine endogenous retrovirus in patients treated with living pig tissue. Science 285:1236–1241

Patience C, Takeuchi Y, Weiss RA (1997) Infection of human cells by an endogenous retrovirus of pigs. Nat Med 3:282–286

Pitkin Z, Mullon C (1999) Evidence of absence of porcine endogenous retrovirus (PERV) infection in patients treated with a bioartifical liver support system. Artif Organs 23:829–833

Tibell A. (2001) Regulating clinical xenotransplantation in Europe. Graft 4:157–159

United Network of Organ Sharing (1997) 1997 Report of the OPTN: Waiting List Activity and Donor Procurement, UNOS, Richmond, VA, and the Division of Transplantation, Office of Special Programs, Health Resources and Services Administration, U.S. Department of Health and Human Services, Rockville, Maryland.

U.S. Federal Statute (1938) Federal Food, Drug and Cosmetic Act, 21 U.S.C. 321(g), sect. 201(g)

U.S. Federal Statute (1944) Public Health Service Act, July 1, 1944, ch. 373, Title III, 351, 58 Stat. 702, currently codified at 42 U.S.C. 262.

U.S. Public Health Service (1996) Draft Public Health Service Guideline on infectious disease issues in xenotransplantation. Federal Register 61:49920–49932

van der Laan L, Lockey C, Griffeth BC, Frasier FS, Wilson CA, Onions DE, Hering BJ, Long Z, Otto E, Torbett BE, Salomon DR (2000) Infection by porcine endogenous retrovirus after islet xenotransplantation. Nature 407:90–94

Wang L, Sun J, Li L, Mears D, Horvat M, Sheil AGR (1998) Comparison of porcine hepatocytes with human hepatoma (C3A) cells for use in a bioartificial liver support system. Cell Transplant 7:459–468

Wilson CA, Wong S, Muller J, Davidson CE, Rose TM, Burd P (1998) Type C retrovirus released from porcine primary peripheral blood mononuclear cells infects human cells. J Virol 72:3082–3087

Subject Index

A
ABO blood group 10
accommodation 5, 8, 10
acute vascular rejection 5, 7–10, 12
African green monkey 104, 109
AIDS 102, 105, 110–112, 116
alpha-herpesvirus 75–79, 82–84, 89
Asian nonhuman primate 111
ATLL 106–107

B
Baboon 93, 101, 103–112, 114–115
Baboon endogenous retrovirus 109, 111, 114–115
beta-Herpesvirus 75, 84, 90
beta-retrovirus group 111
blood vessel 3–4, 6–7

C
carbon monoxide (CO) 11
CCR5 105
CD4+ T cells 105, 106
CD59 6, 10
cellular rejection 4–5
Cercopithecine herpesvirus 82
chimpanzee 103, 105, 108–109
chronic rejection 5, 11
cloning 9, 13, 15
coreceptor 105
CXCR4 105
cytomegalovirus 75, 84

D
decay accelerating factor (DAF) 6
diagnostic testing 107

E
EBV 75, 90, 93
Endogenous retrovirus 112
Exogenous 104, 111
Exogenous retrovirus 104

F
Food and Drug Administration 103

G
Galα1-3Gal 6, 8–9
gamma-herpesvirus 75, 90
gene knock-in 13
gene therapy 111, 113
genetic engineering 1–4, 8, 10, 12–13, 15
glycosyltransferase 9

H
H. papio (see also Baboon) 93
hemoxygenase 10
hepatocyte 3–4
herpes B virus 82, 84, 89, 105, 112
Herpesvirus 73–75, 78–79, 82–85, 89–90, 94–95, 105, 112, 117
HHV-8 75, 90, 94–95
HIV 1, 2 104–106, 112, 116
HTLV 102, 106–107, 116
human genome 102, 114
Hyperacute Rejection 6–9

I
iatrogenic infection 63
immune system 3–4
infection 23, 26–30, 32–34, 36–38
integration 102, 104

interleukin-2 106
islet 45

J
juvenile baboon 110

L
langur 111
liver transplant 109
Lymphocryptovirus 90

M
maternal antibody 110
membrane co-factor protein 6

N
natural killer cell 16
new epidemic 48, 52
New World monkey 88, 93
nonhuman primate 73–74, 101, 103–110, 112, 114, 116–118

O
Old World monkey 88, 90
Old World primate species 88, 90, 107

P
Papio cynocephalus endogenous Retrovirus 115
Parkinson's disease 4
PcEV 116
porcine endogenous retrovirus 112, 116–117
primate worker 109, 112
public health 23, 25, 29, 32, 34, 36–38
pX region 106

R
RD-114 111
receptor 102, 105–106, 108, 111, 116
recombination 115–116
retrovirus 13, 101–106, 105–117
Rhadinovirus 90, 94

S
Simian endogenous retrovirus (SERV) 112, 115, 116
Simian Foamy Virus (SFV) 108–111, 114, 116
Simian Immunodeficiency Virus (SIV) 104–105, 110, 116
Simian Retrovirus (Type D) 111
Simian T Cell Lymphotropic Virus 106–107, 110, 116
sodium-dependent neutral-amino acid transporter 111
STLV 106–107, 110, 116

T
Talapoin monkey 111
tax 106
transgenic mouse 106, 109
transmission 104–107, 110, 117
type C retrovirus 114, 116
type D retrovirus 105, 111, 114–115

V
vaccine 111
vascular rejection 4
virulence 48, 58–61

X
Xenotourism 103
xenotransplantation 1–5, 10–13, 15–16, 23–25, 27–39, 48, 53, 57, 60–62, 64, 66

Z
zoo worker 109
zoonosis 52, 54, 65
zoonotic 23, 27, 29–30
zoonotic agent 13

Current Topics in Microbiology and Immunology

Volumes published since 1989 (and still available)

Vol. 234: **Frankel, Arthur E. (Ed.):** Clinical Applications of Immunotoxins. 1999. 16 figs. IX, 122 pp. ISBN 3-540-64097-5

Vol. 235: **Klenk, Hans-Dieter (Ed.):** Marburg and Ebola Viruses. 1999. 34 figs. XI, 225 pp. ISBN 3-540-64729-5

Vol. 236: **Kraehenbuhl, Jean-Pierre; Neutra, Marian R. (Eds.):** Defense of Mucosal Surfaces: Pathogenesis, Immunity and Vaccines. 1999. 30 figs. IX, 296 pp. ISBN 3-540-64730-9

Vol. 237: **Claesson-Welsh, Lena (Ed.):** Vascular Growth Factors and Angiogenesis. 1999. 36 figs. X, 189 pp. ISBN 3-540-64731-7

Vol. 238: **Coffman, Robert L.; Romagnani, Sergio (Eds.):** Redirection of Th1 and Th2 Responses. 1999. 6 figs. IX, 148 pp. ISBN 3-540-65048-2

Vol. 239: **Vogt, Peter K.; Jackson, Andrew O. (Eds.):** Satellites and Defective Viral RNAs. 1999. 39 figs. XVI, 179 pp. ISBN 3-540-65049-0

Vol. 240: **Hammond, John; McGarvey, Peter; Yusibov, Vidadi (Eds.):** Plant Biotechnology. 1999. 12 figs. XII, 196 pp. ISBN 3-540-65104-7

Vol. 241: **Westblom, Tore U.; Czinn, Steven J.; Nedrud, John G. (Eds.):** Gastroduodenal Disease and Helicobacter pylori. 1999. 35 figs. XI, 313 pp. ISBN 3-540-65084-9

Vol. 242: **Hagedorn, Curt H.; Rice, Charles M. (Eds.):** The Hepatitis C Viruses. 2000. 47 figs. IX, 379 pp. ISBN 3-540-65358-9

Vol. 243: **Famulok, Michael; Winnacker, Ernst-L.; Wong, Chi-Huey (Eds.):** Combinatorial Chemistry in Biology. 1999. 48 figs. IX, 189 pp. ISBN 3-540-65704-5

Vol. 244: **Daëron, Marc; Vivier, Eric (Eds.):** Immunoreceptor Tyrosine-Based Inhibition Motifs. 1999. 20 figs. VIII, 179 pp. ISBN 3-540-65789-4

Vol. 245/I: **Justement, Louis B.; Siminovitch, Katherine A. (Eds.):** Signal Transduction and the Coordination of B Lymphocyte Development and Function I. 2000. 22 figs. XVI, 274 pp. ISBN 3-540-66002-X

Vol. 245/II: **Justement, Louis B.; Siminovitch, Katherine A. (Eds.):** Signal Transduction on the Coordination of B Lymphocyte Development and Function II. 2000. 13 figs. XV, 172 pp. ISBN 3-540-66003-8

Vol. 246: **Melchers, Fritz; Potter, Michael (Eds.):** Mechanisms of B Cell Neoplasia 1998. 1999. 111 figs. XXIX, 415 pp. ISBN 3-540-65759-2

Vol. 247: **Wagner, Hermann (Ed.):** Immunobiology of Bacterial CpG-DNA. 2000. 34 figs. IX, 246 pp. ISBN 3-540-66400-9

Vol. 248: **du Pasquier, Louis; Litman, Gary W. (Eds.):** Origin and Evolution of the Vertebrate Immune System. 2000. 81 figs. IX, 324 pp. ISBN 3-540-66414-9

Vol. 249: **Jones, Peter A.; Vogt, Peter K. (Eds.):** DNA Methylation and Cancer. 2000. 16 figs. IX, 169 pp. ISBN 3-540-66608-7

Vol. 250: **Aktories, Klaus; Wilkins, Tracy, D. (Eds.):** Clostridium difficile. 2000. 20 figs. IX, 143 pp. ISBN 3-540-67291-5

Vol. 251: **Melchers, Fritz (Ed.):** Lymphoid Organogenesis. 2000. 62 figs. XII, 215 pp. ISBN 3-540-67569-8

Vol. 252: **Potter, Michael; Melchers, Fritz (Eds.):** B1 Lymphocytes in B Cell Neoplasia. 2000. XIII, 326 pp. ISBN 3-540-67567-1

Vol. 253: **Gosztonyi, Georg (Ed.):** The Mechanisms of Neuronal Damage in Virus Infections of the Nervous System. 2001. approx. XVI, 270 pp. ISBN 3-540-67617-1

Vol. 254: **Privalsky, Martin L. (Ed.):** Transcriptional Corepressors. 2001. 25 figs. XIV, 190 pp. ISBN 3-540-67569-8

Vol. 255: **Hirai, Kanji (Ed.):** Marek's Disease. 2001. 22 figs. XII, 294 pp. ISBN 3-540-67798-4

Vol. 256: **Schmaljohn, Connie S.; Nichol, Stuart T. (Eds.):** Hantaviruses. 2001, 24 figs. XI, 196 pp. ISBN 3-540-41045-7

Vol. 257: **van der Goot, Gisou (Ed.):** Pore-Forming Toxins, 2001. 19 figs. IX, 166 pp. ISBN 3-540-41386-3

Vol. 258: **Takada, Kenzo (Ed.):** Epstein-Barr Virus and Human Cancer. 2001. 38 figs. IX, 233 pp. ISBN 3-540-41506-8

Vol. 259: **Hauber, Joachim, Vogt, Peter K. (Eds.):** Nuclear Export of Viral RNAs. 2001. 19 figs. IX, 131 pp. ISBN 3-540-41278-6

Vol. 260: **Burton, Didier R. (Ed.):** Antibodies in Viral Infection. 2001. 51 figs. IX, 309 pp. ISBN 3-540-41611-0

Vol. 261: **Trono, Didier (Ed.):** Lentiviral Vectors. 2002. 32 figs. X, 258 pp. ISBN 3-540-42190-4

Vol. 262: **Oldstone, Michael B.A. (Ed.):** Arenaviruses I. 2002, 30 figs. XVIII, 197 pp. ISBN 3-540-42244-7

Vol. 263: **Oldstone, Michael B. A. (Ed.):** Arenaviruses II. 2002, 49 figs. XVIII, 268 pp. ISBN 3-540-42705-8

Vol. 264/I: **Hacker, Jörg; Kaper, James B. (Eds.):** Pathogenicity Islands and the Evolution of Microbes. 2002. 34 figs. XVIII, 232 pp. ISBN 3-540-42681-7

Vol. 264/II: **Hacker, Jörg; Kaper, James B. (Eds.):** Pathogenicity Islands and the Evolution of Microbes. 2002. 24 figs. XVIII, 228 pp. ISBN 3-540-42682-5

Vol. 265: **Dietzschold, Bernhard; Richt, Jürgen A. (Eds.):** Protective and Pathological Immune Responses in the CNS. 2002. 21 figs. X, 278 pp. ISBN 3-540-42668-X

Vol. 266: **Cooper, Koproski (Eds.):** The Interface Between Innate and Acquired Immunity, 2002, 15 figs. XIV, 116 pp. ISBN 3-540-42894-1

Vol. 267: **Mackenzie, John S.; Barrett, Alan D. T.; Deubel, Vincent (Eds.):** Japanese Encephalitis and West Nile Viruses. 2002. 66 figs. X, 418 pp. ISBN 3-540-42783-X

Vol. 268: **Zwickl, Peter; Baumeister, Wolfgang (Eds.):** The Proteasome-Ubiquitin Protein Degradation Pathway. 2002, 17 figs. X, 213 pp. ISBN 3-540-43096-2

Vol. 269: **Koszinowski, Ulrich H.; Hengel, Hartmut (Eds.):** Viral Proteins Counteracting Host Defenses. 2002, 47 figs. XII, 325 pp. ISBN 3-540-43261-2

Vol. 270: **Beutler, Bruce; Wagner, Hermann (Eds.):** Toll-Like Receptor Family Members and Their Ligands. 2002, 31 figs. X, 192 pp. ISBN 3-540-43560-3

Vol. 271: **Koehler, Theresa M. (Ed.):** Anthrax. 2002, 14 figs. X, 169 pp. ISBN 3-540-43497-6

Vol. 272: **Doerfler, Walter; Böhm, Petra (Eds.):** Adenoviruses: Model and Vectors in Virus Host Interactions. Virion and Structure, Viral Replication, Host Cell Interactions. 2003, 63 figs., approx. 280 pp. ISBN 3-540-00154-9

Vol. 273: **Doerfler, Walter; Böhm, Petra (Eds.):** Adenoviruses: Model and Vectors in Virus Host Interactions. Immune System, Oncogenesis, Gene Therapy. 2003, 33 figs., approx. 280 pp. ISBN 3-540-06851-1

Vol. 274: **Workman, J. L. (Ed.):** Protein Complexes that Modify Chromatin. 2003, 38 figs., XII, 296 pp. ISBN 3-540-44208-1

Vol. 275: **Fan, Hung (Ed.):** Jaagsiekte Sheep Retrovirus and Lung Cancer. 2003, 63 figs., XII, 252 pp. ISBN 3-540-44096-3

Vol. 276: **Steinkasserer, A. (Ed.):** Dendritic Cells and Virus Infection. 2003, 24 figs., X, 296 pp. ISBN 3-540-44290-1

Vol. 277: **Rethwilm, A. (Ed.):** Foamy Viruses. 2003, 40 figs., X, 214 pp. ISBN 3-540-44388-6

MIX
Papier aus verantwortungsvollen Quellen
Paper from responsible sources
FSC® C105338

If you have any concerns about our products, you can contact us on
ProductSafety@springernature.com

In case Publisher is established outside the EU, the EU authorized representative is:
Springer Nature Customer Service Center GmbH
Europaplatz 3, 69115 Heidelberg, Germany

Printed by Libri Plureos GmbH
in Hamburg, Germany